BODY & SOUL

A NATIONAL BLACK WOMEN'S HEALTH PROJECT BOOK

BODY & SOUL

The Black Women's Guide to Physical Health and Emotional Well-Being

LINDA VILLAROSA, EDITOR

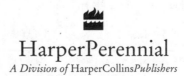

HarperPerennial

A Division of HarperCollins*Publishers*

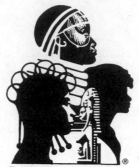

The National Black Women's Health Project

The National Black Women's Health Project (NBWHP), founded in 1981 by health activist Byllye Avery, is a national and international self-help and health advocacy organization committed to improving the health of Black women.

Headquartered in Atlanta, Georgia, the NBWHP has over the past decade crafted all of its programs within the context of a self-help/empowerment model. A model that first carves out individual and personal liberation to move and change the society as a whole.

NBWHP has nine chapters and members in forty-one states. For more information on NBWHP and/or membership write or call:

NBWHP
1237 Ralph David Abernathy Boulevard, SW
Atlanta, Georgia 30310
(404) 758-9590•1-800-ASK-BWHP•FAX (404) 758-9661

BODY & SOUL. Copyright © 1994 by Linda Villarosa. All rights reserved. Printed in the United States of America. No part of this book may be used or reproduced in any manner whatsoever without written permission except in the case of brief quotations embodied in critical articles and reviews. For information address HarperCollins Publishers, Inc., 10 East 53rd Street, New York, NY 10022.

HarperCollins books may be purchased for educational, business, or sales promotional use. For information, please write: Special Markets Department, HarperCollins Publishers, Inc., 10 East 53rd Street, New York, NY 10022.

Designed by Jessica Shatan

Library of Congress Cataloging-in-Publication Data
   Body & soul : the Black women's guide to physical health and emotional well-being / Linda Villarosa, editor.
      p. cm.
   Includes bibliographical references and index.
   ISBN 0-06-055359-6 — ISBN 0-06-095085-4 (pbk.)
   1. Afro-American women—Health and hygiene. 2. Afro-American women—Mental health. I. Villarosa, Linda. II. Title: Body and soul.
   RA778.B67 1994
   613'.04244'08996073—dc20   94-13140

95 96 97 98 ❖   10 9 8 7 6 5 4 3

Contents

Contributors

Contributing Writers
Allison Abner
Karen Carrillo
Danella Carter
Rachel Jackson Christmas
Frances Jemmott
Tenley-Ann Hawkins
Toni Y. Joseph
Benilde Little
Angela Mitchell
Retha Powers
Linda Villarosa
Elsie B. Washington
Evelyn C. White
Teresa Wiltz
Patricia Mason Woods
Antronette K. Yancey, M.D., M.P.H.

Research and Reporting Ruth Manuel-Logan, chief
Tonya M. Adams
Nana A. Agyemang-Badu
Maya Browne
Evette Porter
Margie Shaheed
Joy Rankin
Bette Vargas
Jan A. Wyche

National Black Women's Health Project Education Committee
Byllye Y. Avery
Joy Church, M.D.
Sheila Cort, M.P.H.
Pauline D. Hicks, Ph.D.
Jean R. King, Ph.D.
Arlene Vincent Mark
Cynthia I. Newbille
Beverly Guy-Sheftall, Ph.D.
Watrina Watson
Lisa Diane White
Valerie Boyd
Abigail Pennington, M.D.

Medical Advisors
Denise Bell-Carter, M.D.
Freda C. Lewis-Hall, M.D.
Melody T. McCloud, M.D.
Antronette K. Yancey, M.D., M.P.H.

Art Coordinators   Mark Gabor, chief
Judy Watson Remy

Acknowledgments

I wish to thank the following people:

The staff of the National Black Women's Health Project, with extra gratitude to the members of the NBWHP Education Committee, who gave up many Saturdays to help create and critique this book.

The women who told their personal stories in order to heal others and the many writers, researchers, and advisors for their dedication and attention to detail.

Each and every one of my colleagues at Essence Magazine, especially the senior editors, Tonya M. Adams and Deborah Gregory.

The women who have done this work before and who have greatly influenced this book, including Byllye Y. Avery, The Boston Women's Health Book Collective, Angela Y. Davis, and Evelyn C. White.

Everyone at HarperCollins, with special thanks to Janet Goldstein and Betsy Thorpe for their attention and care.

My agents, Barbara Lowenstein and Madeleine Morel, for pulling this project together and sticking with it beyond the end.

Dwight Carter, for the wonderful cover photography; Michaela Angela Davis for styling, Miriam Jiminez-Boland for hair and makeup; and Hafeezah Basir, Janice Carter, Jake-ann Jones, and Soukaina Mafundikwa for being the cover models.

Mark Gabor, for giving his all and more.

Allison Abner, Michelle Adams, Benilde Little, Martha Southgate, and Jacqueline Woodson for being my friends.

Those who believed in me throughout the years: Patti Adcroft, Marc Bloom, Jane Chesnutt, Audrey Edwards, and Susan L. Taylor.

Clara Villarosa, Andres Villarosa, Alicia Villarosa, and in memory of my grandparents—the best family anyone could ask for.

And most of all, to Victoria Starr for keeping the books, paying the bills and every other little thing.

Dedicated to
Audre Lorde, Toni Y. Joseph, DorisJean Austin,
Danitra Vance, Ebun Phillips Bowen,
and all of the other Black women who
have died before their time.

Foreword

by Angela Y. Davis and June Jordan

"The Black woman is the mule of the world," wrote Zora Neale Hurston. We are expected to take care of everyone but ourselves, carry everyone's load but our own. How do we stop devaluing our bodies and our psyches? There ought to be a way, says the song June wrote for Sweet Honey in the Rock, that we can sit down and break down and know how to put ourselves back together.

Body & Soul offers us much-needed guidance as we try to put ourselves back together. This book leads Black women back to ourselves, urges us to stay close to ourselves, to take our health needs seriously and to try to think about good health as being much more than the mere absence of disease. *Body & Soul* challenges us to let go of the narrow definitions of health imposed on us by people who don't care about us—who don't know how we live or how we die. This book maps the terrain of Black women's health consciousness, marking a moment when we finally give ourselves permission to be concerned about ourselves and to look at the range of issues implied by our quest for physical, spiritual, and emotional health.

We cannot conceptualize healthy bodies, psyches, and communities without addressing problems that have always been taboo. This means that we must go beyond the civil rights framework that privileges men over women and the public sphere over the private. Now we have to raise hard questions about the relationship between our public and private lives.

Public violence is no more deserving of our protests than is private violence. Just as we move to end police brutality, we must oppose and terminate all such crimes, including the brutality of Black men against Black women and Black parental violence inflicted upon Black children.

The beating of Rodney King, as important as it was in sparking our anger about police crimes, does not mean we ignore the beatings Rodney King inflicted on his wife. The eradication of violence—at home as well as in the streets—is an absolute precondition for building healthy communities.

In our quest for wellness, we cannot forget about the potential of profound connections across sexual and racial boundaries. Homophobia hurts those of us who are lesbians and leads to deep psychic disease among those who are its bearers. As Black women, we are also women of color, and we need to devote more energy to working with our Latina, Native American, and Asian-American sisters. For we cannot pretend to achieve social sanity if we hold on to racist stereotypes about other women and men who also bear the marks of this country's racist history. These are some of the important messages of *Body & Soul.*

Wellness also means that we take seriously our capacity to love. Learning to fearlessly love and respect our individual and collective bodies and souls, we can become warriors against cancer, AIDS, high blood pressure, and the pervasive violence and stress that afflict our communities. We can also more forcefully demand social respect for our reproductive rights. *Body & Soul* urges us to take care of those bodies and souls we love and to act on the political implications of that love.

This love, therefore, is not without accountability. It is self-love forged in a collective embrace, in which we all seek protection and hope. It is a collective, sisterly embrace that brings us all together, including those of us who are otherwise rendered invisible and denied respect and material well-being.

The National Black Women's Health Project (NBWHP), the driving force behind this book, has deepened and complicated our ideas about physical, emotional, and spiritual health. Now *Body & Soul* legitimizes the strategies of self-empowerment and self-help that NBWHP has long advocated as a necessary component of our political activism, our community organizing, and our personal lives. We urge you to read and reread this book and share it with women who need to sit down, break down, and put ourselves back together.

Introduction

I remember the day I became acquainted with the National Black Women's Health Project. Several years ago I attended a one-day conference sponsored by the New York City chapter called "Empowerment, Health, Reproductive Rights: An Agenda for Women of All Colors." More than two hundred participants showed up early that Saturday morning, people of all ethnicities, men and women, gay and straight, all jammed into the auditorium at John Jay High School in Brooklyn. I settled deep into my seat, notepad in hand, ready to be talked at.

Instead the organizer informed us that we were to divide into race/gender groups, go into separate rooms, and talk about times in our lives when we had felt empowered and healthy and had enjoyed reproductive freedom and times when we had felt the opposite. This seemed like a highly unusual move. This was a conference; I had expected some experts with lots of letters after their names to sit up on the stage and tell me what to think. What did my life and what I felt have to do with an agenda for reproductive rights?

There were about fifty of us in my group, which was one of two groups of Black women. Before anyone spoke, we sat together in a circle, quietly getting to know one another. I looked around at the beautiful, calm, intelligent faces and hoped I would make some new friends.

But I was unprepared for what was about to happen. One sister jumped in with the first of many tales of disempowerment. She had had to be rushed to the emergency room because blood was gushing from her vagina. She begged the doctors to remove the IUD that was imbedded in her tissue, but they refused. Hysterical, she yanked the IUD out herself, causing pain more excruciating than she had ever felt. "I am now sterile," she said quietly.

Another woman was told that she might have cancer, and that she needed to come into the clinic for tests. With her legs spread on a table and with no anesthetics, a young white doctor cut out a cone-shaped piece of her cervix. When she screamed out in pain and terror, he looked at her and said, "What's that all about? You have no nerve endings there." Retelling the story, she began to sob so hard that two sisters got up to hold her.

Another woman had been raped repeatedly by an angry boyfriend, another had been sexually abused, another had watched her uncle beat her aunt to death, and still another had been sterilized without her consent.

I was stunned by the pain that lay behind the faces of these serene, intelligent women. I volunteered to be the historian for the group, needing a task to distance myself from the grief that was being deposited in the room. When it was my turn to speak, I felt subdued and constrained, overwhelmed by what I had heard from the other sisters. Haltingly, I talked about my mother, how I felt blessed to have learned about my body, sex, sexuality, and reproduction from her at an early age. At ten, I was unbearably embarrassed to have to listen to her, but she forced me to sit still and made sure I understood. After I told the story, I began to cry, no longer able to hold back the sorrow I felt for the other women. The sister next to me held my hand until it stopped shaking.

Yet when I left that room, rather than feeling sad, I felt empowered, proud to be in the company of survivors. I will never forget that day; the emotions I experienced as I listened to the sisters share will stay with me for the rest of my life. But it made me think about what NBWHP founder Byllye Avery calls our conspiracy of silence. Most of the women in the room had never felt safe enough to share those experiences with anyone, and maybe they never have again.

I think of how the conspiracy existed among the women in my life, because we never talked about our "personal business." At age thirty-six, my mother went into the hospital to get her tubes tied. But during the operation, the surgeon punctured one of her ureters and severed the other. She ended up having a hysterectomy, needed another operation, and had to be hospitalized for three months. For three more months she had to wear a bag strapped to each thigh to collect urine that couldn't be collected into the bladder. It took me years to ask my mother why she needed a hysterectomy in the first place or how she felt. Why hadn't I ever asked her if she was angry about the two large scars that stretch across her belly? When we finally talked about her ordeal, she said that she had been terrified she would die and wouldn't be able to raise my sister and me.

When I was a teenager, my grandmother used to ask me to massage the pain out of her hip, but it wasn't until she died that I found out she had suffered through months of excruciating bone cancer. She had put off going to the hospital because she didn't want to die before she could attend my high school graduation. She never shared her sadness or her fear of dying. Eventually I talked to my mother about it, and she told me that my grandmother had also had breast cancer and had had to have a breast removed. She also had an illegal abortion in the 1940s. I had never known.

Last year I read an essay my best friend wrote and learned that as a little girl, she had endured seven years of sexual abuse. I felt sad and ashamed to realize that I hadn't known of the anguish and anger she felt over having her childhood stolen from her.

The first large gathering of Black women dealing with health issues was inspired by the need to break this conspiracy of silence. Two simple sentences buried somewhere in a health atlas motivated Byllye Avery to organize the 1983 National Conference on Black Women's Health Issues: "A survey reported that more than half of Black women 18 to 35 years old rated themselves in psychological distress. That distress was rated higher than that of diagnosed mental patients."

That startling finding illustrated the kind of emotional pain so many of us carry with us as we move through our lives and pointed to a conspiracy of silence so many Black women have when it comes to our personal and health problems. The conference was organized to give sisters permission to talk about how we felt—physically, emotionally, and spiritually—and to understand that there is no shame in being afraid, no shame in reaching out to grasp another woman's hand for support. It was also created so that we could develop our own approaches to healing ourselves, rather than having some great white father somewhere deciding what is best for us.

From the energy and ideas generated by that conference the National Black Women's Health Project (NBWHP) was born. It began in 1983 as a few scattered self-help support groups in Atlanta, Philadelphia, and New York, arranging for three or more Black women to meet monthly to "take the stress off." There are now nearly 150 such groups around the country and throughout the world. With the women trained by the Project to guide themselves, the discussions range from rapes and abuse the women have quietly suffered to how to do a breast self-examination and where to get a Pap smear.

But even as hundreds of thousands of us have torn down that invisible wall of silence, many problems remain.

- Black women live fewer years than white women.
- Our breast cancer is caught later, and we are more likely to die from it.
- The majority of women and children infected with HIV disease are Black.
- Our children are more likely to be born small, and they die more frequently before reaching one year of age.
- We have heart disease at younger ages, a heart attack is more likely to prove fatal, and we have twice as many cases of high blood pressure as whites.
- Nearly 50 percent of us are overweight.
- We are more likely to smoke, and we are less likely to quit than white women.
- We have higher rates of sexually transmitted infection and pelvic inflammatory disease.
- Over half of us have been beaten, been raped, or survived incest.

As I looked at these statistics, I thought about how little had changed since that first Black women's health conference in 1983. With this thought in mind, I drove up to Pennsylvania to talk to Byllye Avery. I needed to ask her what we can do—as individual Black women and collectively—to change this.

As we sat in Byllye's home surrounded by her beautiful African artifacts in a room painted her favorite color—purple—I realized the first thing we can do: Find our spiritual homes. Make the places where we live reflect ourselves, so that whatever healing needs to be done can begin. Fill it with people who affirm who we are and respect what we need to do with our lives.

Byllye and I spent the next few hours talking about ourselves and our sisters. Too many Black women are like empty wells that never get replenished. We give and give, but get little back. Many of us are dying inside. Unless we are able to go inside, to touch ourselves, to breathe fire and life into ourselves, we can never be healthy or even know what good health feels like.

Good health starts with self-esteem. In order to be healed, we must all believe that we are worthy of it. We must love and trust ourselves and know that feeling good is something we deserve and we can have.

Good health is about power. We have the power to understand how our bodies work and how they feel, and we are empowered to heal our bodies and our souls. Too often we don't know the power we have within ourselves. Instead we give up that power to other people. We need to stop letting doctors get away with piling up all this money, buying all these machines. All this foolishness is putting money back into their pockets on the treatment end instead of the prevention end. This can stop only when we take care of ourselves and avoid the illnesses that keep the medical system in business.

Good health is about intuition. That means being in tune with everything and everyone around us. In this scientific world we don't give credence to the idea that our intuition can lead us to the right place. When faced with health challenges, we must collect all the information, talk to all the doctors, and then go inside ourselves and take direction from our inner voices. We have to believe in ourselves and believe in our ability to make the decision that will lead to healing.

Finally, good health is about talking. We can no longer afford to participate in silence. We have to talk to our children about their bodies and their sexuality. We have to talk to our men to let them know that when they hurt us, they hurt themselves. And we have to talk to each other, to be willing to share our stories, rather than pretend that we haven't had to struggle or face challenges. With talking goes listening, sitting quietly, and understanding and learning from the experience of other women.

I still struggle when I have to talk about myself and how I feel. When I can't make the words come out of my mouth, I put them on paper. That's what this book has been about for me and for all of the women who worked on it. It is written by Black women, for Black women as a way for all of us to grow and learn as we work to improve our personal and collective health.

Reading this book may be your first step toward good health or one of many steps in a long journey. Take this information and use it. This book is no more than you're willing to put into it. Take it with you to the doctor. Share it with a friend or neighbor. Discuss it with your daughter or your mother. Talk about it in your support group.

We couldn't cover every subject about Black women's health in depth here, but where we fall short, we've provided the titles of books you can read and the names of organizations with phone numbers and addresses for you to contact.

As you read this book, look for yourself on each page and in the experiences of other women. Examine your reactions, attitudes, and feelings to the things you read. What are you willing to do to make changes in your life, in order to be a different, more healthy person physically, emotionally, and spiritually? Are you willing to clean your mind and your body of whatever is holding you back?

This book should be part of your growth. There is no such thing as being grown up, because we are in a continual process of growth. You will be in a different place after you read this book. Make that a place where your healing can begin. Imagine that place bathed in your favorite colors and covered in bright African fabric. It is yours, and you deserve it.

—LINDA VILLAROSA
Brooklyn, New York

PART I

OUR BODIES

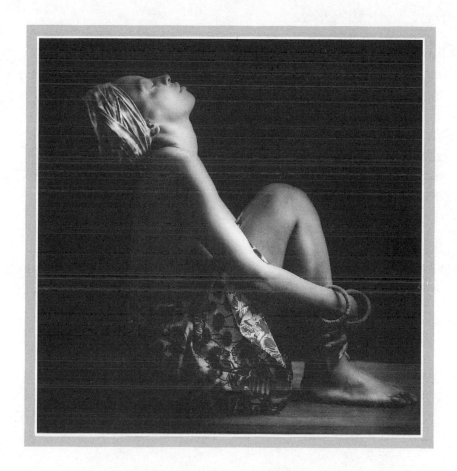

1

Body Weight and Image

Although Black women come in all shapes and sizes, in our community we have an abundance of large women. We often celebrate a wealth of Black female flesh, but being large has also caused many of us an undue amount of pain—both physical and emotional. Along with all of the other derogatory names that we have been called, put "fat" in front of the insult and the injury intensifies.

Each woman deals with issues of weight in her own way. Singer Etta James proudly flaunts her abundant size across the stage. College professor and *Essence* magazine writer E. K. Daufin describes herself as "large and lovely," and she sometimes practices belly dancing in her spare time. Others, however, have been damaged by society's perceptions. They jump from diet to diet, become anorexic or bulimic, and quietly struggle with sorrow and self-loathing.

It's important for large women to take a hard look at their bodies. It's okay to be big, if you're healthy both physically and emotionally. But if weight is causing health problems or if you're hiding pain under layers of fat, it's time to face up, get help, and lose weight.

The Bigger the Better?

According to the National Center for Health Statistics, more than 30 percent of the Black population is overweight. About 45 percent of

Black women are obese, or 20 percent above the ideal body weight for their height, frame, and age. An alarming 60 percent of Black women between the ages of forty-five and seventy-five weigh far more than they ought to.

Though these facts stand, we do have reason to question how overweight and obesity are defined in this country. In the past, physicians used insurance-company tables to measure "ideal" body weight, and these ideal weights were largely derived from the insurance records of white males. In 1990 the government updated the tables as part of its Dietary Guidelines for Americans. Now, for example, the new tables say a person five feet four inches tall should weigh between 111 and 146 pounds if she or he is aged nineteen to thirty-four, and 122 to 157 pounds if she or he is over thirty-five. Despite the update, the tables remain controversial because ideal weights are nearly impossible to estimate. Plus, the guidelines don't distinguish between men's and women's bodies! Rather than relying on tables, it's best to pay attention to your own health—both physical and emotional—to determine whether or not you want or need to lose weight.

The Black community has always been more likely to accept large and voluptuous women than white Americans have been. In all traditional African societies, largeness is celebrated, particularly in women. In contrast to the pursuit and near-worship of thinness in America, Africans view full-figured bodies as symbols of health, wealth, desire, prosperity, and fertility.

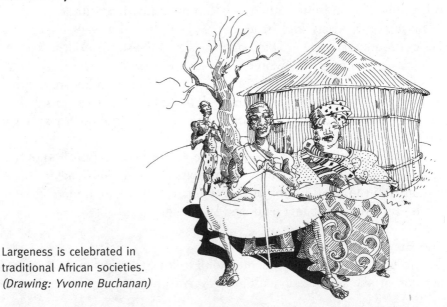

Largeness is celebrated in traditional African societies.
(Drawing: Yvonne Buchanan)

This cultural appreciation for and comfort with large women remains in the African-American community today. Large Black women are seen as capable and nurturing, holding up the world on their steady shoulders. Fat "mammies" like Hattie McDaniel as Mammy in *Gone With the Wind*; Ethel Waters and later Louise Beavers as Beulah, TV's favorite Black maid; and pancake maven Aunt Jemima (although her image has slimmed down in recent years) are a few of the familiar images of fat Black women. Perhaps the most well known and loved contemporary African-American woman of any size, Oprah Winfrey is everywoman, a kind, caring, nurturing symbol to our community and to the larger society. We accept her and find comfort in her size, even as it fluctuates.

Alice Walker has explained that in our community, thinness, not fatness, is rejected "because we don't have a tradition of skinniness in any sense—not in our food, not in our bodies. The sense of roundness . . . is a very precious thing we share with the majority of peoples in the world. The whole thing about being angular and linear . . . it's not our culture, it's not our tradition."

Embracing our African roots can be a positive and affirming process for Blacks throughout the diaspora. Yet it is vital that we examine and change the undeniably negative consequences of obesity among Black women. More than a matter of aesthetics, excess weight puts us at a higher risk for diabetes, stroke, coronary heart disease, and hypertension—all debilitating, life-threatening health problems. Already at greater risk for all maladies ranging from headaches to heart attacks, Black women can ill afford to ignore any problem that shortens our life span, as obesity has been proven to do.

Why So Much Fat?

According to some experts, there is a direct correlation between heredity and body weight. One researcher has noted that if both your parents were obese, you have an 80 percent chance of being obese, while the risk drops to 18 percent if neither parent was obese. Other researchers suggest that obesity is a physiological phenomenon that is influenced by our metabolic and nervous systems. They say that overweight people often have a slow metabolism (the process that turns food into energy) that hinders the ability to burn up the calories they consume.

African-Americans may carry a specific gene from our African forebears that predisposes some of us to excess weight, according to Lorraine Bonner, M.D., a physician who practices in Oakland, California. "There is evidence to suggest that the Africans who survived the Middle Passage to this country were those who were best able to utilize and retain the meager scraps of food they were fed," explains Dr. Bonner. "People who are in an environment of famine maintain fat as a means of selective survival. I think it's safe to say that many African-Americans today have retained this genetic marker from their African ancestors who were brought here as slaves."

The food we eat also plays a part in how big we are. Soul food, a tradition that has been handed down from generation to generation, is high in fat, sugar, and calories. Much of it is fried in grease, and fatty pork parts add to the flavor of many dishes. What's more, poverty also helps determine who's fat and who's not. Poor women are twice as likely to be overweight as their more affluent sisters, and the Black community has more than its share of poor folks. Low-fat, low-calorie foods and fresh fruits and vegetables are often expensive or unavailable in poor communities. Many people are left with high-fat, high-calorie, processed choices simply because these are the only foods they can afford or find.

Unspoken Pain

Tradition, heredity, metabolism, and poverty are major factors in Black obesity, but that is still far from the whole story. Recent studies indicate that for Black women, overeating and excessive weight gain are often triggered by deep-seated and painful psychological problems. Women are socialized to be around food—planning meals, cooking them, serving them, and cleaning up—especially in our culture. Food is a socially acceptable, controllable, legal, cheap addiction.

Obsessed with food, many Black women are trapped on a physical and emotional roller coaster that leaves them filled with self-hatred, hopelessness, and despair. "All too often people are not eating for nutrition; rather, they're eating for comfort," notes Gladys Jennings, Ph.D., associate professor emeritus of food science and human nutrition at Washington State University in Pullman, Washington.

Sociologist Becky Wangsgaard Thompson, Ph.D., of Princeton University is among a handful of experts who has conducted research on the emotional aspects of compulsive eating among women of color. In her study, Dr. Thompson found that many Black women overeat to quell the fear, rage, grief, and disappointment that pervade their lives.

The title of Dr. Thompson's research paper, "Raisins and Smiles for Me and My Sister," was prompted by a poignant story an African-American woman shared with her. As the story goes, Rosalee (not her real name) grew up in a violent home. Whenever she would hear her parents fighting, she would sneak a box of crackers, a jar of grape jelly, and raisins from the kitchen. She would spread the jelly on the crackers, arranging the raisins in the shape of a happy face, a ritual that always made her younger sister smile. As their parents screamed at each other in the next room, the sisters would stuff themselves with one "happy-face cracker" after another.

"At the age of four, Rosalee was already using food to protect herself from the pain of her family," Thompson explains. "Compulsive eating is a mechanism many Black women have devised to cope with hardship. Food is a cheap, legal, and accessible commodity women use to combat oppression."

Compulsive Eating: The Impact of Sexual Abuse

For many Black women, overeating is a response to the loss of childhood innocence that has been stripped from them in the form of physical and sexual abuse. Indeed, the sexual abuse of children is one of the country's most frequent and widespread crimes, affecting as many as 25 percent of female children before they reach the age of thirteen, according to the Federal Bureau of Investigation.

Gail E. Wyatt, Ph.D., an African American professor at the University of California at Los Angeles, cites studies that suggest that African-American females between the ages of nine and twelve are more frequently victims of sexual abuse than are white females. Most abuse occurs in a home and is perpetrated by someone known and trusted by the victim, such as a family member, neighbor, baby-sitter, or minister. Princeton researcher Thompson reports that two-thirds of the women in her study had been sexually molested by family members or friends.

"People are just beginning to make the correlation between sexual abuse and eating problems," Dr. Thompson explains. "Sexual abuse is such a traumatic and wounding event that it is often repressed deep in the psyche. It often takes a long time before women can come to terms with the experience and understand how the sexual abuse is connected to their eating."

Dr. Bonner has also seen the link between her obese Black female patients and sexual abuse. "A large number of them are incest survivors," she says. "Compulsive eating is a form of pain management for these women. They use food as a drug to anesthetize themselves from the pain they've experienced."

Ardena Shankar, chair of the Santa Cruz, California, County Task Force on Self-Esteem, says she firmly believes that her overeating was

"Eating has let
me get the
nurturing I
wanted but
couldn't find any
other place."

—JOYCE DELANEY,
LEGAL ASSISTANT, LOS
ANGELES, CALIFORNIA

It's hard to say it, but I've thought I was very ugly since puberty. A lot of my body image has to do with my father. Every woman in the street had to meet with his approval. He also directed comments toward me, and I've really internalized things he said about me.

I guess I was twelve or thirteen when I got really depressed and gained thirty-seven pounds. I said to myself, "If I'm large, no one—especially my dad—will look at me this way." It would stop if I got big enough because he seemed to have an aversion to overweight women. But he would still say things. My dad used to call me "Biggin" and put me down all the time because I was gaining weight, but he would still touch. I remember we were at a family picnic. My father got drunk, and my dad's cousin drove. We were in the backseat, and he opened up my blouse and said, "Look, titties," and no one said anything. I'm overweight by about fifty pounds. I eat a lot all the time and when I'm not hungry. I eat when I'm upset, when I'm depressed, under pressure, and especially when I'm bored. You get that instant gratification; it tastes good. No matter how quick, it's pleasurable; it's always there. It's something that's been there when other things haven't.

Eating has let me get the nurturing I wanted but couldn't find any other place. Emotionally my family is very distant, very closed. I know my mother is aware of something. You can't live in a house and have these things happen and not know what's going on. But she's not well, and this problem is the last thing this woman needs. My father can't own up to anything. I don't ever anticipate saying anything to him. He knows I have a hard time dealing with him, so we're very distant.

I'm very angry. That's been a big problem; how I deal with anger. I've always been taught you just don't get angry, you hold everything in. I'm angry about the lies. I feel like I'm protecting all these things.

prompted by the sexual abuse she suffered as a child: "I wasn't always fat. I was a thin child until I started getting molested. My weight just took off after that."

Eating Disorders
It has long been assumed that Black women didn't suffer from eating disorders such as anorexia nervosa and bulimia. But recent reports have proven that assumption wrong.

While the majority of those who suffer from eating disorders are white women, growing numbers of Black women may also be affected. Wrote Maya Browne in the June 1993 *Essence* magazine article "Dying to Be Thin," "I had been suffering from anorexia with intermittent episodes of bulimia for almost two years. Because I was a dancer, people expected me to be thin, and because I am Black, no one suspected an eating disorder."

Essence followed up Browne's article with a survey of its readers conducted by the University of South Carolina School of Medicine and Arizona State University researchers. They found that:

- 71.5 percent were preoccupied with the desire to be thinner.
- 71.5 percent were terrified of being overweight.
- 64.5 percent were preoccupied with fat on the body.
- 52 percent were preoccupied with food.

Noted the researchers: "African-American women are at risk for and suffer from eating disorders in at least equal proportions to their white counterparts. [They] have adopted similar attitudes towards body image, weight and eating as their white counterparts, thus contributing to their high risk for these disorders."

Binge-purge behavior or bulimia was surprisingly common among the survey's respondents. It is characterized by massive, uncontrolled food bingeing, which is then followed by purging through vomiting or the use of laxatives. Some bulimics also exercise compulsively to "burn off" the large amounts of food they have consumed. Though bulimics also fear becoming fat, unlike anorexics, they generally don't become thin. In fact, family and friends often can't detect this eating disorder, because bulimics are secretive about their vomiting and often appear physically normal.

Anorexia nervosa is less common but more serious. It is a form of severe and deliberate self-starvation that can sometimes lead to death. Though they become skeleton-thin, many anorexics continue to think they look fat, even as they stop menstruating and become weak and ill. Some also overexercise in an attempt to rid the body of any and all fat.

As with their white counterparts, Black females who suffer from anorexia and bulimia often have low self-esteem, repressed anger, and a high probability of having been physically, emotionally, or sexually abused. Most harbor an intense and irrational fear of gaining weight and have a distorted body image. Many come from families that place heavy emphasis on achievement, perfection, and looks. Many are dancers, models, and actresses who rely on their physical appearance for their livelihoods. Food—eating it or not eating it—may be the one area in their lives they feel they can control.

Maria P. Root, author of *Bulimia: A Systems Approach,* has noted that striving women of color are under tremendous pressure as role models, many times feeling that they must be perfect (and perfectly thin) in order to counteract negative racial stereotypes. Just as some large Black women overeat in order to have something they can control, anorexics and bulimics may also be trying to find a sense of control in an oppressive world.

Here are some signs that point to disordered eating.

- Making repeated comments about being fat or feeling fat—even when weight is below average
- Eating in secret
- Compulsively overeating
- Eating only tiny portions
- Seeming depressed
- Vomiting, taking large amounts of laxatives, diuretics, or diet pills
- Constipation or lack of menstruation
- Purposeless, excessive physical activity that is not part of a training program
- Light-headedness, weakness, or dizziness not accounted for by illness
- Mood swings

Several professional organizations that can help Black women recognize the symptoms of and recover from eating disorders are listed at the end of the chapter.

Loving Yourself Versus Losing Weight: Making the Healthy Choice

There are many full-figured Black women who are happy, healthy, and comfortable with their weight, who have made peace with their bodies, refusing to let their size or shape dominate their lives.

If you are a large, fit Black woman with a history of good physical, mental, and spiritual health, focus on learning how to love and celebrate yourself as you are. There is no need to become entangled in the "yo-yo" dieting and endless weight-loss regimes that obesity experts now say are detrimental to both physical and emotional health. Be realistic and *loving* when you evaluate your body and your well-being. No amount of drastic dieting or exercise will transform a naturally full-figured body into a thin one. Work to achieve and accept *your* best body, not that of someone else.

On the other hand, if excess weight is exacerbating your health problems and causing you psychological distress, the problem needs to be addressed. An improved, nutrition-filled diet can help obese Black women shed unwanted fat. Nutritionist Gladys Jennings suggests experimenting with a simple formula: Begin to cut back on the *S's* in your life—sugars, snacks, spirits, salt, seconds, and sitting. Dr. Bonner advises her overweight patients to make beans, rice, vegetables, and fruit the core of their diet. For more information on nutrition, see chapter 4, "Eating Right."

No matter what size you are, you should definitely add physical activity to your daily routine, and exercise is a key component of any weight-loss plan. (Be sure to check with your health-care provider before beginning an exercise program.) Brisk walking is a safe, easy, convenient form of exercise, especially for larger women. For specific information on exercise and large women, see chapter 3, "Moving Our Bodies."

Even when motivated, many of us may have difficulty with traditional weight-control programs. Researcher Shiriki K. Kumanyika, Ph.D., notes that "weight-control programs [such as Weight Watchers] may be inherently biased toward the needs and values of the dominant culture and, therefore, may be less attractive to or less successful with those who are not members of the majority." Instead she points to more appropriate models

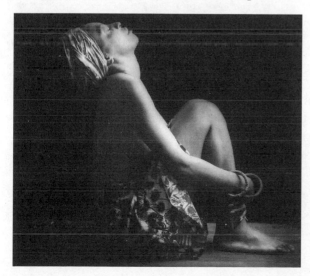

We must look inside ourselves to deal with problems that are causing overweight and eating disorders.
(Photo: Debbie Egan-Chin)

"When I was angry, I would go to the refrigerator."

—STUDENT,
NEW YORK CITY

Since the age of twelve I've been trying to diet, but it hasn't worked. A lot of people in my family are big, and when I was younger, they bothered me about my size. My mother had been small, but later gained a lot of weight. She'd say to me, "You don't want to end up like me, do you?" I wish I'd listened. Right now I weigh 190 pounds and wear a size 16.

I don't hate myself, but I think if I were smaller, things would be easier. I could find clothes, my feet wouldn't hurt, and men would accept me immediately. I feel that they are attracted to me but are holding back. One guy said we didn't go together because I had a stomach. My dream is a flat stomach. I don't like the way my stomach looks when I don't have any clothes on.

Eventually I began to read things in magazines about compulsive eating, and I started paying attention to my patterns. I noticed that when I was angry, I would go to the refrigerator. And plenty of times I was eating when I wasn't hungry. I realized boredom is why I eat two Skor bars before lunch. But I also noticed that if I start to do something and I'm really into it, I can look up and I haven't eaten anything for hours.

I have compared myself to an alcoholic. It bothers me that I sit down and say I'm not going to eat something, and I eat it anyway. I want to be able to eat just to live, for my health. It bothers me that I have to use food to deal with problems. If I have to eat something every two seconds and every time I eat I feel worse afterward, I'm no better than the drug addict on the corner.

such as the Baltimore Church High Blood Pressure Program's series of two-hour counseling/exercise sessions, called Lose Weight and Win. In that eight-week program, 184 Black women and 3 white women from ages eighteen to eighty-one lost—and maintained—an average of six pounds. At least as important, it was a community-based, collective effort.

Still, some Black women find success in groups like Overeaters Anonymous (see the list below). Based on the principles of Alcoholics Anonymous, OA is a nonprofit organization that aids the compulsive overeater. Thousands of people of diverse ethnic backgrounds attend the free meetings held daily in most cities.

Managing Stress/Improving Your Self-Esteem

It's very important to pay attention to the connection between stressful events and your eating habits. So many of the unhealthy choices Black women make are spurred by the unexamined stresses and strains in our lives. Ask yourself, "Am I eating because I'm hungry or because I feel bad and food makes me feel better?" If it's the latter, step back and try to feed your inner hunger with love and understanding rather than food.

Compulsive eaters can also work on improving their present rather than remaining victimized by the past. If you suspect that you were sexually abused at any point in your life, seek professional help as soon as you can. Chances are high that unhealthy eating patterns will change as you begin the process of healing from your abuse.

Anything you do that boosts your self-esteem and makes you feel better about yourself can be an antidote to overeating. If you've always wanted to go to school, learn a particular craft, or pursue a different career, try to put your plans into action. Taking charge of your life and becoming productive can help change the sense of helplessness and lack of control that dominates the relationship some Black women have with food.

For More Information

ORGANIZATIONS: Body Awareness and Weight Control

NATIONAL ASSOCIATION TO ADVANCE FAT ACCEPTANCE, P.O. Box 188620, Sacramento, CA 95818; (916) 443-0303 or (800) 442-1214. NAAFA has fifty chapters in the U.S. and Canada and distributes information and literature.

THE MELPOMENE INSTITUTE, 1010 University Ave., St. Paul, MN 55104; (612) 642-1951. The Institute helps girls and women link physical activity and health through research, publication, and education. Call for a group of articles in its "larger woman" packet.

OVEREATERS ANONYMOUS WORLD SERVICE HEADQUARTERS, P.O. Box 92870, Los Angeles, CA 90009; (310) 618-8835. Call a local chapter for free twelve-step meetings in your area.

ORGANIZATIONS: Eating Disorders

AMERICAN ANOREXIA BULIMIA ASSOCIATION, 418 E. 76th St., New York, NY 10021; (212) 734-1114.

CENTER FOR THE STUDY OF ANOREXIA AND BULIMIA, 1 W. 91st St., New York, NY 10024; (212) 595-3449.

NATIONAL ANOREXIC AID SOCIETY, 1925 E. Dublin-Granville Rd., Columbus, OH 43229; (614) 436-1112 (hotline).

NATIONAL ASSOCIATION OF ANOREXIA NERVOSA AND ASSOCIATED DISORDERS, Box 7, Highland Park, IL 60035; (708) 831-3438.

BOOKS

A Hunger So Wide and So Deep, Becky W. Thompson, University of Minnesota Press, 1994.

Breaking Free from Compulsive Eating, Geneen Roth, New American Library, 1990.

Freeing Someone You Love from Eating Disorders, Mary Dan Eades, M.D., Perigee Books, 1993.

Fat Is a Feminist Issue, Susie Orbach, Berkley Publishers, 1982.

Great Shape: The First Fitness Guide for Large Women, Pat Lyons and Debby Burgard, Bull Publishing, 1990.

The Hungry Self: Women, Eating and Identity, Kim Chernin, Harper & Row, 1986.

The Black Health Library Guide to Obesity, Mavis Thompson, M.D., with Kirk A. Johnson, Henry Holt, 1993.

Sizing Up: Fashion, Fitness and Self-Esteem for Full-Figured Women, Sandy Summers Head, Fireside Books/Simon & Schuster, 1989.

When Food Is Love: Exploring the Relationship Between Eating and Intimacy, Geneen Roth, New American Library, 1992.

Why Weight? A Guide to Ending Compulsive Eating, Geneen Roth, New American Library, 1989.

MAGAZINES AND ARTICLES

Radiance, The Magazine for Large Women, P.O. Box 30246, Oakland, CA 94604; (510) 482-0680.

"Living Large, Getting Fit," E. K. Daufin, *Essence,* August 1990.

"Unhealthy Appetites," Evelyn C. White, *Essence,* September 1991.

"Coming Home: One Black Woman's Journey to Health and Fitness," Georgiana Arnold, in *The Black Women's Health Book: Speaking for Ourselves,* ed. Evelyn C. White, The Seal Press, 1990.

"Heavy Burden," Rosemary L. Bray, *Essence,* January 1992.

"Heavy Judgement," Deborah Gregory, *Essence,* August 1994.

2

Our Skin, Hair, Eyes, and Teeth

Black is beautiful. That goes for our dark and lovely skin, our full, thick hair, and our many-shades-of-brown eyes. But too many of us don't believe this. Our vision has been crowded with images of white women with alabaster complexions, long, straight hair, aquatic blue eyes, and even, white teeth. We look into our mirrors, scan our dusky skin, feel the mass of lamb's wool nesting atop our scalp, check large, gap-toothed smiles, and with disillusionment in our plain brown eyes, wonder where we went wrong.

However, thanks to the Black Power movement and, more recently, the celebration of Afrocentricity, we are able to recognize and honor our own beauty—to a point, that is. Old habits die hard. Although Black models grace the covers and pages of mainstream magazines, most are light-skinned, their look "exotic." And although the natural has reemerged, although dreadlocks are flowing and Black *and* bald are also beautiful, companies that make chemical relaxers are certainly *not* going broke.

This chapter is not about developing a particular ideal of beauty. It is a guide to keeping your skin, hair, eyes, and teeth healthy so that your own inner—Black—beauty shines through.

Skin

We have an obsession with skin color in our community. Though we currently refer to ourselves as Black, in the past, to call someone black was to insult, something akin to "yo' momma." The phrase "If you're white, you're all right. If you're brown, stick around. But if you're black, get back" rang all too true. *Black* was too intense a word to toss around unless you aimed to provoke. *Black* spelled pain. *Colored* was a gentler term.

We have an endless array of terms to describe our various shades, such as "half-white," "high yaller," "redbone," and "tar baby," to name a few. But no one shade of "black"—from eggshell to blue black—is better than any other. The palette of beautiful hues is endless.

And Black is healthful: Dark skin is firmer and smoother and resists aging better than white skin does. (The saying "Good black don't crack" is true!) Sun-damaged white skin contains large amounts of degenerated elastic tissue that the body must constantly reabsorb and replace. This process decreases the total amount of skin, eventually causing shrinkage and wrinkling. Because dark skin holds a higher content of melanocytes, granules within the skin cells that produce a dark pigment called melanin, there is little or no skin wrinkling. In Black skin these melanocytes are larger, thus preventing the upper layers of skin from degenerating with time and cumulative sun damage. The higher content of melanin also protects against skin cancer, though we are by no means immune. So to rework an old phrase: "The blacker the berry, the *healthier* the juice."

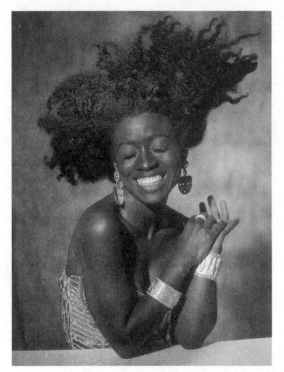

This image of performer Alva Rogers, which appeared on the cover of Essence, proves that Black is beautiful. *(Photo: Matthew Jordan Smith)*

Caring for Our Skin

We were blessed with gorgeous skin, and we have to take care of it.

The body needs to be washed frequently to remove dead cells, superfluous oil, perspiration, and dirt from the skin surface. Compared with white skin, Black skin is dryer, and an accumulation of dead skin cells— "ash"—shows up more against our dark skin. To slough off dead cells, use a loofah or cleansing grains. Be careful not to rub too vigorously or use extra-coarse grains; this could lead to irritation and scarring.

My embarrassing introduction to ashy skin came during the preteen years. Asked to give a final report, I shyly approached the front of my sixth-grade class. As I nervously read, I could hear snickers coming from around the room.

When the report was over, I sat down, then turned and asked my best friend, Marisol, what had been so funny.

"Your knees," she answered, still giggling.

"Were they shaking?"

"No," Marisol whispered. "They're white."

Sure enough, my twelve-year-old knees were white as chalk. And it didn't stop there. Upon pulling my knee socks down, I found my legs to be just as white. The same went for my elbows, the backs of my arms, even my cheeks and chin.

"Here," she said, handing me a tiny jar of petroleum jelly.

It was my induction into the ranks of shining dark-skinned girls. But I didn't want to shine. I wanted to be ash-free.

Years and hundreds of lotions, oils, and poultices later, I have still not beaten the ash thing. Many over-the-counter products soak right into my skin, leaving it as dry as it was before. Eight glasses of water a day leave me feeling healthier but with the same knees I had in sixth grade. A temporary solution, baby oil, slathered onto shower-damp skin, allows me to face the public with minimal embarrassment. Otherwise, I'm still searching.

> *"I didn't want to shine. I wanted to be ash-free."*
>
> —JACQUELINE WOODSON, WRITER, BROOKLYN

Be gentle with the delicate skin on your face. You need to wash your face at least twice daily with a mild cleanser and rinse with cold water to close the pores. Don't use cleanser that contains perfume or deodorant or that makes the skin feel dry. A cleanser like this doesn't have to be expensive; check stores where natural products are sold.

After you wash, moisturize your skin to replenish the natural oils that are lost with bathing and the environment. For your face, use a moisturizer to protect against the sun's damaging rays; and given the sorry state of the ozone layer, be sure that the product contacts a sunscreen with an SPF (sun protection factor) of at least 15. We get skin cancer less than white folks do, but we do get it. At night, also use moisturizer.

Choose moisturizing products carefully: Traditional Black hair- and skin-care products often contain heavy oils that can block the pores and cause the skin to break out. Though acne is generally milder in Black skin, it can still result in dark spots and scars.

It is wise to give yourself an at-home facial about once a week. It's also a nice treat—and good for the skin—to have a professional facial once in a while if you can afford it. Facials deep-clean, slough off dead skin, unclog dirt and oil from the pores, and stimulate facial muscles. You can purchase at-home scrubs and masks at drugstores or health-food stores or make your own. One sister swears by her grandmother's recipe for smooth skin. (Granny had a glowing, unlined face well into her sixties.) She opened up her pores by placing a steaming washcloth on her face, then very gently scrubbed with a concoction of uncooked oatmeal, finely ground almonds, and water. Next she applied a facial mask made of egg whites, left it on for a half hour, then rinsed with cold water.

The right food also has to go *into* your body. Supermodel Beverly Johnson knows this is true. When she first started her career, she was a self-professed junk-food addict. "When I say I lived on fast food, I mean f-a-s-t. Candy and cookies and chips, to name a few," she writes in her first book, *Beverly Johnson's Guide to a Life of Health and Beauty*. "I was always tired, and I looked it. My complexion had poor tone, my hair had no luster, and I developed skin irritations. . . . I began thinking that I could only last one or two more years in the business if my health stayed so poor."

Slowly she changed her diet, substituting herbal tea, juices, fresh fruits and vegetables, and natural foods for junk. The new eating plan, she says, did wonders. "It has made my complexion and my hair, a woman's two foundations for beauty, more lustrous and healthy than they ever were. It has improved my circulation and given me more energy."

A well-balanced diet, including plenty of fresh vegetables, fruit, and juice, keeps the skin healthy. To flush out toxins, drink at least eight glasses of water a day. Learn to control stress. Don't smoke or overindulge in alcohol (no more than one drink per day); these habits wreak havoc on the skin.

Some Common Problems of Black Skin

Acne
Acne can be merely annoying, or at worst it can cause shame, insecurity, and depression. It occurs when the oil glands in the skin become inflamed and clogged with oil and dead skin cells. Bacteria can get trapped in the stopped-up oil, and the gland can eventually erupt, creat-

ing sore, swollen areas that we know as pimples. Because the area is infected, white blood cells travel there to aid in healing. When these cells mix with oil, bacteria, and dead cells, a white tipped pustule forms.

Acne first occurs during the teen years, affecting 90 percent of adolescents. The hormonal changes that cause the breasts to develop and pubic hair to grow also stimulate the oil glands in the skin. These same kinds of hormonal changes also occur about two weeks to ten days before our menstrual periods—which explains why so many of us are plagued by premenstrual break-outs. Stress also triggers a hormonal response that stimulates oil glands and can lead to acne.

If acne is severe—your skin is constantly broken out with large, sore pimples and cysts—you'll need to see a dermatologist. You may receive a prescription for an oral antibiotic such as tetracycline. You might also be given antibiotics in cream, ointment, or roll-on form.

For very stubborn cases, doctors can prescribe a medication called accutane, which closes down the body's production of oil. Though this drug works well for some people, it is also highly toxic. Accutane can cause birth defects and is never prescribed for women who are pregnant or even considering pregnancy. Some people who take the drug experience side effects such as very dry, peeling skin, very chapped lips, dry genitals, and sun sensitivity.

If you use over-the-counter acne preparations, such as lotions and astringents, don't leave them on overnight, because they can be too drying. You might like to try over-the-counter products that contain alphahydroxy acids (AHA's). Made from fruit, AHA's loosen dead skin and help open the pores. Read labels carefully, and choose a product that is oil-free.

Everyone who suffers from acne can minimize its effects by following these tips:

- Keep your face clean. Use a mild, oil-free cleanser, and avoid harsh scrubs that are too abrasive for skin that scars easily.
- Find ways to reduce stress, such as meditation, exercise, and writing in a journal.
- Use oil-free skin-care products. Read labels and look for the word *noncomedogenic,* which means "nonclogging."
- Keep hair-care products that contain oil away from your face. Don't use the products around your hairline, and wear a scarf when you sleep to keep hair off your face.
- Eat properly. Iodides—found in salt, salty snacks, fast food,

processed foods, shellfish, and some vitamin supplements—irritate acne. Also stay away from peanuts and chocolate. Drink six to eight glasses of water a day.
  ▪ Keep your hands off your face. Picking causes scarring and irritation.

Atopic Dermatitis

The familiar word *eczema,* often used to refer to atopic dermatitis (AD), is actually a general term for all types of dermatitis, the medical name for "inflammation of the skin." All types of eczema cause itching, redness, and often blisters and peeling. Atopic dermatitis tends to be the most severe and long-lasting kind of eczema. It can cause itchy, swollen skin and generally affects the insides of the elbows, backs of the knees, and the face. In some cases it can cover the entire body.

AD generally affects people who either suffer from asthma and/or hay fever or have family members who do. That puts Blacks at particular risk because we are so prone to asthma. AD is not contagious, but it is inherited. It usually begins in childhood—often during infancy—with dry, itchy, scaly skin and rashes on the cheeks, arms, and legs. In many cases the problem fades during childhood, although sufferers have a tendency to develop other problems such as dry, easily irritated skin, eye problems, and skin infections.

AD tends to flare up when the sufferer is exposed to certain substances or conditions. To lower the risk of a flare-up, these triggers should be avoided:

Irritating substances, such as skin products that contain alcohol, solvents, detergents, bleach, woolens, paints, fragrances, some soaps, and tobacco smoke.

Dry skin. Keep the skin moist with oils. It's better to choose natural or pure oils; skin lotions tend to have high water content and can sometimes make the problem worse.

Heat and high humidity. Bathe and shower in warm rather than hot water, and try to avoid drastic changes in temperature.

Stress. Find ways to control it, such as meditation, exercise, writing in a journal, talking about problems in a support group or with a therapist.

Cortisone or steroid creams are generally recommended as treatment. They can be purchased over-the-counter, or stronger products can be dispensed by prescription.

For more information contact the Eczema Association for Science and Education, 1221 S.W. Yamhill St., suite 303, Portland, OR 97205; (503) 228-4430.

Hyperpigmentation

Though melanin protects the skin and keeps it looking young, it can also create unstable pigmentation. Any type of irritant of the skin—acne, insect bites, hair bumps, or eczema—can cause unwanted changes in the skin. Dark spots, irregular patches, and discoloration are fairly common and often take months to fade. The hormonal changes caused by pregnancy and birth control pills, medication, and sun exposure can also cause hyperpigmentation in some women. To avoid these problems:

- Don't squeeze pimples.
- Avoid abrasive cleansers and harsh soaps on your face.
- Be careful not to scratch or irritate the skin.
- Always wear sunscreen of at least SPF 15, especially if you're pregnant or on the Pill.
- Ask your doctor if your prescription medication causes an allergic action in the sun.

Many Black women use over-the-counter fade creams to lighten dark spots and discoloration, but those products have recently come under fire. Hydroquinone, the active ingredient of these creams, has been linked to cancer, and consumer activists have attacked the manufacturers for exaggerating their marketing claims. Instead, try a body lotion containing alphahydroxy acids.

Keloids

Our skin is tough and heals more quickly than white skin does. But sometimes it heals too well. This overhealing produces raised scars known as keloids. Keloids tend to run in families, and they can develop after any trauma to the skin—surgery, cuts, scrapes, burns, severe acne, vaccinations, and insect bites.

Keloids can be difficult to treat. A dermatologist may prescribe a drug similar to cortisone, which is a type of steroid. It comes in cream or ointment form and can help soften or shrink the lesion. Sometimes it is injected directly into the scar. Surgery can also be used to treat keloids.

Because treatment is tricky, it's best to try to prevent keloids. If you are keloid-prone, avoid any kind of trauma that might produce a wound, including ear and nose piercing. Don't pick or scratch at scars. If you notice a keloid forming, see a dermatologist early on. Keloids are sometimes easier to treat when they are new.

Dermatosis Papulosa Nigra

Over half of all Black women have dermatosis papulosa nigra (DPN), dark growths that generally crop up on the face and neck. They look like moles and generally become more numerous with age. DPN is not serious, but you should have your doctor check your growths to make sure. Some women don't like how they look or find them itchy and irritating, so they have them removed. They can be burned off with an electric needle (electrosurgery) or frozen off using liquid nitrogen. However, treatment can be uncomfortable, and they can grow back.

Vitiligo

Vitiligo is a frightening and mysterious disease in which patches of skin (or all of it) lose pigment due to the destruction of melanocytes. This disease made news recently when singer Michael Jackson said that he had it. A Black person stricken with it can literally turn white.

Vitiligo generally begins with the fingers, feet, and around the mouth and eyes, giving the sufferer two-toned skin. The effect is much more marked in dark-skinned people because of the contrasting skin colors.

Experts are not sure what causes vitiligo; some think the body develops an allergy to its own pigment cells, while others believe that the cells simply destroy themselves during the process of pigment production. There is no cure for vitiligo, but several treatment options exist. One is to repigment the depigmented cells through a combination of drugs and ultraviolet light. Another, used in cases of extensive pigment loss, is to "bleach" the normal skin with a specific prescription preparation so that the dark skin looks similar to the depigmented skin. With no real cure, many sufferers have become expert in using makeup to cover contrasting skin tones.

Vitiligo can be emotionally crushing to the person who has it. For support and more information, contact the National Vitiligo Foundation, P.O. Box 6337, Tyler, TX 75711; (903) 534-2925.

Hair

Women of African ancestry have found many creative ways to style and adorn their lush hair by braiding it, wrapping it, and gracing it with shells and beads. African-American women have adapted those styles in fascinating, inventive ways. Imagine Patti LaBelle and one of her wild, imaginative styles, and you know it's true. But our hair is also beautiful in its simplest form: a close-cropped, short 'fro. And Caribbean women and men have helped popularize long, thick, natural dreadlocks.

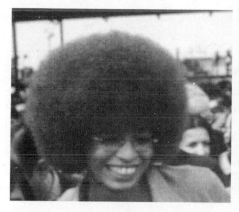 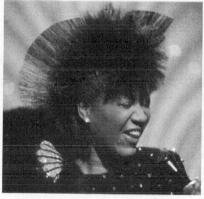 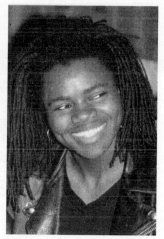

There's no end to our creative hairstyles. From left to right, Angela Davis and singers Patti LaBelle and Tracy Chapman. *(Photos: Globe Photos, Inc.)*

For too long, however, Black women have been wrapped up in the pathology of the term "good hair." "I used to think only Black women with so-called 'good hair' were the luckiest women in the world," wrote Lonnice Brittenum Bonner in her witty book *Good Hair: For Colored Girls Who've Considered Weaves When the Chemicals Became Too Ruff.* "You know what I mean. Hair that's naturally straight, loosely curled, or waved. Those of us with springy African hair were banished to 'bad hair' purgatory, doomed to spend eternity trying to make it look 'good.'" After chemical straighteners, dark burn marks from the curling iron, wigs, a greasy jheri curl, wearing a stocking cap to bed, the author has come to terms with her "Nappy Hair Phobia." "What does good hair mean?" she writes. "It means hair that is the best it can be, hair that's healthy-looking, a natural adornment. Notice that I *didn't* refer to hair of a certain texture or 'grade' as if our hair should be graded like a piece of USDA choice meat. If you can manage and enjoy your hair without going through major changes, then I'd say it's pretty good."

Caring for Black Hair

Our hair is thick and full of body, unique in shape and structure. Some of us have soft, cottony hair; others' is coarse and wooly. It can be tightly wound, close to the scalp, or looser and more curly. But whatever the texture, everyone's Black hair has one thing in common: It breaks easily. Compared to straight hair, curly hair weakens at every turn and must be treated gently. Always use a pick or wide-toothed comb when grooming your hair. And forget about being admonished for being tender-headed as a child: Treat your hair gently; don't yank or pull.

"I now know I'm a great person— with or without hair."

—Mali Michelle Fleming, journalist and African dancer/teacher, Washington, D.C.

My hair affair began early, when I was four years old. All of my mother's efforts to tame my spongy, sandy brown hair were short-lived and futile. And it's been a tug-of-war, literally, ever since.

From the tender age of five, I started the ritual of getting my hair straightened. Like most young Black girls, I started out getting it pressed with a straightening comb. By the time I was ten, I graduated to the chemical perm, so my hair could stay straighter longer—since that was the ultimate goal.

When I was sixteen, I was tired of getting the regular perm and having to hot-curl it. So I figured I'd try the newest thang—the jheri curl. It proved to be a mixed blessing. Once I went through the long procedure for those ready-made, moist, loose curls, I was elated. I tossed my hot curlers aside, grabbed my activator, and simply washed and went. I loved this "easy to care for" hair. But touch-up time came, as it invariably does for all perms, and that's when my curly perm fell out, literally. Clumps of my hair tumbled into the tub as I washed it. It had broken off at the back of the crown, leaving only the roots.

There was nothing left for me to do but shave it into a short, natural Afro. Somehow, I wasn't upset. Something inside me simply reassured my spirit that it wasn't the end of the world and life would go on. And it did. Most folks thought that I looked really attractive with it cut so short. And the men! Honey, I got more play with a short natural than I ever did with my permed 'do.

But since I was still in a predominantly white, all-girl high school, peer pressure kicked in, and as soon as my hair was strong enough, I went and got my hair relaxed again.

I went through a couple more hair changes until I decided to get in touch with who I really was—a natural kind of sister. But I still liked that long-hair feeling, so I dabbled in Afrocentric hairstyles like cornrows and braids until I decided to lock my hair. I envisioned having locks hanging down my back and wearing them in a myriad of beautiful styles. But not long after I started twisting and grooming, my hair started falling out again. The perms, the jheri, the braids had all taken their toll: I had worked my hair to death.

I was really emotionally hurt. I'd put a lot of physical and spiritual energy into grooming my hair. But I told myself that I'd just have to deal with this. I cut off what was left of my hair, and now I am back to a near-bald, short 'fro. I had a small, spiritual ceremony and prayed for peace and guidance about all facets of my life and most of all, to be a strong, African woman. I now know I'm a great person—with or without hair.

Black hair also tends to be dry, so you mustn't wash it too often—generally only about once or twice a week—using a gentle shampoo. Follow that with an oil-based conditioner. After shampooing and between washings, apply a light oil, hairdressing, or moisturizer to the hair, especially on the ends, to keep it soft. Light coconut oil is a nice option. Deep-condition the hair once or twice a month, and trim off the dead ends every two months to keep it looking and feeling healthy. Also, massage the scalp daily to increase circulation and stimulate natural oils and growth.

If you relax your hair—the majority of African-American women do—you need to be even more strict about proper hair care. The best relaxers on the market don't contain lye and do contain conditioners, but they're chemically based nonetheless. Most experts recommend having your hair relaxed in a salon by a professional who understands how the chemicals work and is experienced applying them. But if you can't afford a salon and do your own hair at home, be extra careful. Overprocessing can lead to severe damage and hair loss. And never apply chemicals to hair that has already been chemically treated (don't relax hair that has been dyed or jheri-curled) or if your scalp is cut or irritated.

Dreadlocks are an easy-to-care-for natural option for sisters. Long, beautiful dreadlocks symbolize a "natural" person who is in touch with her African ancestry. Locks can be difficult to start. It helps to find a friend who also wants to start dreadlocks; you can do each other's hair.

Some people start them by separating freshly washed hair into tiny sections and placing a small amount of a waxy pomade, aloe vera, or styling gel on each section. Then twist the section in one direction, avoiding overtwisting, which can cause the hair to break off. The hard part is waiting for the hair to "lock." Most folks say it's best not to wash your hair as you're waiting for it to lock—about a month. Instead, massage your scalp, moisturize it with a light, natural oil, and gently retwist any locks that unravel. After a month, gently wash and deep-condition your hair about every three weeks, and continue to retwist and massage and moisturize the scalp. Be patient: It can take a while—as long as a year—for the hair to lock.

If you don't want to go to the trouble to lock your own hair, many salons will start it for you, but given the popularity of the style, be prepared for the cost.

Regardless of the style you choose, diet plays a major part in the health of your hair. Eat lots of fruits and vegetables, and drink plenty of water to keep the hair from becoming dehydrated.

Hair Loss

Alopecia, hair loss, is caused by stress, poor diet, scalp infection, illness, and medication. Black women often suffer hair loss due to the strong chemicals we use on our hair. We can reverse the problem by changing or discontinuing the product.

Alopecia areata is another story. It is a rare dermatologic disorder in which the body identifies its own hair as foreign and works to immunize itself from the follicles by removing the hair from the body. Mostly the hair falls out in round or oval patches, but it can also affect the entire body. Some folks with the disorder are totally bald and without lashes, brows, or pubic hair.

It is not a nervous disorder, nor is it disabling. In fact, most persons with alopecia are in excellent heath. But from a psychological standpoint it can be extremely traumatizing.

For support, contact the National Alopecia Areata Foundation, P.O. Box 150760, San Rafael, CA 94915-0760; (415) 456-4644.

Hair Pulling

About 8 million people—mostly women—suffer from a little-known impulse disorder called trichotillomania. Sufferers compulsively twist, twirl, or tug at their hair, eyebrows, and even pubic hair, generally as a reaction to stress. It is so serious in some people that they end up with bald spots and try to cover the condition under wigs or hats. It can be a source of shame for sufferers, many of whom are too embarrassed to talk about it or have no idea that others also pull their hair.

For more information or to find out about therapists and support groups, contact the Trichotillomania Learning Center, 1215 Mission St., suite 2, Santa Cruz, CA 95060; (408) 457-1004; or the Obsessive Compulsive Foundation, P.O. Box 70, Milford, CT 06460; (203) 878-5669.

Eyes

The eyes are two of the most delicate parts of the body and should be handled with extreme care. The eyebrows and eyelashes serve to catch particles of dirt before they fall into the eyes, and the eyes themselves have their own defense system. They are well nourished with blood vessels, and to wash away dirt and bacteria, they are bathed in a clear fluid called tears. When anything jeopardizes the eyes, they react defensively. In many cases the defense reflex produces reddening or bloodshot eyes.

Your Vision

Contrary to the popular myth, eating carrots won't keep your eyes healthy; only proper eye care will. That means an eye exam at least every other year or more often if you're over thirty-five, if you have eye problems, or on your doctor's advice.

Many, many Americans require corrective lenses—either eyeglasses or contacts. The American Optometric Association points to these reasons:

Myopia (nearsightedness). About 30 percent of Americans are nearsighted, which means they can see clearly up close but not at a distance. Myopia usually begins during the school years and can become progressively worse, although most times it stabilizes.

Hyperopia (farsightedness). Approximately 60 percent of Americans are farsighted to some degree, and the condition has probably existed since their childhood. Farsighted people can see better at a distance than close up.

Astigmatism. Sixty-five to 70 percent of Americans have some degree of this condition, which results from an irregular-shaped cornea (the clear, front surface of the eye). It causes blurred or distorted vision, headache, eye fatigue, and irritation.

Presbyopia, also known as "aging eyes." This gradual decline of the ability of the eyes to focus sharply and clearly on near objects occurs when the convex disk that sits over the colored portion of the eye loses its flexibility. Most people notice that during their forties they have to hold reading matter farther and farther away from the eyes. It is not a disease and should not be confused with farsightedness. Most folks with

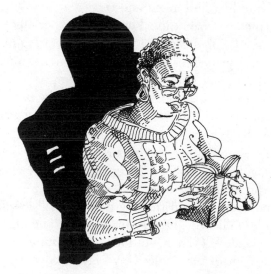

Half-glasses correct age-related farsightedness. *(Drawing: Yvonne Buchanan)*

this condition wear reading glasses, bifocals, or bifocal contact lenses.

Some people choose surgery, the newest trend in vision correction. The most common surgery is radial keratotomy (RK), which is used to correct nearsightedness. In this procedure, the ophthalmologist makes four to sixteen incisions in the cornea, depending on the amount of correction needed. About 60 percent of those who have undergone this treatment achieve 20/20 vision.

RK carries the potential for risks and complications. In some cases the surgery can induce farsightedness, glare, halos, fluctuating vision, and an inability to wear contact lenses. For some people a second operation is necessary to further correct vision. Complications are rare but include infection, cataracts, or rupture of the wound.

For more information, talk to an ophthalmologist, and then get a second opinion.

Avoiding Serious Eye Disease

Glaucoma occurs when the internal pressure in the eye rises so high that the optic nerve is damaged. Over 2 million Americans have this disease, which is four to five times more common in Blacks than in whites; most sufferers are forty years of age or older. Compared with whites, we contract the disease earlier and are more likely to go blind as a result of it. Diabetes doubles the risk of glaucoma, and Black women are especially prone to diabetes: The rate of diabetes is 50 percent higher for Black women than for white women.

The best way to avoid a chain reaction of health problems, including glaucoma, is to keep yourself healthy and avoid and treat diabetes. The best direct defense against glaucoma is an annual eye exam, especially if you know you have diabetes or a family history of glaucoma. Waiting for symptoms is dangerous because glaucoma generally has none. (Some sufferers do report blurred vision that comes and goes, seeing colored rings around lights, a loss in side vision, and pain or redness in the eye.)

Doctors usually treat the disease with prescription eyedrops to lower eye pressure and sometimes with surgery.

Cataracts also occur with age, and diabetes is also a risk factor. No one knows exactly what causes cataracts, but we've all seen elders whose eyes are cloudy and opaque and who can't see well.

Again, keeping healthy and avoiding and treating diabetes will lessen the risk of cataracts. Ultraviolet radiation (present in sunlight) and cigarette smoke should also be avoided. (When outdoors, wear sunglasses that screen out at least 95 percent of ultraviolet [UV] rays. Federal law mandates that all sunglasses must be marked with the amount of UV protection; look for a sticker.)

Surgery is also an option. The procedure takes only about an hour and is done under local anesthesia. A small incision is made in the cornea, and the surgeon pushes the clouded lens out of its capsule in the eye. In most cases an artificial replacement lens is inserted. It is then held in place by spring hooks. Most patients can go home the same day, wearing an eye patch for twenty-four hours. By the next day, they can return to normal activities.

However, in some cases cataract surgery is done on patients who don't need it. Doctors can make several thousand dollars per operation, and cataract-surgery mills that prey on the elderly have sprung up in recent years. If you feel that you are being pressured to have surgery, get a second or even third opinion. Be sure to choose a surgeon who has performed the operation many times.

For more information on this condition, read *Cataracts: The Complete Guide from Diagnosis to Recovery for Patients and Families* by Dr. Julius Shulman.

Diabetic retinopathy, which can lead to blindness, has a direct link to our high rate of diabetes. If you know or suspect that you have diabetes, it is imperative that you see an eye doctor. A Martin Luther King Jr./Charles Drew Medical Center study showed that by the time Black diabetics visited an eye clinic for help, almost 40 percent of them already had severe retinopathy. Less common but just as serious is hypertensive retinopathy. So be sure to keep your blood pressure in check to avoid blindness.

Teeth

Though we are known for our big, beautiful smiles, many Blacks also have serious dental problems. One-fourth of African-Americans over age forty-five have lost *all* of their teeth, and we are more likely than whites to wait several years before making a trip to the dentist's office. Part of the problem is dental insurance: 65 percent of us don't have it, and dental bills can add up.

But the best way to avoid the dentist and the buzzing, sadistic drill is to keep your teeth healthy between the two visits you *must* make every year.

The Dentist

A trip to the dentist can be unpleasant. Even a simple checkup can involve some pain. But grit those teeth and bear it: Good dental health calls for a cleaning and checkup every six months. You'll also need to have a set of X rays taken every three to five years to reveal conditions within the teeth and bones. (Make sure that you are covered fully with a lead apron when the X rays are taken, especially if you are pregnant.)

Not long ago a Florida woman, Kimberly Bergalis, died of AIDS supposedly contracted from her dentist. Despite the hysteria that followed, it is extremely unlikely that you would ever contract the AIDS virus in the dental setting. Still, you should make sure that your dentist and hygienist wear gloves (they'll probably also wear masks and eyewear to protect themselves), that disposable items are changed after each patient, and that equipment is sterilized.

Nobody really likes going to the dentist; some people, however, get extremely nervous. But try to relax because tensing up makes any discomfort worse. And take along some soothing music to listen to on a personal stereo; it generally won't disturb the dentist or hygienist doing work in your mouth.

Tooth Care

Even though during our lifetimes we'll brush our teeth about fifty thousand times, practice doesn't make perfect: Too many people brush incorrectly. You should do it at least twice a day, after breakfast and before bed; if you can brush after lunch, all the better. Use a soft toothbrush, and replace it every three to four months. Tip your toothbrush at a 45-degree angle, and brush gently with a short up-and-down motion. Don't scrub too hard; this can cause gum damage. Brush just a couple of teeth at a time on the outside, inside, and on chewing surfaces.

You should also floss at least once a day, before or after brushing. Insert the floss between your teeth, and gently rub it up and down the tooth surface to dislodge food and plaque.

Eating right also keeps the teeth healthy. You should avoid candy and sticky, gooey foods that get caught between the teeth. If you do snack, clean the teeth thoroughly afterward. Eat fruit and raw vegetables as a substitute for sweets.

Protect your baby's mouth by avoiding "rock-a-bottle-teeth syndrome." This occurs when a child sucks on a bottle constantly or falls asleep with it in her or his mouth. The sugar in the milk or other liquid can harm teeth and gums. Though their teeth will fall out, children should still see a dentist, and if possible, one who specializes in pediatric dentistry. The first visit should be at age three.

Healthy Gums

When bacterial plaque, the sticky, colorless film that forms on the teeth, builds up, periodontal or gum disease ensues. At worst it leads to periodontitis, an infection that can cause the teeth to loosen and fall out. This problem is more common in Blacks than in whites.

You can prevent gum disease by brushing, flossing, and visiting the dentist every six months. If you notice that you have unexplained bad breath, loose teeth, or red, swollen, or bleeding gums, alert your dentist right away. Brushing with baking soda and peroxide is a good home remedy for the beginning signs of gum disease.

Where to Get a Dental Exam and How to Pay for It

Though some people are covered by dental insurance, 65 percent of Blacks are not. If you are covered, the insurance should pay for all or part of your exam. It should run about $50, depending on where you live, and you will have to pay an additional cost for the X rays. Depending on where you live, Medicaid may pay for your dental exam. Medicare doesn't cover preventive dental care.

For More Information

ORGANIZATIONS: Skin

AMERICAN ACADEMY OF DERMATOLOGY, Communication Dept., P.O. Box 4014, Schaumburg, IL 60168-4014; (708) 330-0230. Ask for the pamphlets about Black skin, vitiligo, and hair loss.

THE AMERICAN SKIN ASSOCIATION, INC., 150 E. 58th St., 32nd floor, New York, NY 10155-0002; (212) 753-8260. ASA generates support for skin research and provides information and education to the public on the skin and its disorders.

CENTER FOR SKIN RESEARCH, INC., 818 18th St. NW, suite 940, Washington, DC 20006; (202) 857-0383.

NATIONAL ORGANIZATION FOR PERSONS WITH ALBINISM AND HYPOPIGMENTATION (NOAH), 1500 Locust Street, Philadelphia, PA 19102; (800) 473-2310 or (215) 545-2322.

NATIONAL ARTHRITIS AND MUSCULOSKELETAL AND SKIN DISEASES INFORMATION CLEARINGHOUSE, P.O. Box AMS, 9000 Rockville Pike, Bethesda, MD 20892; (301) 495-4484. Provides information, resources, and patient education.

SKIN CANCER FOUNDATION, 245 Fifth Ave., suite 2402, New York, NY 10016; (212) 725-5176. The SCF offers nationwide distribution of pamphlets, brochures, and other informational materials.

SOLUTIONS CENTER, 530 E. Eighth St., suite 103, Oakland, CA 94606; (510) 893-7546. This clinic can provide informational materials on Black skin care.

ORGANIZATIONS: Eyes

AMERICAN ACADEMY OF OPHTHALMOLOGY, P.O. Box 7424, San Francisco, CA 94120-7424; (415) 561-8500.

AMERICAN DIABETES ASSOCIATION, 1660 Duke St., Alexandria, VA 22314; (703) 549-1500.

AMERICAN OPTOMETRIC ASSOCIATION, 243 N. Lindbergh Blvd., St. Louis, MS 63141, Attn. Communication Center; (314) 991-4100.

BETTER VISION INSTITUTE, 1800 N. Kent St., suite 904, Rosslyn, VA 22209; (703) 243-1508. For information on prevention, detection, and treatment of eye diseases.

NATIONAL EYE CARE PROJECT HELPLINE, (800) 222-3937. Provides information about eye diseases and free eye exams for the financially disadvantaged or people over sixty-five.

NATIONAL EYE INSTITUTE, INFORMATION OFFICE, Building 31, room 6A32, Bethesda, MD 20892; (301) 496-5248. A division of the National Institutes of Health, this agency distributes information on cataracts, glaucoma, and diabetic retinopathy.

NATIONAL EYE RESEARCH FOUNDATION, 910 Skokie Blvd., suite 207A, Northbrook, IL 60062; (800) 621-2258 or (708) 564-4652. Recorded information for eye patients.

NATIONAL SOCIETY TO PREVENT BLINDNESS, 500 E. Remington Rd., Schaumburg, IL 70143; (800) 331-2020 or (708) 843-2020. This organization provides information on eye injuries, diseases, and prevention.

ORGANIZATIONS: Teeth

AMERICAN DENTAL ASSOCIATION, 211 E. Chicago Ave., Chicago, IL 60611; (312) 440-2500.

NATIONAL DENTAL ASSOCIATION, 5506 Connecticut Ave. NW, suite 24, Washington, DC, 20015; (202) 244-7555. Black dentists.

NATIONAL INSTITUTE OF DENTAL RESEARCH, National Institutes of Health, 9000 Rockville Pike, bldg. 31, room 2C35, Bethesda, MD 20892; (301) 496-4261.

BOOKS: Skin

All About Health and Beauty for the Black Woman, Naomi Sims, Doubleday, 1976.

Beverly Johnson's Guide to a Life of Health and Beauty, Beverly Johnson, Times Books, 1981.

The Color Complex: The Politics of Skin Color Among African-Americans, Kathy Russell, Midge Wilson, and Ronald Hall, Harcourt Brace, 1992.

Fornay's Guide to Skin Care and Makeup for Women of Color, Alfred Fornay, Fireside Books, 1989.

The New Medically Based No-Nonsense Beauty Book, Deborah Chase, Henry Holt, 1989. (This book is not specifically for Black women, but it has some good general information.)

True Beauty: Secrets of Radiant Beauty for Women of Every Age and Color, Beverly Johnson, Warner Books, 1994.

Women of Color: The Multicultural Guide to Fashion and Beauty, Darlene Mathis, One World, 1994.

BOOKS: Hair

Accent African: Traditional and Contemporary Hairstyles for the Black Woman, Valerie Thomas-Osborne and Carla Brown, Cultural Expressions Inc. (New York), 1992.

All About Health and Beauty for the Black Woman, Naomi Sims, Doubleday, 1976.

Beverly Johnson's Guide to a Life of Health and Beauty, Beverly Johnson, Times Books, 1981.

Black Hair Is . . . The Complete Hair Care Guide for Today's Black Woman, Marilyn Singleton, Image Perfect Communications Inc. (Marietta, Ga.), 1992.

Good Hair: For Colored Girls Who've Considered Weaves When the Chemicals Became Too Ruff, Lonnice Brittenum Bonner, Crown Books, 1994.

True Beauty: Secrets of Radiant Beauty for Women of Every Age and Color, Beverly Johnson, Warner Books, 1994.

Women of Color: The Multicultural Guide to Fashion and Beauty, Darlene Mathis, One World, 1994.

3

Moving Our Bodies

Black women define athleticism in the world. Among the preeminent female superstars of sport, African-descended women are certainly well represented. Think about basketball players Cheryl Miller and Harlem Globetrotter Lynnette Woodard, pro tennis player Zina Garrison, Olympic skaters Surya Bonaly and Debi Thomas, track stars Gail Devers and Jackie Joyner-Kersee, and swift African long-distance runners as well as such legends as Wimbledon tennis champion Althea Gibson, sprinter Wilma Rudolph, and volleyball great the late Flo Hyman.

Millions of Black women of all ages and sizes take advantage of the many health benefits of exercise by running, playing tennis, swimming, dancing, taking aerobics classes, walking, and participating in many other sports activities. Nonetheless, many of us don't exercise at all. In fact, Black women are less likely to exercise than white women and Black men. We have a variety of reasons, many of which *sound* valid, including "I don't have time," "I don't know how," "I don't have anyone to watch my children," "I'm too fat," "I'm too old," "I'm tired," or "I don't have access to facilities."

Yet for every obstacle, there's a solution. In the words of one health practitioner who treats the ailments of many women who *don't* exercise, "Sisters find someone to look after their kids when they want to go out

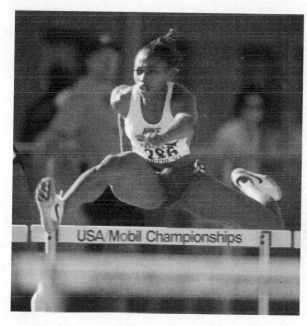

American Gail Devers is
one of the world's top
athletes.
(Photo: Victah, New York)

to a club. We make time to have our hair done. We aren't too tired to go
to the mall and shop. Exercising and taking care of our bodies is about
commitment to good health."

Given the startling fact that exercise is the cheapest, easiest, safest way
to avoid serious illness such as heart disease, that it can stave off the
effects of aging, speed weight loss, and help us look and feel good physically and emotionally, each and every one of us must find a way to
include regular physical activity in our lives. If you haven't started to
exercise, it's never too late: According to Walter M. Bortz II, M.D.,
author of *We Live Too Short, We Die Too Long: How to Achieve and Enjoy
Your Natural 120-Year-Plus Life Span,* "A fit person of 70 is equivalent to
an unfit person of 30."

The Benefits of Exercise

The physical and emotional benefits of exercise are numerous and well
documented. Exercise:

Fights disease. According to a study conducted by the Cooper Institute
in Dallas, unfit women have a 5.33 times greater premature death rate
than fit women. Exercise can help lower cholesterol levels and blood
pressure to prevent cardiovascular diseases such as heart attack and
stroke. In fact, the American Heart Association now classifies physical
*in*activity as a risk factor for cardiovascular disease on par with smoking

and high blood pressure. Moderate exercise can also lower the risk of diabetes and build up the immune system to fight colds and flu.

May fight cancer. Harvard University researchers have demonstrated a decreased incidence of breast cancer in former collegiate athletes as compared with nonathletes. Experts attribute this finding to two factors: the effects of exercise on the hormonal balance at a critical time in the early development of the cancer (several decades before a mass is evident) and the greater likelihood of lifetime exercise participation. Recent studies in Sweden link sedentariness to an increased risk of colon cancer. This may be related to the *anticonstipation* effect of vigorous exercise—contractions in the colon or large intestine are stimulated if food material is present.

Promotes weight loss. A number of studies have proven that diets don't work for most women. In the long run most dieters don't end up at a lower weight or even at the same weight, but at a higher one! Instead, the best way to lose weight and keep it off is by eating high-fiber, low-fat foods and exercising regularly. Exercise burns fat and calories and increases the metabolism (the rate at which the body burns calories) for up to thirty-six hours after exercise is finished.

Builds bones. At about age thirty-five, a woman's bones begin to thin. But women who have exercised before that age have denser bones so that bone loss doesn't affect them as much. But even older women who begin an exercise program can restore some of the bone that has been lost. Only weight-bearing exercise such as walking, running, or lifting weights builds bones.

Eases some reproductive health problems. Both anecdotal and scientific reports indicate that women who exercise have fewer menopausal and premenstrual symptoms. Pregnant women who work out moderately report fewer backaches and less shortness of breath and fatigue, and they bounce back more quickly after delivery.

Relieves stress and depression. Exercise can help cope with the everyday slights and pressures that so many of us have to live with. A good workout eases hostility, anger, tension, and anxiety, which may be especially beneficial for women with hard-driving, competitive personalities—as long as they don't make "work" of exercise by being too goal-oriented. Exercise can also relax the mind and body and erase a bad mood.

Boosts self-esteem. People who are fit look and feel stronger and healthier than those who are sedentary. Being able to run or walk two miles, cycle around the park, or bounce through an African-dance class provides a sense of accomplishment and pride.

I grew up in rural Georgia with three older brothers, so competition was always the name of the game. I felt that I always had to be twice as good to justify my brothers' faith in choosing me—a girl!—to be on their team when we played football. Many times, though, I was the superior athlete.

When it came time for college, I chose Tennessee State University because it was one of the few schools offering "scholarships" (really work-study jobs) to female athletes in track and field. It didn't hurt that Wilma Rudolph [winner of three gold medals in the 1960 Olympics] was a senior there when I was being recruited.

At this point in my life, I'm just interested in being healthy. I've always liked to feel fit, and I've worked to remain the same size for the past ten years. I like fresh air and the outdoors, so walking, tennis, and calisthenics are my chosen activities. And I'm a morning person, so I reserve an early hour or so for myself.

My motto is "Don't overdo!" Paying attention to your body lets you know what you should and shouldn't do. The important thing is to pick something you can do regularly—for me, that means every day. That "no pain, no gain" mentality is just not a healthy one. Exercise makes me feel better, think better, get more done. And there's a side benefit: I've always transferred the "don't quit" mentality that I learned in track competition to other areas of my life.

> *"I've always transferred the 'don't quit' mentality that I learned in track competition to other areas of my life."*
>
> —WYOMIA TYUS, YOUTH COUNSELOR, MOTIVATIONAL SPEAKER, 1964 AND 1968 OLYMPIC GOLD MEDALIST IN THE 100 METERS FOR TRACK AND FIELD, LOS ANGELES

What Is Fitness?

Fitness has three components: strength, flexibility, and stamina.

Strength. Your muscles get stronger when they contract against resistance. The resistance may be a weight or your own body weight, as when you increase leg strength by running up hills or build your arms with push-ups.

Strength training doesn't necessarily mean lifting massive weights in order to develop bulging muscles. In fact, because of hormonal differences, women have less muscle mass and cannot ever pump up to become Incredible Hulks. And contrary to popular mythology, weight training does not cause body fat to turn into muscle, nor does muscle turn into fat when you stop training. Fat cells and muscle cells are very different, and you can't transform one into the other. But if you do a nonstop twenty-to-thirty minute weight-training workout, your body will burn calories, which leads to loss of fat, plus you'll build up your muscles. This will make you look trimmer and leaner.

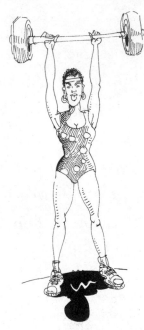

Weight training builds strength and muscle tone. *(Drawing: Yvonne Buchanan)*

To build strength, start out slowly. If you're working out in a club, ask for instruction. If you'd rather use weights at home, consult one of the many books and videotapes on the market.

Flexibility. This is the ability to bend, stoop, and reach without straining or pulling muscles. The joints and muscles of women are generally more flexible than those of men, and children are more agile than adults because flexibility declines with age. You can increase flexibility by doing stretching and yoga exercises.

Endurance. Also known as aerobic capacity, endurance is the most important component of fitness, at least as far as good health and weight loss are concerned. Some women may consider themselves fit if they can make it up the steps without getting out of breath, while others don't feel in shape unless they can run five miles without stopping.

Endurance is the ability to persist in an exercise. It depends on the ability of the heart to pump blood efficiently through the lungs and the circulatory system to supply oxygen to the muscles. As you exercise, the body demands energy in the form of calories, and calorie burning leads to loss of fat.

You must do an aerobic activity—such as walking, running, skating, tennis, basketball, or aerobic dance that gets your breath going and your heart pumping—for twenty to thirty minutes three times a week in order to get in shape and stay in shape. You also have to exercise at a brisk enough pace to reap cardiovascular benefits. A slow stroll through the park isn't going to strengthen your heart and lungs. To get what is called the "training effect," you must get your heart pumping at about 70 percent of its maximum for twenty to thirty minutes. Experts note that for the average woman, the maximum is about 180 to 190 beats per minute. That means that your target heart rate should be about 125 to 135 beats per minute.

To make sure you are exerting yourself enough to reap fitness benefits, check your pulse during your exercise session:

Place two fingers (not your thumb) on the big artery on the side of your neck or the artery in your wrist.

Count the number of beats for ten seconds.

Multiply that number by 6 to determine the number of beats per minute.

Remember, you should be aiming for a sustained rate of 125 to 135 beats per minute. If you aren't there, pick up the pace a bit.

With some fitness activities, such as swimming, you can get an aerobic, strength, and flexibility workout: Your muscles grow stronger as they push against the resistance of the water, your joints and muscles become more flexible as you stroke your arms and kick your legs, and as you exert yourself, your heart and lungs grow more powerful. Other forms of exercise, such as yoga, increase flexibility only and don't provide a cardiovascular workout. It's best to mix up your workouts: Do an activity that increases your aerobic capacity three times per week, and on other days, stretch or do yoga or try to get in a day of strength building each week.

An Adaptable Exercise Prescription

Too many of us are all talk and no walk: Although 99 percent of Americans identify physical activity as a good health habit, a much smaller percentage of folks are out there "just doing it." But all of us can profit, even at low to moderate intensities of activity. In fact, the greatest health benefits are derived when those who are the least fit get busy.

The key is a flexible program of *gradually* increased activity, tailored to your individual lifestyle and preferences. If you're thirty-five or over or have one or more cardiovascular-disease risk factors (smoking, diabetes, high blood pressure, high cholesterol, obesity, family history of heart attack or stroke before age sixty), have a thorough medical evaluation by your doctor before beginning a fitness program. It is important to begin at a level appropriate to your age, physical condition, and overall health. Here are a some tips for getting started and keeping going:

Start out slowly. If you don't, you may end up with an overuse injury resulting from too much, too soon. If you're a walker, begin with a ten- or fifteen-minute walk, and then increase your distance and speed week by week. It's best to judge your distance by time—try walking for twenty to thirty minutes per session—rather than trying to count blocks or miles. As a beginner, walk fast enough to get your heart pumping, but not so fast that you're panting. As you walk, you should be able to carry on a conversation. If you want to increase the intensity, build up to a brisk walk and then a slow jog.

Be sure to stretch early in your workout, preferably after a few minutes of low-intensity exercise. Stretching loosens up your muscles to help prevent injury. Your warm-up should include at least ten minutes of stretching exercises, and at the end of your workout, cool down with another five to ten minutes of stretching.

Get the right equipment. If you're a runner or walker, get a pair of sturdy, well-cushioned athletic shoes. If you don't know which kind to buy, go to a sporting-goods store and ask the clerk for help. (Many are knowledgeable and helpful.) Wear clothing that lets the skin breathe, and in the winter, wear layers. If you're roller-skating, get knee pads, wrist protectors, and a helmet, and always wear a helmet if you're cycling.

Keep consistent. It's easier to stay in shape than to get into shape, stop working out, then have to start all over. Get your heart pumping at least three times a week for twenty to thirty minutes each session. If you start to get bored, try something new, like a gospel or funk aerobics class if you can find one in your area.

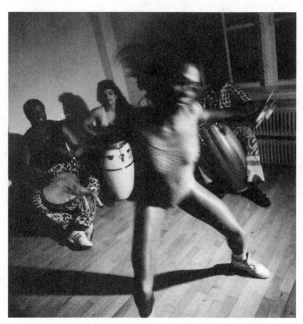

African-inspired aerobic dance is a great way to get in shape.
(Photo: N. Stephen Chin)

Work out at the same time each day that you exercise. That way you will think of exercise as part of your daily routine. For variety, change your activity: Cycle one day, walk the next, take an aerobics class two days later. And choose the time of day that suits you best: If you're a hard-core night owl, you may not be able to drag yourself out of bed for an early-morning skate. So take a walk at lunchtime instead.

Exercise with a friend, your mate, or your child. This will keep you motivated, and the two of you can inspire, encourage, and support each other. Try organizing women in your building or your community to exercise together, especially if you feel unsafe in the neighborhood. Another suggestion: Make workout dates. Instead of meeting a friend over dinner or going to a movie, meet in the park for a walk or skate, or take an exercise class together.

If you have a VCR, try an exercise video. Many Black women instructors, such as Victoria Johnson and Donna Richardson, offer aerobic workouts on video that you can do at home in front of your TV set. This works well during the winter and in the heat of the summer.

If you're pregnant, don't be afraid to exercise, but don't overdo it. Pregnant women should not participate in contact sports such as soccer or basketball and should not do extremely strenuous activities that could cause the body temperature to increase dramatically—like road racing. Instead, try activities such as low-impact aerobics (the YWCA and some hospitals and health clubs have special classes for mothers-to-be), walking, and swimming.

Set a goal. Build up gradually to participate in a walkathon, bikeathon, fun run, or tennis tournament. This will keep you interested and focused.

Walking for Wellness

Brisk walking is the best exercise for most people because it's easy, safe, and fun. With this in mind, sisters are taking to parks, shopping malls, beaches, and streets in record numbers. In 1992, The National Black Women's Health Project launched "Walking for Wellness," a campaign to encourage African-American women to get together and form walking groups. Pilot programs began in Atlanta, Los Angeles, Boston, and Gainesville, Florida, and have since spread to other cities.

Anyone in a community can start a program by organizing friends, family members, and neighbors. If you would like to start a Walking for Wellness group in your community, call NBWHP at (800) ASK-BWHP. The national organization will provide your chapter with training and information to get started.

As you're walking, keep in mind the Walking for Wellness pledge, written by Dr. Marcia I. Wells-Lawson:

In the spirit of those who came before me, and in those whose image I have been created, I pledge, here and now, to commit my life to wellness of mind, wellness of spirit, and wellness of body. As I walk along this pathway to wellness, I realize that I, and sisters like me, stem from greatness. As I walk with my head held high, to the stride and the beat set by my ancestors, I pledge to give myself permission to be free, free from oppression of all kinds, free from abuse and misuse of all kinds, free from all that hinders me from being and becoming.

"If you really want to walk, you can make the time for it."

—Watrina Watson, student, volunteer coordinator for the Walking for Wellness Program at the Center for Black Women's Wellness, Atlanta, Georgia

I live with a lot of stress in my life: I'm twenty-three, attending school, raising a three-year-old on my own, and trying to exist on public aid in Atlanta. Before I started exercising on a regular basis, it seemed like money, school, and even everyday living would stress me out. I really couldn't handle the stress. I kept it bottled up inside. And if something ticked me off, I would get real upset or hysterical.

I was also seriously overweight. Heart disease runs in both sides of my family. I wanted to lose the weight, because I don't want to have a heart attack before I'm thirty years old. I don't want my son to have health problems either. And the more I learn about health issues, the more it makes me want to eat right and do right. Still, even though I talked about exercising all the time, I never did it. I figured I just didn't have the time.

So I entered a Walking for Wellness program at the Center for Black Women's Wellness where I study and work as a volunteer. Now every Tuesday and Wednesday from eleven-thirty to noon, me and about twenty other women at the Center get out and walk. We walk at least two or three miles. These days, I can put in three or four miles.

Walking is great exercise. If you're walking at an upbeat pace, you're really doing something. But you're not overstraining yourself. You're walking at your own pace, and you're feeling really comfortable. Sometimes I listen to music on my Walkman. Other times I walk to clear my head when my week's been really rough. I never get bored. Sometimes I walk around the park. I try to walk in new and different places. That way you get to see all sorts of new things.

Walking has changed my life: I'm much calmer than I used to be. I have more energy. I've learned that you can make time for anything you want to do. If you really want to walk, you can make the time for it.

As I walk, with my head held high, I pledge to include walking as a necessary part of my routine activities and not allow anyone or anything to keep me from honoring this pledge. My walking time is mine. It is something I do for myself. I earned it, and I deserve it.

I know that there are those who will not be supportive nor seek to understand my decision to commit to wellness as a way of life; but my response to this negativity and my determination to persevere are guided by the words of the poet Maya Angelou:

You may shoot me with your words,
You may cut me with your eyes,
You may kill me with your hatefulness
But like dust, and like air I'll rise, I'll rise, I'll rise!

Exercise and Larger Women

No one is too fat to exercise, so don't let anyone ever tell you that. Exercise is great for larger women. For large women who are happy with their size, exercise can tone muscles, increase stamina and strength, and make you feel relaxed and good about yourself. For women who want to lose weight, physical activity combined with high-fiber, low-fat eating is the only sensible way to take it off and keep it off—for good.

The first step away from a sedentary lifestyle should be a trip to your doctor for a comprehensive medical evaluation to make sure that you don't have any health problems that should be treated before beginning an exercise program.

Walking and swimming are two good options. Both of these activities are easy on the joints, which is important for large women whose weight can sometimes put extra stress on the knees, hips, and ankles. Choose your athletic shoes carefully; larger women need plenty of cushioning and support to absorb the impact of the weight and avoid injury. Don't be shy: Ask the shoe salesperson to recommend shoes that are designed with a bigger body in mind.

In some cities there are exercise clubs and groups that cater to large women. For more information, see Resources for Large Women, below.

Exercising Caution

It's important to be enthusiastic about working out, but you must also exercise caution in order to prevent injury. Sports injuries can leave you watching from the sidelines if you're not careful. To prevent all kinds of sports injuries:

Warm up properly. If you don't loosen your muscles and joints with ten to fifteen minutes of stretching, your risk of suffering both chronic and acute injury increases. And don't forget to cool down after your workout.

Get the proper shoes. Many women sprain ankles or develop shin splints or stress fractures by wearing the wrong kinds of shoes—or no shoes. You must wear shoes when doing aerobics, preferably a pair with plenty of cushioning and support. If you like to walk or run, you should also have the proper footwear to support your feet and cushion the force

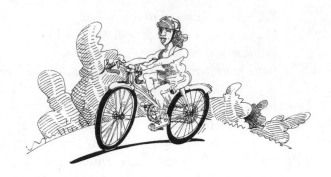

Biking provides strength
and cardiovascular
fitness—and it's fun.
*(Drawing: Yvonne
Buchanan)*

of your weight. Your best bet may be cross-training shoes, which you can wear for a variety of fitness activities. Ask the shoe salesperson about this option.

Start out slowly. Doing too much too soon is the easiest way to get injured. Work into a higher level of exercise intensity by building gradually.

Listen to your body. If you feel pain, that means something is wrong. Don't try to be tough and exercise through pain. Instead, stop and try to get at the root of the problem by paying attention to the signals your body is sending. You may need to get new shoes, switch sports, slow down, stop running or walking on pavement, switch to low-impact aerobics, or make other adjustments in your routine.

If you sustain a serious injury, you may need to see a sports doctor. Podiatrists and orthopedic surgeons generally specialize in sports-related injuries. Ask your general practitioner to recommend someone, or call a local recreational sports team or health club for a referral.

Swimming, walking, and biking are three of the safer sports around. All are relatively easy on the joints. If you do sustain an injury, especially a chronic problem, you may need to switch to swimming as you rehabilitate.

For more detailed information on injuries and injury prevention, read *The Complete Sports Medicine Book for Women* by Mona Shangold, M.D., and Gabe Mirkin, M.D.

For More Information

ORGANIZATIONS

AEROBICS AND FITNESS ASSOCIATION OF AMERICA, 15250 Ventura Blvd., suite 200, Sherman Oaks, CA 91403; (800) 233-4886. AFAA answers questions from the public regarding safe and effective exercise programs and practices and offers certification programs in aerobics and personal training.

AFRICAN AMERICAN ASSOCIATION OF FITNESS PROFESSIONALS, 1507 E. 53rd Street, Suite 495, Chicago, IL 60615; (312) 854-5843. Provides information and networking for Black fitness professionals. Publishes a quarterly newsletter.

AFRICAN AMERICAN ATHLETIC ASSOCIATION, INC., 355 Lexington Ave., 16th floor, New York, NY 10017; (212) 953-3100. Founded by Arthur Ashe in 1990, AAAA is an advocacy, support, and resource organization for Black athletes.

THE BLACK WOMEN IN SPORT FOUNDATION, P.O. Box 2610, Philadelphia, PA 19130; (215) 763-6609. This nonprofit group encourages and promotes the involvement of Black women in sports.

THE MELPOMENE INSTITUTE, 1010 University Ave., St. Paul, MN 55104; (612) 642-1951. Helps girls and women link physical activity and health through research, publications, and education.

WOMEN'S SPORTS FOUNDATION, Eisenhower Park, East Meadow, NY 11554; (516) 542-4700 or (800) 227-3988. Provides information, advocacy, and support for women athletes.

WOMEN OF COLOR IN SPORTS, c/o Adrienne R. Lotson, 10236 W. 96th St. #A, Overland Park, KS 66212; (913) 541-1864. This organization supports, encourages, and promotes professional women of color in the sports industry.

BOOKS

The Bodywise Woman, staff and researchers of the Melpomene Institute for Women's Health Research, Human Kinetics (Champagne, Ill.), 1993.

Complete Book of Fitness Walking, James M. Rippe, Simon & Schuster, 1990.

A Hard Road to Glory: The History of the African-American Athlete, Arthur Ashe, Amistad Press, 1993.

The Joy of Walking: More Than Just Exercise, Stephen Christopher Joyner, Betterway Books (Cincinnati), 1992.

Prevention's Practical Encyclopedia of Walking for Health, Mark Bricklin and Maggie Spilner, Rodale Press, 1992.

Walk for Life, David Balboa and Deena Balboa, Perigee Books, 1990.

Walk It Off!: 20 Minutes a Day to Health and Fitness, Suzanne Levine, Plume Books, 1991.

Walking—The Pleasure Exercise: A 60-Day Walking Program for Fitness and Health, Mort Malkin, Rodale Press, 1986.

Victoria Johnson's Attitude: An Inspirational Guide to Redefining Your Body, Your Health, and Your Outlook, Victoria Johnson, Penguin Books, 1993.

Resources for Large Women

WOMEN AT LARGE FITNESS CLUBS has locations in about twenty cities. To find out whether there's one in your area, call (509) 965-0115.

SMART MOVE, INC., in New York City offers exercise classes with the big woman in mind. Contact them at 131 West 72nd St., New York, NY 10024; (212) 721-4590.

Also in New York City, FirSTep Fitness offers exercise classes for the large woman that focus on cardiovascular and strength training. Call (212) 982-1825.

THE NATIONAL ASSOCIATION TO ADVANCE FAT ACCEPTANCE may also be able to steer you toward local exercise classes for large women. You must first become a member of the National Chapter (for $35 per year) before joining a local group. Contact NAAFA at (916) 558-6880 or (800) 442-1214, or write to P.O. Box 188620, Sacramento, CA 95818.

THE MELPOMENE INSTITUTE, a nonprofit organization, offers useful articles in its "larger woman" packet as well as quarterly seminars. Call (612) 642-1951, or write to 1010 University Ave., Saint Paul, MN 55104.

FOR HELPFUL EXERCISES AND INFORMATION READ *Great Shape: The First Fitness Guide for Large Women* by Pat Lyons and Debby Burgard, Bull Publishing, 1990.

CHECK OUT THESE VIDEOTAPES: *IDREA Presents: The Larger Woman's Workout* (Great Changes, 12516 Riverside Dr., N. Hollywood, CA 91607; [818] 769-4626. This company also has workout apparel and lingerie for the larger woman.). This tape features African-American participants. Women at Large Fitness Center offers *Breakout* and *Sharlyne Powell's 30-Minute Workout,* which are available by mail for $14.95 plus $4.50 shipping and handling. Write to 1020 S. 48th Ave., Yakima, WA 98908, or call (509) 965-0115. Call for information on the training school in Yakima for those interested in starting their own fitness centers, and ask about the newly opened spa for the larger woman located in Maui.

4

Eating Right

For centuries, African-Americans have had a love affair with food. Black men and women are many of the world's best chefs, not to mention your grandmother, great aunt, mother, and even you—folks who can create magic in the kitchen.

But the way we prepare our delectable food has its downside: Our traditional meals, which are often high in fat, cholesterol, salt, and sugar, have helped fuel disproportionately high rates of health problems such as cardiovascular disease, obesity, diabetes, and cancer. These medical woes result in lower life expectancy for African-Americans compared with our white counterparts.

The Food We Love

Soul food is rich in history and culture, reflecting the spirit of our ancestors both here and in the motherland. In fact, what we eat, why we eat it, and how these foods affect our health is being examined by African-American physicians, scientists, historians, and nutritionists who are only beginning to piece together our four-century relationship with food.

Slave traders shipped yams, rice, corn, black eyed peas, peanuts, okra, a melon similar to watermelon, and other crops to America with their slave cargo. The traders may have been heartless and cruel, but they weren't stupid: They provided slaves with foods that they were accustomed to in order to keep them alive.

Once our ancestors reached these shores, Africans from different parts of the continent were thrown together, and they exchanged folk tales, tribal songs, and recipes. Although it has long been believed that slaves subsisted almost solely on scraps left over from the master's kitchen, our descendants were much more enterprising than that. They hunted, fished, and cultivated small vegetable gardens, just as they had in Africa.

Many dishes now enjoyed by African-Americans and others are rooted in the food traditions of western and sub-Saharan Africa. The preslavery method of roasting meats in in-ground pits, for example, evolved to the modern-day backyard barbecue. Savory stews and one-pot meals such as gumbo and jambalaya can be traced directly to African coastal communities. Candied yams and sweet-potato pie, holiday favorites, are derivatives of the crop that helped our ancestors survive the Middle Passage. The Windward Coast of Africa contributed the red or cayenne pepper and the melegueta pepper, spices to this day responsible for the pleasant burn of many African-American dishes.

When our slave ancestors did have to dine on leftovers from their masters' meals, they cooked creatively. "Soul food is survival food," cookbook author Jessica B. Harris has said. "Slaves made the best of a bad lot."

While the whites ate "high on the hog," eating bacon, ham, and sausage, slaves were given the fattier parts of the pig such as the neck, shoulder, stomach, and intestines. The master's family ate turnips, and the slaves were left with the tougher turnip greens. Thrown together, however, ham hocks and turnip greens made a tasty, although less than healthy, meal. Other dishes such as chitlins (pig intestines), cracklin' corn bread (corn bread with bits of fried pig skin), and blackeyed peas cooked with ham hocks also relied heavily on fatty cuts of pork.

Unhealthy Eating

Many of us haven't let go of the traditional way of eating. It's comforting and familiar and tastes good. We know how we *should* be eating. Each day, Americans are bombarded with public-service announcements from government agencies and organizations such as the American Cancer Society and the American Heart Association. In the past two decades, nearly every newspaper, magazine, TV, and radio station has greatly expanded coverage of health, fitness, and nutrition. The media, health organizations, and the government urge us to eat right, exercise, and

Put a piece of cake, a pint of ice cream, or a bag of potato chips in front of me, and I would dive for them. Potato chips were my hugest weakness, and cake still is. I was always trying to eat with my mind on my health, but too often I would consume too much and eat the wrong kinds of foods.

I've never been overweight, but I'm really afraid of getting fat. My mother had been a small woman all of my life, but then she started putting on weight after she turned forty-two. She's not really fat now, but her metabolism slowed, and I knew it would eventually happen to me. I also became more aware of the health problems that run in my family—heart disease, cancer, hypertension, and high cholesterol—and decided that I wanted to get myself on a path of healthy eating.

I felt like I needed to be in control of my eating. I don't like to cook, so I wasn't eating meals regularly. I was grabbing something here and something there—usually junk food or whatever was easy. I decided to become aware of everything I put in my mouth. So I started to keep a diary of everything I ate. I felt this would retrain me in my eating habits. I made columns listing foods consumed, calories, grams of fat and cholesterol, and milligrams of sodium.

With everything down in front of me on paper, I realized that what I thought was a small, hardly filling, harmless breakfast of two toasted, buttered English muffins was actually almost surpassing the daily limits I had set for myself. I divided the limited amounts among breakfast, lunch, and dinner so that I wouldn't eat to my maximum limits before the end of the day. Then at the end of the day, I would total the amounts for a satisfactory or unsatisfactory score. After about the first week, I always got good scores.

Now I eat much more regularly. For breakfast I generally have plain yogurt and low-fat granola with a glass of orange juice. Lunch is my biggest meal of the day. I often go out, but now I choose healthy restaurants that serve salads or vegetarian dishes. I usually have a piece of fruit or a scoop of frozen yogurt to get me through the afternoon. My dinner is generally small, like fruit or salad or whatever is left over from lunch.

I feel different now when I eat. I used to sit down and eat until my stomach felt like it would burst or I felt like I could just roll over and fall asleep. Now I eat until I'm satisfied. I feel much more energetic—and less guilty. My body also seems much more healthy, and I have the feeling that I'll live to be very old.

"I felt like I needed to be in control of my eating."

—TONYA ADAMS, MAGAZINE EDITOR, NEW YORK CITY

visit our physicians for regular checkups, emphasizing that serious ailments can often be prevented through proper nutrition and early intervention. The food industry has adjusted to this health boom with a proliferation of healthful offerings—low-salt, low-fat, low-cholesterol, and sugar-free.

Yet all of this information has failed to create a marked nutritional consciousness among African-Americans. Many of us still cling to the old familiar high-fat, high-salt, high-cholesterol, sugar habits. What's more, many Black women have more than we can handle—jobs, family, volunteer work, and so on. When time is short, it's easy to fall prey to poor eating habits and become junk-food junkies. And our nutritional shortcomings have an effect: An alarming number of Black women are obese, leading to a more than 50 percent higher rate of diabetes than that of white women. Far too many of us are dying young of diseases that can be prevented by following a healthy diet.

Eating Right

The American Cancer Society has developed general guidelines to help you reduce your risk for cancer and other so-called "lifestyle" illnesses, diseases that are affected by what we eat. (Scientists estimate that 35 percent of all cancer deaths may be related to what we eat.) The steps, each of which can be gradually adapted, include:

- Avoiding obesity, which is defined as weighing 20 percent or more than what is considered to be the maximum desired weight.
- Eating fewer foods that have high cholesterol levels. Meat, butter, egg yolks, and some types of oils are all high-cholesterol foods.
- Cutting down on total fat intake, especially animal fats that come from meat and dairy products.
- Eating bulkier, high-fiber foods such as vegetables and whole-grain breads and cereals.
- Eating at least five servings of fruits and vegetables each day, especially those that are rich in vitamins A (apricots, broccoli, carrots, peaches, sweet potatoes, and spinach) and C (cabbage, red and green peppers, broccoli, strawberries, and citrus fruits such as oranges and grapefruit).
- Consuming only moderate amounts (if any) of salt-cured, smoked, and nitrite-cured foods such as bacon, ham, and smoked fish.
- Limiting alcohol intake, if you drink at all.
- Cutting down on salt. That means reading labels carefully to detect

canned goods and packaged items that contain sodium, as well as putting away the salt shaker. Instead substitute other kinds of seasonings such as herbs, onions, garlic, pepper, and lemon juice to give food flavor.

- Reduce intake of sugar. Eat fewer sweets, especially heavy, packaged desserts. Rather than relying on sugar substitutes that are made of chemicals that may be dangerous, adjust your "sweet tooth." You don't have to give up sugar—just cut down.
- Reducing fat intake may be the most important recommendation for Black women. Eating fatty foods contributes to high blood pressure, heart disease, stroke, cancer, and obesity, a problem that plagues an alarming number of us. With that in mind, remember the following guidelines for fat intake:
- Choose food items with less than one gram of fat per thirty calories.
- Keep fat to 30 percent or less of total calories as recommended by health and medical organizations. Even better, reduce fat even further.
- Keep saturated fat (found in animal products and many prepared and packaged foods) to less than 10 percent of total calories.
- Calculate the percentage of calories from fat using this formula: calories x .30 = number of calories from fat.

> ## *Cooking Tips for Cutting the Fat*
>
> - Cook with nonstick pans to cut down on added fats.
> - Brown and sauté with chicken broth or nonstick spray instead of oil, butter, or margarine.
> - Use skim milk instead of cream or whole milk when the recipe allows.
> - Eat low-fat dairy products.
> - Create sauces and toppings from fresh fruit, vegetables, and herbs instead of oil and butter.
> - Dress salads with lemon juice, fresh herbs, or low-fat yogurt instead of mayonnaise or oil-based dressings.
> - Use olive, safflower, or canola oil rather than lard or butter.

For help in deciding what to eat and what not to eat—and how much—review the food pyramid on the following page.

Sorting through the many guidelines can be a challenge in itself, but the bigger challenge is to make the choice to eat healthfully. Many people are rooted in unhealthy eating habits, such as consuming too many fatty foods, because they are afraid to try to change. You may feel unprepared to make a dramatic change in the way you and your family eat. Maybe you're worried that you don't know how to cook healthfully, that it's too complicated, or that you can't afford the foods you need. Or maybe you resent having to deprive yourself of an activity you love—eating.

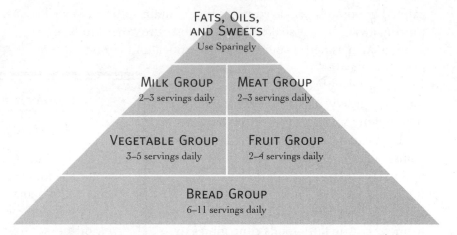

The food pyramid suggests the best way to balance your diet. The largest proportion of your diet should consist of the foods at the base of the pyramid. *(Chart: Adapted from the American Dietetic Association)*

The Food Guide Pyramid

Experts say that for most people, it's best to make adjustments, rather than to suddenly unload a dramatic new menu on yourself and your family. Start by increasing your intake of fruits, vegetables, and grains and trimming all visible fat from meat before you bake it or broil it on a rack.

You really can alter your eating habits. Think of it this way: Picture your body, the body that keeps your mind and spirit alive. Do you really want to put greasy, salty, sugary foods inside of the temple of your soul? Consider the time and money you put into making yourself look good—clothes, hair, creams, lotion, makeup. Why go to all of that trouble to make your outer body look good, then throw just anything inside? Think about it.

Reading Labels

Reading labels is critical to choosing healthy foods. As of May 1994, food labels became standardized. Labels must reveal the following information as shown on the package for macaroni and cheese on page 53.

The government also restricts the use of nutritional claims. For example, if the label says "low-fat," the item cannot have more than 3 grams of fat per serving. If the serving size is small (50 grams or less), it must have fewer than 3 grams of fat. This rule prevents a very small serving of a fatty food from being called low-fat.

If the label says "less" or "reduced" (such as "reduced salt" or "less fat"), the amount of the reduction must be at least 25 percent and the percentage has to be included on the label.

More things to watch out for on labels:

If an item has more than 500 milligrams of sodium per serving, don't buy it. (Remember that some foods that contain sodium don't necessarily taste salty.)

If the list of ingredients on the label contains a number of long words that you don't recognize, they're probably additives or preservatives, and you're better off without the product.

Avoid foods that are high in fat. Especially steer clear of foods high in saturated fats, such as animal fat, palm and coconut oil.

Grocery stores and fast-food restaurants often stock leaflets describing a food's nutritional value. If the information is not displayed, ask for it.

If you have any difficulty interpreting the connection between vitamins, minerals, and your body, get more information by reading books and articles, or ask a doctor or dietitian.

Larger food manufacturers often print toll-free phone numbers on their packaged foods. Call for an explanation. Newspapers, which traditionally have focused their food coverage on recipes, now concentrate on nutrition and often print results of the latest nutrition research. Stay abreast.

Nutrition Guide

Serving Size ½ cup (114g)   Servings per Container 4

Calories 260 (Calories from fat 120)

Per serving	% Daily Value	Daily Value
Fat (13g)	17%	Less than 75g*
Saturated Fat (5g)	20%	Less than 25g*
Cholesterol (30 mg)	10%	Less than 300mg
Sodium (660mg)	28%	Less than 2,400 mg

Per serving	% Daily Value	Daily Value
Carbohydrate (31g)	10%	352g*
Complex Carbohydrate (26g)		
Sugars (5g)		
Dietary Fiber (0g)	0%	25g
Protein (5g)		50g

Vitamins & Minerals   % Daily Value

Vitamin A 4%	Vitamin C 2%	Calcium 12%	Iron 4%

*For a 2,350 calorie diet. Your Daily Value may be higher or lower, depending on your calorie intake.

Meat or No Meat?

The quest for sound nutrition has led some sisters to completely eliminate meat and meat products from their diets. Some folks are afraid of the chemicals used to eradicate animal diseases and preserve meat, others voice ethical objections to animal slaughter (this fits into an Afrocentric lifestyle for many who note that some of our ancestors were vegetarians who worshiped some animals and considered them sacred). Others are worried about their health: Meat is high in fat and cholesterol.

Studies show that vegetarians have lower levels of cholesterol and triglycerides (fatty acids in the bloodstream) than meat eaters. They are also less inclined toward obesity, high blood pressure, and coronary heart disease—serious health threats among our people. Cutting down on or eliminating meat can aid in weight loss. Depending on how they're cooked, vegetables and fruit are lower in calories and fat than meat is.

"Being a
vegetarian gives
me a sense of
being involved
in my life
processes and the
functioning of
my body."

—Trina Moore, caterer,
Sunfired Foods,
Takoma Park, Maryland

I became a vegetarian at a young age. When I was sixteen, I had a teacher who told me about vegetarianism, and it all just made sense to me. I was a strong-headed teenager, so when I got home from school that day, I told my mother I was not going to eat meat anymore, and I didn't.

I dove right in and started out by fasting for seven days, drinking only juice and water. In doing this, I lost ten pounds of what I considered to be body waste. My body cleansed itself of toxins. I felt light-headed and had headaches for the first three days, but by the fourth day, I felt more energized than I had ever felt before.

At first my family thought that becoming a vegetarian was a drastic move, but after seeing the positive results I experienced, they all became more health-conscious of what they ate. Three (out of six) of my sisters are also vegetarians. Being a vegetarian gives me a sense of being involved in my life processes and the functioning of my body.

After a few years, I made the move to "live" foods only—fresh fruits, vegetables, and nuts. I started reading about vegetarianism and fasting and found that meat, dairy, flour, white sugar, and certain grains produce mucous in the body. Mucous lodges in the weak areas of the body and creates disease. I believe that if you only eat foods like fruit, nuts, and vegetables that do not produce mucous, you can ward off disease and illness a lot more easily.

For example, when I was ten years old, I had a cataract and had to wear eyeglasses. After being on a live-foods diet, the cataract went away and I no longer wear glasses. That's just an example of controlling your body and health through a vegetarian diet. My two daughters have never eaten meat in their lives and have no desire to do so. I took them step-by-step through the process of preparing meat for consumption, from the farm to the slaughterhouse to the supermarket and finally to the plate. This little educational trip confirmed for the girls that they did not want to even try meat.

Although vegetarianism is a viable and healthful alternative, before eliminating all meats and dairy products from your diet, read some of the abundant research on vegetarian diets. For more information on vegetarianism, contact the Vegetarian Resource Group, P.O. Box 1463, Baltimore, MD 21203; (410) 366-VEGE. The group, which publishes the *Vegetarian Journal,* can offer resources and cooking tips.

Raw and lightly steamed vegetables are a good alternative to boiled, mushy ones. High heat can break down vitamins to components small enough to wash away In cooking water. Vegetables should be cooked so that they retain their bright color, an indication that nutrients remain.

The Trouble with Milk

Black folks figure disproportionately among the 50 million Americans who can't digest milk products. The National Dairy Board estimates that 75 percent of us may have a problem with milk, compared with 21 percent of whites. Lactose intolerance, a resistance to milk consumption, can cause gas, which can lead to bloating, abdominal cramping, and diarrhea.

Our inability to digest milk may be a good thing: Even some mainstream experts are beginning to question whether milk and other dairy products are good for us at all. A 1992 report by the Physicians Committee for Responsible Medicine (a group that also advocates strict vegetarianism) questioned the nutritional value of cow's milk, linking it to a number of health problems including diabetes, ovarian cancer, cataracts, iron deficiencies, and allergies. Scientists and regular people alike also worry about the hormones and antibiotics given to the cows that produce the milk we drink.

On the other hand, milk and other dairy products are high in protein and calcium, which are important for growing children. Calcium is crucial for women because it helps prevent bone thinning, which affects women later in life.

It's up to individual families to decide what to do about dairy products. At minimum, we should cut down on dairy products, and when we do eat them, we should always choose low-fat dairy products such as skim or low-fat milk. You can also find healthy substitutes for dairy products, such as soy, rice, or nut milk. You can buy soy ice cream and soy cheese. These products are available in health food stores, but be aware that they cost more than dairy products. (A note about soy and nut substitutes: They aren't necessarily low-fat, so check labels carefully.)

As for calcium, other foods are high in that mineral. Nuts, seeds, and beans are high in protein, and greens, black-eyed peas, canned sardines and salmon with bones, oysters, dates, and figs are high in calcium. You can also try hijiki, a black sea vegetable that contains fourteen times more calcium than milk does.

For those who are lactose-intolerant, many products can help the body digest milk products. You can take digestive aids that contain lactase, a natural enzyme that breaks down lactose into its simpler component sugars. It comes in tablets that can be taken along with food. You can also try lactose-reduced dairy products, which are widely available.

For more information, contact the Food Allergy Network, 4744 Holly Ave., Fairfax, VA 22030; (703) 691-3179; the National Digestive Disease Information Clearinghouse, P.O. Box NDDIC, 9000 Rockville Pike, Bethesda, MD 20892; (301) 654-3810; or *The Newletter for People with Lactose Intolerance and Milk Allergy,* P.O. Box 3074, Iowa City, Iowa 52244; (800) 356-8501. Or read *No Milk Today: How to Live with Lactose Intolerance* by Steve Carper.

Healthy Soul Food

The saying "Today is the first day of the rest of my diet" hangs in a little frame in Sheral Cade's office at Parkland Memorial Hospital in Dallas. A one-pound rubber replica of yellow fat sits on the edge of her crowded desk. The chair that faces her is where sisters come when they are ready or they have been ordered to change their eating habits and, in the process, improve their health.

In the sixteen years she's counseled patients, registered dietitian Cade has learned that a big part of our resistance to proper nutrition is the notion that we have to eliminate down-home foods, soul food, the food so many of us love. Some of her clients have told her they believe that greens, potatoes, and breads are fattening.

It's not the foods, however, that are unhealthy. Cade has one word she repeats: preparation. The salt pork and ham hocks that flavor the greens make them fatty and salty, and the grease that potatoes are fried in make them unhealthy. Slathering butter or margarine on bread and rolls adds fat and calories.

Cassondra Armstrong is the chef and owner of the Dining Table, a popular Dallas restaurant and caterer that specializes in "new Southern cuisine." When preparing her flavorful dishes, she strives to balance good food and good nutrition and has learned to adjust traditional recipes. For example, she substitutes fresh, homemade chicken stock for ham hocks and salt pork when seasoning cabbage, string beans, and greens. She also uses less salt than she grew up with when cooking, and only at the customer's request will she serve sugar with iced tea and other brewed beverages. Her potato salad contains low-calorie, cholesterol-free mayonnaise, and she uses cholesterol-free stick margarine whenever a dish calls for butter.

Darmone Holland, a sister from Brooklyn who became a strict vegetarian in 1989 because she was afraid that her "toxic diet" contributed to her ovarian cysts, goes a step further: She cooks soul food with no meat or dairy products. "I make barbecue tofu, black-eyed peas, collard greens with no meat seasonings, steamed sweet potatoes, and I use sea salt or lemon juice instead of overprocessed table salt," she explains.

New Orleans Red Beans (MAKES 8 SERVINGS)

1 pound dry red beans   *3 tablespoons chopped garlic*
2 quarts water   *3 tablespoons chopped parsley*
1 1/2 cups chopped onion   *2 teaspoons dried thyme, crushed*
1 cup chopped celery   *1 teaspoon salt*
4 bay leaves   *1 teaspoon black pepper*
1 cup chopped sweet green pepper

Pick through the beans to remove any bad ones; rinse thoroughly. In a 5-quart pot, combine the beans, water, onion, celery, and bay leaves. Bring to a boil; reduce heat. Cover and cook over low heat for about 1 1/2 hours or until the beans are tender. Stir and mash the beans against the side of the pan.

Add the green pepper, garlic, parsley, thyme, salt, and black pepper. Cook, uncovered, over low heat until creamy, about 30 minutes. Remove bay leaves. Serve over hot cooked brown rice, if desired.

PER SERVING:

calories: 171   dietary fiber: 7.2 g
sodium: 285 mg   carbohydrates: 32 g
total fat: 0.5 g   cholesterol: 0
saturated fat: 0.1 g   protein: 10 g

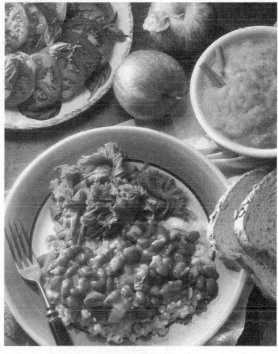

(Courtesy: National Cancer Institute)

Our food can be more healthful. The above recipe, an alternative to a meal that can be high in fat, is recommended by the National Cancer Institute.

Caffeine

Some people believe that caffeine is our society's most commonly used drug. On average, Americans consume one to three cups of coffee a day, and others who don't drink it find ways to get caffeine—from tea, chocolate, soft drinks, cold/allergy medication, weight-loss drugs, and pain relievers.

No one really knows whether or not caffeine is harmful, although most experts suspect that it is. Studies linking caffeine with heart disease and other health disorders have proven inconclusive. Still, women with stomach trouble, lumpy breasts, kidney problems, and nervous disorders or who are pregnant should avoid coffee and other caffeinated beverages. If you're already feeling stressed out and overwhelmed, caffeine is the last thing you need.

Caffeine is addictive, and millions of us—even casual coffee drinkers—may feel that we can't get through a day without it. We're used to the jolt we get from it in the morning and accustomed to drinking it in the afternoon to get through the day. Try skipping a day to see what happens. If you are addicted, you won't feel well. Subjects in a recent study reported headaches, drowsiness, depression, fatigue, and severe flulike symptoms once they gave up their cup-a-day habits. Caffeine withdrawal was too severe for 13 percent of the subjects, who broke down and took over-the-counter pain medicine that contained caffeine and which was forbidden under the terms of the study.

Though scientists don't know whether or not caffeine is bad for us, being addicted to anything can't be healthy. Wean yourself away from caffeine, or go cold turkey. As far as decaffeinated beverages, the jury is still out: The process that removes the caffeine may be harmful. Instead, substitute herbal tea or sparkling water for hot and cold caffeine drinks.

For More Information

ORGANIZATIONS

AMERICAN HEART ASSOCIATION, 7272 Greenville Ave., Dallas, TX 75231; (800) AHA-USA1 or (214) 706-1508. In cooperation with the American Assocation of Retired Persons, AHA sponsors "Eating for Healthy Tomorrows." This program features nutrition education for older African-Americans.

AMERICAN DIETETIC ASSOCIATION, 226 W. Jackson Blvd., suite 800, Chicago, IL 60606-6995; (800) 366-1655. Call the toll-free number for answers to questions about healthy eating or to request nutrition brochures.

CENTER FOR SCIENCE IN THE PUBLIC INTEREST, 1875 Connecticut Ave. NW, suite 300, Washington, DC 20009-5728. Write for publications and posters that discuss nutritional issues.

FOOD AND NUTRITION INFORMATION CENTER, U.S. Dept. of Agriculture, National Agricultural Library Bldg., room 304, Beltsville, MD 20705; (301) 504-5719. A resource center for nutritional information.

HUMAN NUTRITION INFORMATION SERVICE, Public Information Office, U.S. Department of Agriculture, Federal Bldg., 6505 Belcrest Rd., room 244, Hyattsville, MD 20782; (301) 436-7725. Distributes information on nutrition and contacts for outreach programs targeted to African-Americans.

NATIONAL MEDICAL ASSOCIATION, 1012 10th St. NW, Washington, DC 20001; (202) 347-1895. Distributes a fact sheet called "Nutrition and Blacks."

NATIONAL URBAN LEAGUE, 500 E. 62nd St., New York, NY 10021; (212) 310-9000. Distributes booklets and posters about nutrition and health for African-Americans.

U.S. FOOD AND DRUG ADMINISTRATION, Office of Consumer Affairs, 5600 Fishers Lane, room 16-85, Rockville, MD 20857; (301) 443-5006. Provides information and outreach programs specifically targeted to African-Americans.

For a complete listing, including local programs, request *The Directory of African-American Nutrition Programs,* Lori George, Account Supervisor, Porter/Novelli, 1120 Connecticut Ave. NW, 11th floor, Washington, DC 20036-3902; (202) 973-5864.

Black Cookbooks with Healthy Recipes

The Black Family Dinner Quilt Cookbook: Health-Conscious Recipes & Food Memories, Dorothy Height and the National Council of Negro Women, Inc., The Wimmer Companies (Memphis, Tenn.), 1993.

The Dooky Chase Cookbook, Leah Chase, Pelican Publishing, 1990. Has a section devoted to low-sodium, low-cholesterol Creole dishes.

A Healthy Food and Spiritual Nutrition Handbook, Keith T. Wright, K. T. Wright Health Masters (Philadelphia), 1989.

Heal Thyself Cookbook: A Complete Guide to Natural Living through Vegetarian Cooking and Holistic Juicing, Diane Ciccone, A & B Book Publishers (Brooklyn), 1992.

Kwanzaa: A Celebration of Culture and Cooking, Eric V. Copage, William Morrow and Company, 1991.

(Note: There are also dozens of mainstream cookbooks, available in bookstores, that feature healthy recipes that you can choose from.)

5

Killing Us Softly: Cigarettes and Alcohol

We have grown almost numb to negative images of ourselves in the media—Black teen girls surrounded by screaming babies, or men in handcuffs. Except in cigarette or liquor advertisements. In these we are beautiful, confident, well-dressed, happy, wealthy, in love—and killing ourselves.

Smoking is the top cause of preventable deaths. The Centers for Disease Control Office on Smoking and Health estimates that every year 434,000 people die from smoking-related diseases such as lung cancer, emphysema, and heart disease. That translates to twelve hundred deaths per day and fifty deaths an hour. We are more vulnerable to these health problems because Blacks smoke more than whites and quit less. Lung cancer is six times more common in Blacks than in whites.

As for alcohol, drinking leads to a number of serious health concerns such as cirrhosis of the liver, sexual dysfunction, and fetal alcohol syndrome. According to a Department of Health and Human Services report and other studies, heavy drinking also causes Blacks more social problems than it does whites. These include violence, run-ins with the police, high-risk sexual behavior, motor-vehicle accidents, trouble at work, and spouse problems—all of which are often triggered or exacerbated by drinking.

But while health messages targeted at us are few and far between, smoking and liquor ads abound. Tobacco manufacturing is a dying industry, and statistics show that consumption of alcoholic beverages is on the wane. With fewer people to entice, cigarette and liquor companies have managed to hone in on one population—us. Tobacco and liquor rely heavily on billboards, primarily in neighborhoods where Black and Latino people reside. A 1987 survey by the city of St. Louis, for example, found three times more billboards in Black neighborhoods than in white neighborhoods. Another study reported that 76 percent of billboards in communities of color advertise alcohol and tobacco products, as compared with 42 percent in white communities.

Tobacco and alcohol companies also advertise heavily in periodicals aimed at Black folks, making smoking and drinking look sexy and glamorous. Advertising is the bread and butter of consumer magazines, and publications such as *Essence, Ebony,* and *Jet* rely more on tobacco and liquor advertising than do mainstream publications. Part of the problem is that some manufacturers of cosmetics, athletic shoes, and other products avoid buying ads in Black magazines, either afraid of being mistaken as a "Black product" or wrongly believing that we don't have enough money to purchase their wares.

Tobacco and liquor companies, however, have become masters at marketing their products to the Black community. We found out how closely tobacco companies study us during the controversy over Uptown, the ill-fated cigarette that was designed to appeal to Blacks. A 1990 *New York Times* article stated that Uptown was to be a mentho-

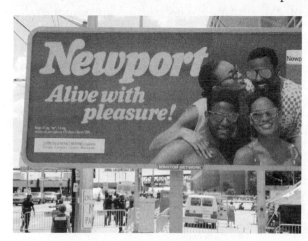

Tobacco companies advertise disproportionately in our communities.
(Photo: Albert Trotman/Allford Trotman Associates)

lated brand (which, incidentally, made it higher in tar and nicotine) because 69 percent of Black smokers prefer that flavor, that the cigarettes would be packed facing down because Blacks open the packs from the bottom, and that the name Uptown was chosen after it scored high in consumer surveys of African-Americans. Fortunately, Uptown was extinguished thanks to the outcry from a number of prominent Blacks and African-American community groups. We have also fought back against the high-octane brands of malt liquor dumped in our communities. Writes David Grant in *Scope,* the newsletter of the Institute of Black Chemical Abuse: "'Powermaster,' a brand of malt liquor created by G. Heilman that epitomized the sexual come-ons, racial stereotyping, and promise of a bigger alcoholic 'punch' typical of malt liquor advertising, was still-born due to a firestorm of community protest."

How Dangerous Is Smoking?

Over 40 million Americans have wised up and quit smoking, but African-Americans, especially women, quit at a rate that's lower than the national average. That's why cigarette companies are targeting us. Smoking is so dangerous that it's banned by law in many public places, and smokers have an increasingly difficult time finding places where they *can* indulge in their habit. The hazards of smoking can hardly be overstated.

While homicide, AIDS, and drugs grab the spotlight, cigarette smoking quietly kills our people. According to Reed Tuckson, M.D., the former commissioner of public health for the District of Columbia, cigarette smoking accounted for an estimated 40 percent of all deaths among adult Black men living in Washington. Also:

- Six times as many people die from smoking as from automobile accidents.
- Cigarette smoking is the number-one cause of lung cancer (the number-one cause of death by cancer in women), and smoking also contributes to breast cancer and other cancers.
- Cigarette smoking accounts for one-third of all deaths from heart disease.
- Cigarette smoking is the major cause of emphysema and chronic bronchitis.
- Smoking during pregnancy increases the risk of spontaneous abortion, stillbirths, and infant death. Babies born to women who smoke during pregnancy weigh an average of nearly a half pound less than babies born to nonsmokers.

- A woman who smokes and takes birth control pills is ten times more like to suffer a heart attack and twenty times more likely to have a stroke compared with a woman who does neither.
- Combined with air pollution, smoking contributes to asthma, a serious and growing problem among African-Americans.
- Secondhand smoke or environmental tobacco smoke is also very dangerous, especially to children. Exposure to smoke is tied to 150,000 to 300,000 ailments a year in children, and the risk of lung cancer is 30 percent higher for spouses of smokers than for spouses of nonsmokers.

Added to these serious health hazards, smoking is just plain nasty. When folks smoke, their hair and clothing smell, not to mention their breath. Smokers are also more likely to have red eyes, yellow teeth, a gray pallor about their skin, and wrinkles, especially around the mouth, as they age. And what could be worse than listening to someone's hacking cough, a common side effect of cigarettes? The habit is also expensive: A tobacco addict may put thousands of dollars up in smoke each year.

Why Smoke?

The title of Terry McMillan's best-selling novel, *Waiting to Exhale*, has nothing to do with smoking, but like many Black women, her characters use cigarettes to ease their stress, anxiety, and sorrow. McMillan's Bernadine finds herself craving a smoke after her husband has left her for a white woman. ". . . it had been 106 days since she'd quit smoking. But damn, that was what she needed right now. A cigarette. A cigarette would help her believe this. A cigarette would help her understand that her life has just been revised. A cigarette would help her decide exactly what to do next."

Regardless of how people started or why they continue to smoke, it's extremely hard to quit. Nicotine is a highly addictive substance, and the vast majority of smokers are physically addicted to it. That means that the nervous system has adapted to nicotine, and over time the brain and nervous system require nicotine to function normally. Thus, after sleeping eight hours deprived of nicotine, the typical smoker wakes up irritable, restless, and craving a smoke. Addiction may be even more powerful for Blacks, because we tend to smoke brands that are high in nicotine.

Smoking is also psychologically addictive. Smokers become accus-

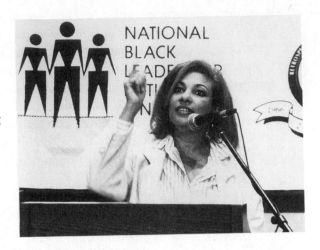

Speaker at an antismoking leadership-training workshop. *(Photo: J. V. Evers Photography, Los Angeles; courtesy Regina M. Penna, Women and Girls Against Tobacco, Berkeley, Calif.)*

tomed to the movements of smoking, holding a cigarette between the fingers, drawing smoke in, blowing it out, and so on. They may need to smoke in certain settings, such as at work, in bars, or in times of stress and anxiety.

How to Quit

As the old saying goes, "It's easy to quit smoking. I know because I've done it a thousand times." The fact is it's not easy to quit. If someone tells you that all it takes is self-control, that person has never tried to kick the habit. Withdrawal symptoms can be wicked. Along with intense craving, people trying to quit will have headaches, irritability, difficulty concentrating, and slight weight gain.

But you can do it. And when you do, you can reverse some of the havoc smoking has wreaked on your body—regardless of how long you smoked or how old you are when you quit. One study found that women who quit faced about the same cancer-death risk as those who never smoked.

Of smokers who make a serious attempt at quitting, only about 20 to 25 percent manage to stop for more than a year. (The Surgeon General reports that Blacks are more likely to try to quit smoking, although whites more often manage to stay off cigarettes for a year or more.) But if you've tried and haven't been able to quit, don't think you've failed. Quitting is a process; previous attempts aren't failures, they're rehearsals. In fact, these rehearsals may increase the chance of success on the next attempt.

There are many ways to quit, and statistics vary widely as to their suc-

I tried quitting smoking a number of times over the past thirty-one years. Usually, I'd stop for a week or two and then start right back. The reality of developing lung cancer and heart disease was always present in my mind, but somehow I always found a way to rationalize my smoking habit. Every time I came down with a cold, I'd swear up and down cancer was forming in my lungs. My throat became so raw during these episodes that it forced me not to smoke. After my colds cleared up, I'd say to myself, "Oh, I feel much better now, so I must not have cancer." And I'd start smoking all over again.

One day it was announced at work that employees could no longer smoke at their work stations. My employer offered all smokers in the company an opportunity to quit through the American Cancer Society's "Freshstart" smoking-cessation program. As an added incentive, my company agreed to foot the bill.

A coworker and I decided to join the program together. We had been talking on and off about quitting smoking, and it seemed only natural that we should support each other now. It worked. Within a month both of us had quit. The first thing I learned following the program is that habits are deceptive. You don't realize the depth of them until you break them. I never really thought of myself as a heavy smoker, but after I quit smoking, I couldn't move my bowels without a cigarette. Can you believe it? For a short while I had to take an unlit cigarette into the bathroom with me.

It's two years later, and I feel great about myself for having stopped smoking. I've just committed to a regimen of exercise and proper dieting so that I can lose the twenty-five pounds I've gained since. In spite of the unwelcome weight, I'm happy to know that I found the inner force within that has allowed me to add years to my life. I will now invoke that same power as I strive to conquer my next feat. And I will win again.

"I feel great about myself for having stopped smoking."

—SHIRLEY D. JENKINS, COMPUTER TECHNICIAN, BROOKLYN

cess rates. Some people manage to quit by enrolling in structured smoking-cessation programs such as Smokenders. For a fee of about $300, you can join a group that meets once a week for six weeks and gradually withdraw from cigarettes. (Check your phone directory for a local listing.) The American Cancer Society sponsors Freshstart, a four-session group program (check your local branch for possible applicable fees). Both Freshstart and Smokenders have about 25 to 30 percent success rates. Sponsored by the Seventh Day Adventist Church, the Five-Day Plan has also proven effective for some people. For no fee or a low fee, participants meet for five consecutive days after stopping cold turkey. The program offers counseling, stressing eating fresh fruit and drinking water and juices. For more information, contact Seventh Day Adventist, Community Health Services, 85 Long Island Expressway, New Hyde Park, NY 11040; (516) 627-2210.

Others swear by hypnosis, during which the subconscious mind is trained to quit. Though some hypnotherapists claim success rates of 40 to 80 percent, more realistic studies estimate about 15 to 20 percent. (Hypnosis isn't cheap: You may end up paying up to $100 per hour.) For more information or referrals, contact the American Society of Clinical Hypnosis, 2200 E. Devon Ave., suite 291, Des Plaines, IL 60018; (708) 297-3317; or the Society for Clinical and Experimental Hypnosis, 128A Kings Park Dr., Liverpool, NY 13090; (315) 652-7299.

Acupuncture is another option, but quit rates are fairly low—only 5 to 15 percent according to the American Council on Science and Health. Over-the-counter aids such as filters that gradually remove tar and nicotine from cigarettes are even less effective; don't bother.

Nicorette, a nicotine gum, has proven more useful. Prescribed by a doctor, it releases a small hit of nicotine into the lining of the mouth to help the smoker deal with the physical side effects of nicotine withdrawal. Gradually, use of the gum is eliminated. It works best for people who are also enrolled in smoking-cessation programs or receiving counseling. Plus it's not extremely expensive, costing about $50 for ninety-six pieces of gum (you can chew up to twenty pieces per day, but the average is eight to ten). Nicorette has its drawbacks, though: Some people become addicted to it, and others get tired of chewing it and go back to smoking.

More recently, physicians have begun to prescribe transdermal patches, which administer a small amount of nicotine through the skin (it is generally worn on the upper arm), gradually reducing the dose over a ten-week period. The results of studies of the patch seem promising, and this method is gaining in popularity. However, at $60 to $75 per two-week supply (depending on the dosage), it can be too expensive for some folks. Again, it works best for people who are enrolled in smoking-cessation programs or receiving counseling.

You'll have to pick and choose the method that's right for you. However, Sue F. Delaney, the author of *Women Smokers Can Quit: A*

Different Approach, who quit after forty years of smoking two packs a day, offers this general advice for those who've decided to quit:

Make a list of the reasons you want to quit. Be sure it's personal; you must quit for yourself, not for others. Instead of writing, "My friends and family are worried about my health," write, "*I* am worried about my cough, my blood pressure, my fatigue."

Set a quit date. Choose a time that is less stressful than others. For instance, a Friday is better than a Monday, which is generally overloaded with work.

Tell everyone you know that you plan to quit. Ask family and friends to support your decision. Draw up a stop-smoking contract, sign it, and place it in plain view.

Face up to the fact that you may gain weight after you quit. With nothing to do with their hands and mouth, many smokers who are trying to quit substitute eating and end up putting on pounds. However, no one should anticipate massive weight gain after quitting. The Office on Smoking and Health notes that the average weight gain after quitting is only five pounds. The best thing you can do for your body is to substitute exercise for smoking.

The day before you quit, smoke heavily. Spill ashes on the floor. Make yourself sick of your disgusting habit.

The night before, get rid of all cigarettes. Wash ashtrays, and throw away matches and lighters.

On quit day, change your routine. Take a bath instead of a shower, drive a different way to work, eat lunch standing up, change your radio station—shake up your day.

Find things to do with your hands and mouth. Chew gum, eat carrot sticks, or drink water. Squeeze a tennis ball, knit, doodle, or do crossword puzzles.

Avoid temptation. Don't sit in the smoking sections of restaurants, don't go out to smoky clubs, and avoid friends who are smokers.

When a craving hits, wait for it to pass, generally a few minutes. Call an encouraging friend or walk around the block when you feel it coming. Or try deep-breathing exercises to calm yourself.

Fighting Unhealthy Advertising

Like the coalition of prominent African-Americans, church groups, and community organizations that snubbed out Uptown cigarettes, others are fighting back against unhealthy advertising. In 1992 Harold P. Freeman, M.D., director of surgery at Harlem Hospital, created an anti-

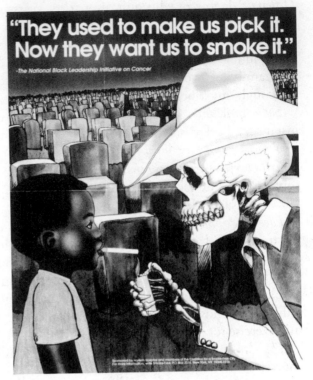

"They used to make us pick it. Now they want us to smoke it."
—The National Black Leadership Initiative on Cancer

This award-winning poster, sponsored by Harlem Hospital and the Coalition for a Smoke-Free City, appeared in the New York City subways. (*Courtesy: SmokeFree Educational Services, Inc.*)

smoking subway poster aimed at the Black community in New York. It is a drawing of a skeleton dressed in cowboy clothing, lighting up the cigarette that is clenched between the teeth of an African-American youngster; the backdrop is a cemetery. The copy reads: "They used to make us pick it. Now they want us to smoke it."

The Reverend Calvin O. Butts 3d of Abyssinian Baptist Church led a group that whitewashed cigarette and alcohol billboards in Harlem. Mandrake, an anonymous Black single father, won an award for guerrilla activism from *Emerge* magazine for painting over tobacco and liquor billboards.

Alcohol Abuse

Approximately 10 percent of adult Americans either abuse alcohol or are dependent on it, and women make up one-third of alcoholics in the U.S. Interestingly, data also indicates that compared with white women, a larger percentage of Black women abstain from drinking. Blacks of the early nineteenth century showed a strong support for the American temperance movement and boasted unusually low rates of alcohol problems. Our ancestors participated in a number of groups and societies such as the Women's Christian Temperance Union and the Independent Order of Good Templars. An 1880 U.S. Census Office report noted that "a large proportion of deaths reported as due to alcoholism occur in connection with delirium tremens, and this form of disease is rare in the colored race."

By the early twentieth century, however, our participation in the temperance movement had declined. As we migrated from the rural South to the urban North, nightlife and heavy drinking became the focus of many city dwellers. And for many Blacks, cheap wine, beer, and bathtub gin became a way to cope with the change in environment.

Presently, among Blacks who do drink, a larger percentage of Black men and women are heavy drinkers as compared with whites.

More important than hard numbers are the frightening effects that alcoholism has on our community. African-Americans who drink excessively suffer the most severe consequences. Black rates of cirrhosis of the liver and esophageal cancer, diseases closely associated with alcohol use, are disproportionate to our percentage of the American population. Compared with white women, we have higher rates of fetal alcohol syndrome, a set of physical and mental birth defects in infants born to women who drink heavily during pregnancy. And, frankly put, when we drink we get into more trouble: Alcohol-related violence, sexual activity, and accidents are common in our community.

Besides these serious risks, if you're trying to lose weight, you should cut down on alcohol or cut it out altogether. Liquor has little or no nutritional value aside from calories, and many of the concoctions that are added to alcohol to make mixed drinks are laden with sugar. Remember, too: The term "beer belly" was coined for a reason.

It's easy to spot an obvious alcoholic, the kind of stumbling, slurring drunk that Richard Pryor characterized so well in his comedy routines. But Black women often have different patterns of drinking. Although alcoholism has a hereditary link (twin studies show that genetics may account for 50 percent of the factors that determine vulnerability to excessive drinking), experts note that we often drink to self-medicate, to quell the disappointments, pain, anger, and rage that characterize our lives. Slave owners of the past knew the value of this kind of "escape alcoholism." Black slaves were provided with alcohol on holidays to keep them passive and under control.

What Is Problem Drinking?

Despite the difficulty in defining terms such as alcoholism, problem drinking, and moderation, the U.S. Department of Agriculture and the

*"I've journeyed
from hell to be
among the
living."*

—DEBORAH GREGORY,
WRITER AND ON-AIR
REPORTER,
NEW YORK CITY

At the age of thirteen, I had my first drink. I was at a house party in some-one's basement. I had a few sips of whatever it was before I went into a blackout. I didn't know that at the time. I thought I'd traveled to some mystical place. My sister propped me up on the way home—amused to see me drunk. By the time we got upstairs, I vomited in the bedroom hallway. I think my sister cleaned it up, but I don't really remember.

By the time I hit eighteen, I'd become a social drinker, popping ampheta-mines (to study in college and keep my weight down), smoking joints, and dabbling in cocaine. At twenty-two, my weekend dabbling had progressed to several times a week. Back then we called it "partying." I'd developed a taste for fine wines and champagne accompanied by frequent hits of cocaine and tokes off joints. I loved nothing more than dancing all night—always on the lookout for Mr. Right, of course (that meant someone with an unlimited supply of cocaine).

At twenty-four, I hopped on a plane and headed for Europe in the hopes of becoming a runway model. My wine addiction progressed the moment I landed in Paris. I met my kind of people: Even though we didn't speak the same language, we drank the same—heavy and into the wee hours of the morning. My life became progressively worse. I was in complete denial about my alcohol and drug abuse. (After all, it was all my other problems that caused me to drink!)

Right before my twenty-sixth birthday, I came back to the States from Milan. I had scored some heroin and was sitting in my New York City apartment with all the lights out. I sniffed heroin and coke, drank wine, and smoked cigarettes. Suddenly, I started throwing my dishes against the wall—all the rage pent up inside of me was seeping out. I left the broken dishes scattered on the kitchen floor. My roommate came home and walked through the kitchen to get to the bathroom. He cut his foot. When he said something to me, I yelled at him, "If you don't like it, why don't you clean it up?" I had hit rock bottom.

My therapist presented me with an ultimatum: Either I had to go to Alcoholics Anonymous, or she would no longer see me. I lied and told her I was going. One day I missed my therapy appointment and didn't even call her. She called and repeated her position. This time I knew she was serious. I went to AA with absolutely no intention of getting sober—I just wanted to get my therapist off my back. She was the only person I had let into my small world, and I didn't want to lose her. I went to an AA meeting at the YMCA in New York that day on July 16, 1982—and I got sober. To say that I've journeyed from hell to be among the living over the last ten years wouldn't begin to capture the experience. My recovery has been nothing short of remarkable. I no longer contemplate suicide, I don't have that big black hole inside, I have friends, a poodle, and most importantly, I carry the message of recovery to other still-suffering alcoholics and drug addicts—people who feel just like I did—scared, alone, and desperate. As long as I stay sober, I know in my heart that I will never have to feel that way again, and I continue to live . . . happy, joyous, and free!

U.S. Department of Health and Human Services offer these guidelines to define moderate drinking:

Men: No more than two drinks per day

Women: No more than one drink per day.

The agencies define a drink as 12 ounces of beer, 5 ounces of wine, or 1.5 ounces of 80-proof distilled spirits (hard liquor). Experts also warn that some people shouldn't drink at all, not even moderately. They are:

- Women who are trying to conceive and pregnant women (alcohol can also affect a man's sexual function)
- Recovering alcoholics
- People who are driving or engaging in activities that require skill or attention
- People taking certain medications, including over-the-counter drugs
- People with certain medical conditions, such as peptic ulcers, heart disease, hypertension, diabetes, and liver disease

Use the above guidelines as a general reference point. If you think your drinking may have moved from moderate to problematic, the National Council on Alcoholism and Drug Dependence recommends that you ask yourself the following questions:

When you're out partying, do you often try to have a few drinks behind your friends' backs?

Do you feel uneasy if alcohol isn't accessible?

Do you often want to keep on drinking after your friends have had enough?

Do you often drink alone, away from family and friends?

Are you sometimes drunk for several days at a time?

Do you sometimes have the "shakes" in the morning and find that a little "taste of something" calms you down?

Are you often depressed or anxious before, during, or after a period of heavy drinking?

If you answered yes to any of these questions, it doesn't mean you're necessarily an alcoholic. But it does mean that you should take an honest look at yourself and consider a change in your drinking habits. An additional question to ask yourself: Is there someone in your life who is concerned about your drinking? If so, seek professional advice.

Getting Help

It may be extremely difficult to face up to a drinking problem. In fact, when looking back, most recovering alcoholics can hardly believe how long they were in denial of their problem. Once you do accept that you have a problem and are ready to reach out for help, you may want to look for one of the treatment and detoxification centers that exist throughout the country. Those with very serious problems may need an inpatient program, which can last anywhere from a few days to a few months. This kind of treatment can be very costly, although some short-term programs are covered by health insurance.

More often, people find relief from private counseling, group therapy, or employee-assistance programs (counseling offered at the worksite). And in recent years, Alcoholics Anonymous, a nonprofit, self-help fellowship of people who want to stop drinking or maintain their sobriety, has exploded in popularity. AA has more than a million members in the U.S. who gather regularly in communities from coast to coast. The criterion for membership is a desire to stop drinking, and the primary obligation and responsibility of members is to stay sober and help other alcoholics achieve sobriety.

Though some practitioners have wrongly asserted that AA doesn't work for Blacks, many African-Americans successfully participate in the program. Some folks are more comfortable meeting with other African-Americans, and in some areas, these kinds of groups are available. The Paseo Group of Kansas City, for example, has been meeting for more than forty years and is one of the country's oldest Black AA groups. To find a group in your area call Alcoholics Anonymous at (212) 870-3400, or check your local phone directory.

Although experts who study treatment for Black alcoholics note that many are drawn to AA because it connects with the spirituality that has long been celebrated in our community, others are uncomfortable with the religious overtones that are part of AA's twelve-step process. For those people, groups such as Rational Recovery Systems, Secular Organizations for Sobriety, and Women for Sobriety offer nonreligious alternatives. For contacts, see the list below.

Whichever way an alcoholic chooses to deal with the problem, it's important to get to the root of it. Most people who simply decide to stop drinking without exploring what triggered alcoholism in the first place end up staring straight down into that glass of liquor again. And remember that you don't have to go through the recovery process alone: Practitioners note that because of the very strong kinship ties in our communities, Black women are most successful when recovery includes family and friends.

Help for Family and Friends

It's difficult to admit that a loved one is drinking too much. Experts who have studied alcohol abuse in our community note that because of our painful history in this country, Blacks tend to understand and sympathize with family members and friends who are using liquor to drink away the hurts. Though compassion has been a source of strength, too much can enable an alcoholic to stay addicted longer.

Dealing with an alcoholic friend or relative can be an exhausting, draining experience. And having an alcoholic family member can throw off the dynamic of the family, especially if the abuser is a parent. But help is available; see listing below.

For More Information

ORGANIZATIONS: Smoking

AMERICAN CANCER SOCIETY NATIONAL HEADQUARTERS, 1599 Clifton Rd. NE, Atlanta, GA 30329; (800) ACS-2345; or call your local office. ACS offers a quit-smoking program called Freshstart. A fee, which is refundable upon completion of the program in most areas, may be applicable. Also ask for the brochure "Smart Move: A Stop Smoking Guide." ACS also offers early warning and detection services, treatments, patient and educational services, and screenings.

AMERICAN COUNCIL ON SCIENCE AND HEALTH, 1995 Broadway, 2nd floor, New York, NY 10023-5860; (212) 362-7044. Ask for the publications "Smoking or Health: It's Your Choice" and "Searching for a Way Out: Smoking Cessation Techniques."

THE AMERICAN HEART ASSOCIATION, 7272 Greenville Ave., Dallas,

TX 75231; (214) 373-6300 or (800) AHA-USA1. Ask for the pamphlet "Calling It Quits" or the videotape *In Control.*

THE AMERICAN LUNG ASSOCIATION, 1740 Broadway, New York, NY 10019-4374; (800) LUNG-USA. Two booklets to ask for: "Freedom from Smoking in 20 Days" and "A Lifetime of Freedom from Smoking." A number of other booklets on quitting smoking and how to get help are also available.

THE NATIONAL CANCER INSTITUTE offers a toll-free information service line at (800) 4-CANCER between the hours of 9:00 A.M. and 4:30 P.M. You can get information on how to quit smoking, referrals to area support and help groups, as well as a cessation program and package. NCI also provides over one hundred booklets and pamphlets, with some geared to African-American women and smoking.

THE NATIONAL CENTER FOR HEALTH PROMOTION, 3920 Varsity Dr., Ann Arbor, MI 48108; (313) 971-6077 or (800) 843-6247. This group offers a variety of smoking-cessation kits. Also inquire about both long- and short-term group sessions and classes.

NICOTINE ANONYMOUS WORLD SERVICES OFFICE, 2118 Greenwich St., San Francisco, CA 94123; (415) 922-8575. NA is a self-help group founded in the twelve-step tradition, centered around nicotine addiction. Literature is available.

OFFICE ON SMOKING AND HEALTH, Center for Chronic Disease Prevention and Health Promotion, 4770 Buford Hwy. NE, Mail Stop K-50, Atlanta, GA 30341; (404) 488-5705. Offers a variety of publications and videos including "Out of the Ashes: Choosing a Method to Quit Smoking" and "Pathways to Freedom."

ORGANIZATIONS: Alcohol Abuse

ADDICTION SERVICES, East Orange General Hospital, 300 Central Ave., East Orange, NJ 07019; (201) 266-8425. Holds biannual conference "Alcoholism in the Black Community" in the spring, which raises money to further train and educate members in the field of addiction.

AMERICAN COUNCIL ON SCIENCE AND HEALTH, 1995 Broadway, 2nd floor, New York, NY 10023-5860; (212) 362-7044. Ask for the publication "The Responsible Use of Alcohol: Defining the Parameters of Moderation."

BLACK ALCOHOL/DRUG SERVICE INFORMATION CENTER, 1501 Locust St., Suite 1100, St. Louis, MO 63103; (314) 621-9009. BASIC offers a variety of services, on an outpatient basis, to help combat alcohol and drug problems in the Black community.

CENTER FOR SCIENCE IN THE PUBLIC INTEREST, 1875 Connecticut Ave. NW, Washington, DC 20009-5728; (202) 332-9110. Request "Marketing Booze to Blacks," available in book and video format. The group also offers consumer-advocacy information including how to organize in your area to stop billboards from going up.

CENTER FOR SUBSTANCE ABUSE PREVENTION, National Clearing-house for Alcohol and Drug Information, P.O. Box 2345, Rockville, MD 20847-2345; (800) 729-6686. The Center has more than eight hundred educational and informative items on inventory. Most are free, but there is a cost-recovery charge for all videos.

INSTITUTE ON BLACK CHEMICAL ABUSE, 2616 Nicollet Ave S., Minneapolis, MN 55408; (612) 871-7878. Provides books, articles, and videos on prevention and treatment of alcoholism.

NATIONAL ASSOCIATION OF LESBIAN AND GAY ALCOHOLISM PROFES-SIONALS, 1147 S. Alvarado St., Los Angeles, CA 90006; (213) 381-8524. Sponsors a national conference to discuss alcohol and drug prob-lems. Offers up-to-date research about alcohol abuse in the lesbian and gay community.

NATIONAL COUNCIL ON ALCOHOLISM AND DRUG DEPENDENCE, Inc., 12 W. 21 St., New York, NY 10010; (212) 206-6770 or (800) 475-HOPE. NCADD offers a variety of program services, a self-test for alcoholism, and prevention and education for alcohol and drug abuse. Call the 800 number for the affiliate in your area.

PUBLIC HEALTH SERVICE, ALCOHOL, DRUG ABUSE AND MENTAL HEALTH ADMINISTRATION, Rockville, MD 20857; (301) 656-9161. This group acts as a referral service for those in need of help with addictions. It offers a twenty-four-hour help line and an adult crisis center as part of its services.

RATIONAL RECOVERY SYSTEMS, Box 800, Lotus, CA 95651; (916) 621-2667. A network of self-help groups that offer what it calls "self-inspired, no-higher-power sobriety based on clear thinking and self-reliance."

SECULAR ORGANIZATIONS FOR SOBRIETY, International Clearinghouse, Box 5, Buffalo, NY 14215; (716) 834-2922. S.O.S., which also stands for Save Our Selves, has self-help groups nationwide that emphasize per-sonal responsibility and group support with no spiritual emphasis.

WOMEN FOR SOBRIETY, P.O. Box 618, Quakertown, PA 18951; (215) 536-8026 or (800) 333-1606. A national self-help organization for recovering alcoholic women. Contact the group for a local referral.

WOMEN'S ALCOHOL AND DRUG EDUCATION PROJECT, Women's Action Alliance, 370 Lexington Ave., suite 603, New York, NY 10017; (212) 532-8330. Offers a resource library and holds several workshops for recovering addicts.

ORGANIZATIONS: Alcohol (for Families and Friends)

AL-ANON FAMILY GROUPS (INCLUDING ALATEEN), P.O. Box 862, Midtown Station, New York, NY 10018-0862; (800) 356-9996. Information and support groups for family members of alcoholics or anyone whose life has been influenced by alcoholism.

ADULT CHILDREN OF ALCOHOLICS (ACA OR ACOA) WORLD SERVICES OFFICE, P.O. Box 3216, Torrance, CA 90510; (310) 534-1815. Groups that address the special problems of adults who were raised in an alcoholic or dysfunctional home, have a parent or parents who are alcoholics (or recovering), or who may be alcoholics themselves.

CO-DEPENDENTS ANONYMOUS, P.O. Box 33577, Phoenix, AZ 85067-3577; (602) 277-7991. Help for people who are somehow involved with or influenced by another person's addiction.

BOOKS: Smoking

How Women Can Finally Stop Smoking, Robert C. Klesges and Margaret DeBon, Hunter House (Alameda, Calif.), 1993.

Women Smokers Can Quit: A Different Approach, by Sue F. Delaney, Women's Healthcare Press (Evanston, Ill.), 1989.

BOOKS: Alcohol Abuse

I'm Black & I'm Sober: A Minister's Daughter Tells Her Story About Fighting the Disease of Alcoholism—and Winning, Chaney Allen, CompCare Publishers (Plymouth, Minn.), 1978.

The Invisible Alcoholics: Women and Alcohol Abuse, Marian Sandmaier, Tab Books (Blue Ridge Summit, Penn.), 1992.

Alcoholism: A Guide to Diagnosis, Intervention, and Treatment, Donald M. Gallant, W. W. Norton and Company, 1987.

Goodbye Hangovers, Hello Life: Self-Help for Women, Jean Kirkpatrick, Ballantine Books, 1987.

The Truth About Addiction and Recovery, Stanton Peele and Archie Brodsky, Fireside, 1992.

Problem Drinking, Nick Heather and Ian Robertson, Oxford University Press, 1989.

6

More Than "Just Say No": Coping with Drug Abuse

Far too many Black women are addicted to drugs. Many sisters are medicating themselves with cocaine, heroin, and prescription drugs, using them to quell the stress, pain, disappointment, and abuse that is a part of many of our lives.

Billie Holiday was one of those sisters. Singing brought her fame and at times a bit of fortune. But heroin ate away the fortune and made her infamous. In 1959 she died a junkie at age forty-four, a map of track marks covering her body.

Drugs in Our Community

Drugs made an initial appearance in the U.S. at the turn of the century in the form of over-the-counter miracle cures and Coca-Cola. No one ever thought that the heroin and cocaine traces found in these products could be addictive. They were wrong. By the 1920s, when cocaine and heroin were outlawed by the U.S. government, tens of thousands were already seriously addicted—including many brothers and sisters.

Drugs went underground during the twenties and thirties, enjoying a limited popularity among the hip crowd of Black artists and musicians.

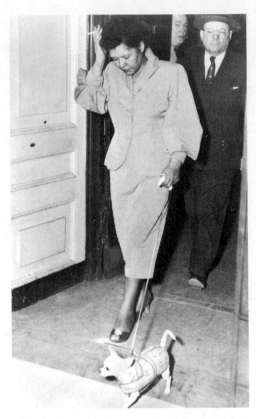

Singer Billie Holiday being released
on bail on charges of narcotic use.
Heroin addiction eventually led to
her death. *(Photo: The Bettmann
Archive)*

But it wasn't until the 1950s, when drugs became plentiful and cheap,
that our people started using in large numbers. By the 1970s, the junkie
subculture was firmly entrenched in our communities. Crime infested
our neighborhoods. Families were destroyed. People killed and were
killed.

Still, no one was prepared for the devastation that the eighties crack
boom wreaked on the inner city. Cocaine, once a ridiculously expensive
drug, was born again in the very affordable form of rock, or crack. For
so many people, one hit of the drug meant instant addiction. Suddenly,
small-time crack dealers sprouted up on virtually every street corner.
And just as suddenly, the prison population increased 150 percent from
1980 to 1990 in Ronald Reagan's and George Bush's War on Drugs.
Black people—in particular African-American men—were overrepre-
sented among those numbers.

African-Americans, especially the poor and disenfranchised, continue
to be ravaged by drugs. Some of us became convinced that the proliferation of drugs in our neighborhoods was no accident.

Drugs exact a toll on our community. Scores of cocaine-exposed babies languish in hospitals. Drugs and AIDS seem to go hand-in-hand: At this writing, 34 percent of Black men with AIDS are intravenous drug users or have partners who are IV drug users. Seventy-four percent of all women with AIDS are IV drug users or have male partners who shoot up. And 62 percent of all Black children with AIDS have mothers who are either IV drug users or have partners who are IV users.

As a nation, we are haunted by drugs. In 1991 there were 1.8 million cocaine addicts and 700,000 heroin addicts in the United States, the highest addiction rates ever. Experts estimate that between 5 and 6 million Americans are in need of serious drug treatment.

Black Women and Drug Abuse

Sisters get hooked for a variety of reasons. Some start out experimenting with drugs or using them recreationally, only to find that they can't stop. Others are trying to escape the combined oppressions of racism and sexism. Instead of talking about the pain or seeking some form of treatment, far too many African-American women self-medicate with illegal drugs. In addition, experts now know that some people are more susceptible than others to addictions of all kinds. For these people, experimenting with drugs can quickly lead to being hooked.

As a group, Black women tend to be drawn to opiates such as heroin, drugs that numb emotional pain. Often sisters turn to cocaine because it gives a false feeling of empowerment; one snort and the user feels ready to take on the world. Overwhelmingly, poor sisters in the inner city turn to crack cocaine, although heroin is making a comeback in some circles.

Once a Black female gets addicted, what plagues her may be quite different from what ails the white female addict or even the brother down the street who's hooked on crack. It may be extremely emotionally difficult to face the problem and then to get off.

Being Black and female in America poses a unique set of problems: We are expected to be superwomen, responsible for the health and well-being of an entire race. We're not supposed to be weak. We're not supposed to need taking care of. Instead, we take care of. Often we're so busy looking after others that we ignore the fact that our own lives are out of control.

And so a woman who's Black and chemically dependent may feel like she's somehow violated the natural order. Many are deeply ashamed. It's further complicated by the fact that as a race, we tend to look askance at psychologists and other mental-health professionals, while many white Americans look at going to therapy as a God-given right. We don't always believe in telling other folks our business. So Black female addicts can end up isolated in misery, seeking treatment only when jobs are threatened or they've been ordered to do so by the courts.

Those who are professionals fear they have even more to lose. They may feel that people look up to them and they have an image to uphold. And so they mask pain and addiction, choosing to sacrifice themselves rather than admit to a problem. Usually, by the time they get help, the illness has progressed to a much greater extent than it does for a white woman in the same boat. Sometimes they never get help.

The Consequences

Let's face it: Most people start using drugs because they make them feel good—temporarily. After all, we live in a feel-good society that encourages people to pop pills or take a drink to ease pain. Some folks dabble with drugs for years and walk away relatively unscathed. But all too often, they get caught up.

And caught: According to a recent *USA Today* special report, though Blacks and whites use drugs at roughly the same rates, Blacks are four times more likely than whites to be arrested on drug charges. A Black person living in Minneapolis is twenty-two times more likely; in Columbus, Ohio, eighteen times; and in Seattle thirteen times. Though we are only 12 percent of the U.S. population, Blacks make up 42 percent of those arrested on drug charges.

Although law-enforcement officials treat drug use as a crime, drug addiction is first and foremost a disease. Someone who misuses drugs may be classified as a substance abuser or as substance-dependent. Substance-abuse victims can't control their drug use. They get high regularly, often just to function on a day-to-day basis. They can't stop using, even though they may have lost everything—family, friends, finances. People who are substance-*dependent* not only can't control their use, but they are also physically addicted. They find themselves needing more and more of their drug of choice to get the same effect, and they suffer withdrawal symptoms when they stop using.

Drugs fall into six major categories: Cocaine, marijuana, opiates, hallucinogens, inhalants, and sedative-hypnotics. (This list doesn't cover nicotine and alcohol, which are discussed in chapter 5, "Killing Us Softly.") Not all drugs are physically addictive, but many are psychologically addictive; that means that the user craves the drug, needing it to function.

Cocaine

Cocaine, also known as snow, blow, coke, toot, and nose candy, causes one of the most potent forms of addiction. It can be snorted through the nose or dissolved and injected into the vein. It also can be chemically altered into the powerful, smokeable crack or freebase.

Cocaine is a seductive stimulant; it gives the user the illusion of power and energy. She feels hyped up and in control of the world. But after a little while that feeling of omnipotence evaporates, leaving the user feeling down and anxious. Next thing she's craving another hit. And that's just the problem: Chasing after that elusive high means that eventually the user gets hooked. Anyone can get trapped by cocaine. It causes chemical changes in the brain that lead to uncontrollable cravings, a jones that will rule every aspect of a person's life. Soon the addict's finances will be shot, and physical and mental health will have deteriorated.

Some addicts use the drug only on weekends, bingeing until they collapse or the supply runs out. Usually, the binge period is followed by a crash that feels like the end of the world. Other users partake on a daily basis, in either large or small doses. In either case, the amount the addict uses will increase over time.

Female addicts resort to desperate means to get the drug. Many sell their bodies, having unprotected sex to finance their next high. Because they are desperate—and high—they don't think about their risk of contracting sexually transmitted diseases, including AIDS. This risky behavior is part of the reason that rates of syphilis, gonorrhea, and HIV have skyrocketed among women.

Cocaine use can be particularly dangerous to the body. It can elevate the blood pressure, heart rate, breathing rate, and body temperature. The pupils dilate and blood vessels constrict. The user loses interest in food and can't sleep. The more she uses, the more she experiences mood swings, upper respiratory infections, and the ubiquitous runny nose.

But these are minor nuisances compared to what else can happen. Using cocaine increases the risk of heart attack or heart failure—even in young people. (Remember the promising basketball star Len Bias who died a few years ago of a cocaine-related heart condition?) The user is more susceptible to brain seizures and strokes, and thinking can become impaired. Some people suffer the violent, erratic, or paranoid behavior known as "cocaine psychosis." Pregnant users can miscarry or deliver a stillborn baby. If she carries the pregnancy to term, the baby can be born cocaine-exposed. Such infants are usually undersized, irritable, and

"I masked my addiction well. People looked at me and didn't see an addict."

—FAVELLA DURDEN, DRUG COUNSELOR, RICHMOND, VIRGINIA

I started using when I was a teenager, in junior high, smoking pot and drinking. I used to drink and throw up and couldn't go to class, but those were not my drugs of choice. It wasn't until I ran into cocaine in college that I knew I was on to something.

Cocaine gave me something I'd never had before: confidence. I didn't think I was attractive. I suffered depression for years. As long as I can remember, I've been depressed. So I tried to feel better any way that I could. One way was by doing well in school and getting praise. The other way was by using cocaine.

I started using when I was a student at Hunter College in New York City. I loved the way it made me feel. It empowered me. It was great. I said, "This is it." I felt secure. I felt I could do anything. And for once, I wasn't afraid.

I would go through these periods when I would stop using. I stayed clean when I got pregnant with my son. I always had these professional jobs that carried a lot of responsibility. I started seeing a man who didn't use. So I didn't either. But every now and then, I'd sneak out and use. And of course, whenever we broke up, I'd start up again. The last year we were together, he started selling coke for financial reasons. That's when my disease blew up. By the time I hit my early thirties, I knew I was an addict. There was just no denying it. I was spending at least $500 or $600 a week on cocaine. I was earning a decent salary, but when you're using, you never have enough money. It's amazing how resourceful you become. And I masked my addiction well. People looked at me and didn't see an addict. I'm creative and resourceful, and I used those traits to get drugs.

But I was a professional person. I felt trapped. I couldn't let people know that I had a problem. By the time I got help, I was very sick. I was totally unmanageable and very suicidal. I had totally fallen apart. Luckily there were people who cared enough to help me go into treatment. When I got out of my drug-rehab program, I didn't go back to work right away. I moved in with my son and my mother. I tried to regroup. Now I'm out on my own again, counseling others.

Still, it's hard. I've had periods of sobriety. And I've had periods where I've gone back and used. It's a constant struggle. When they say one day at a time, it truly is one day at a time. Quitting is never for good. I can say that today I'm sober.

unresponsive, suffer strokes or heart attacks, are at increased risk for crib death (sudden infant death syndrome or SIDS) and can experience emotional and behavioral problems once they get older. Cocaine can also be passed to a baby through breast milk.

Marijuana

Marijuana, reefer, spliff, Mary Jane, or pot, immortalized by the likes of singer Bob Marley, is usually viewed as pretty harmless stuff. Still, it is the most widespread illegal drug in the country. And although you generally don't hear about movie stars checking themselves into the Betty Ford Clinic to cure pot problems, marijuana does present some serious health hazards. Many heavy reefer users go on to harder drugs. It can also be psychologically addictive.

Even in relatively small doses, marijuana will impair short-term memory, concentration, judgment, information processing, perception, and fine motor skills. Driving a car or handling machinery is dangerous for someone stoned on pot. Memory loss can drag on for months. Pot will also increase heartbeat and blood pressure, putting the user with heart or circulatory problems in danger. Heavy users can experience paranoia, chronic anxiety, and depression. Marijuana also carries an increased risk of lung cancer and can disrupt the reproductive system.

Opiates

Opiates, or narcotics, are drugs that are intended for medical use. They are found in pain relievers, anesthetics, and cough suppressants. Such drugs have a high potential for abuse—and addiction. Some opiates, such as opium, morphine, heroin, and codeine, come from resin taken from the Asian poppy. Others, such as Demerol, are synthetic substances that act like morphine.

Heroin is a white or brownish powder that can be snorted but is most often dissolved in water and then injected. On the street, heroin is usually cut with sugar or quinine—even baby laxatives—to extend the supply and increase profits. Opium is found in dark brown chunks or powder that is smoked or eaten. Other opiates are found in tablets, capsules, suppositories, and syrups.

Heroin users account for 90 percent of opiate abusers; half a million Americans are addicted to it. Prescription drugs such as morphine, paregoric (containing opium), and cough syrups laced with codeine are also potentially addictive. Half of the people who abuse opiates will become

"I had no choice but to work like a fiend to pay for my habit."

—IMANI P. WOODS, SUBSTANCE-ABUSE COUNSELOR, SEATTLE

I grew up in Bedford-Stuyvesant, Brooklyn, where there was a lot of discomfort and pain. My mother was a single parent who worked very, very hard and was very, very hard on us. There was a lot of physical abuse. I tried to commit suicide when I was eleven. My grandfather drank; he thought getting me drunk when I was six or seven was funny. I learned very early that drinking was a way to alleviate discomfort.

I started experimenting with other drugs when I was thirteen or fourteen. I was attending Catholic school. I was on the student council. I wanted to change the world. Still, I really felt this need to belong somewhere. I was a real fat kid. I didn't want to be called square.

I started with marijuana. I moved on to cocaine, but I didn't like it very much. One day my senior year of high school, someone gave me heroin. I was totally attracted to how it made me feel. It gave me euphoria. It's like going to an entirely different world where you are present and yet not present. It is total oblivion and total bliss—if you have the right dose. First all the muscles in your body relax. All the troubles and cares in your mind disintegrate. Then you transcend into this sleeplike nod. And there you stay until the drug wears off.

That's where the problems begin. When the drug wears off, you want to get back to that place of peace. And if you are physically addicted, then you have to get back to that place in a few hours, or you'll get withdrawal symptoms. No one knows how bad that feels. The first time you realize you are addicted, you get scared. You get the cold sweats. You get the chills. You get paranoid. You get diarrhea. It's like the worst flu you've ever had in your life. Except you know that if you go out and get some heroin and stick it in your vein, you'll feel better instantly. And so you get this psychological obsession. It's a very, very, very difficult drug to overcome.

Heroin ruled my life. I was not one of those who could steal and prostitute. Not that I didn't try. I was a horrible thief. So I had no choice but to work like a fiend to pay for my habit. I even attended college. I worked in public service. And always, always, I lived in two worlds: I ran the streets and got down and dirty. And then I could be very middleclass.

I tried everything to get off heroin. I tried residential programs. I tried methadone. For ten years I dreamed of getting off drugs. I would get uplifted and think I could make it. I was a star patient. But I failed every time. It didn't work for me until I was ready.

In 1981, I was attending yet another methadone program when I met a woman who was a former addict. She knew exactly what I was talking

about because she'd done it herself. Finally I was able to pull myself out of
the terrible morass I was in—with the help of God and a lot of prayer. I
now have a great sense of gratitude for being able to get out of that hell.

addicted; the drug will become an obsession, and more and more will be
needed to achieve the same high.

Users say they take opiates to relax; witness the heroin junkie
slumped over and nodding out on the street. After injecting opiates,
the user feels an immediate rush. Sometimes she may vomit.
Restlessness is common. If she uses too much, overdose is possible.
She won't be easy to awaken. The pupils become smaller, and the
breathing slows. Her skin becomes blue, cold, and clammy. She may
die.

Opiate withdrawals are legendary and can set in within six hours after
the drug wears off. Withdrawal symptoms include nausea, diarrhea,
abdominal cramps, chills, sweating, runny nose and eyes. Symptoms are
strongest within the first twenty-four to seventy-two hours but can last
as long as ten days. Sleeplessness and cravings for the drug can last for
months afterward.

Everyone knows that using dirty needles is tantamount to volunteer-
ing to get AIDS. But users can also contract liver disease and tetanus.
Using opiates also makes people vulnerable to infections of the heart
lining and valves, congested lungs, and skin abscesses. Experts estimate
that almost half of female addicts suffer from heart disease, anemia, diabetes, pneumonia, or hepatitis during pregnancy and childbirth. They
also have more spontaneous abortions, premature births, stillbirths,
breach deliveries, and cesarean sections. Their babies may suffer serious
withdrawal symptoms. Many babies die.

Hallucinogens

Many of us think of hallucinogens as sixties drugs whose use peaked in
the days when hippies were urged to tune in, turn on, and drop out.
Indeed, LSD, mescaline, and peyote use has declined steadily over the
past couple of decades. Still, these drugs have their fans in folks who use
them for mind-altering hallucinations, or trips. Hallucinogens can also
be found in the form of phencyclidine, known as PCP or angel dust,
which can be smoked or inhaled. In the past, PCP was popular in some

Black communities. Many people freaked out on PCP, becoming violent and out of control.

People who take hallucinogens use them intermittently only. It's hard to function in the real world stoned on acid; the trips are marathon highs that last for hours, greatly impairing cognitive abilities. Because of this, it's rare to see an LSD addict.

Inhalants

Inhalants are breathable chemicals that produce mind-altering vapors. They are inhaled through the nose and, like anesthetics, slow the body down.

Inhalants aren't generally thought of as drugs because most of them

---

Prescription Drug Abuse

The good news: Black women are much less likely to abuse prescription drugs than are white women. Still, roughly 12 percent of Americans abuse prescription drugs at some point. The fact is, just because a doctor prescribes a drug doesn't mean the patient is immune from getting strung out: If someone needs a daily hit of a drug—whether it's cocaine or Valium—just to get through the day, that person is addicted.

It's easy to get hooked. A doctor might have prescribed Valium when work started fraying the nerves. But even small doses of Valium can be addictive. Or a stressed-out sister might have started popping Dalmane, a sleeping aid, after spending too many nights tossing and turning. Morphine took the edge off the pain after surgery; but some people abuse it long after the operation.

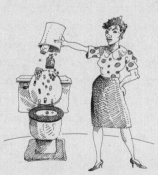

Get rid of any unused or left-over prescription drugs.
(Drawing: Yvonne Buchanan)

Ask yourself whether you or someone you love has any of these most commonly prescribed drugs—Valium, Percodan, Dalmane, Tranxene, Darvon, or codeine—in the medicine cabinet. How often are they used? Further, ask yourself these questions, provided by the American Institute for Preventive Medicine:

Do I need this drug to feel better?

Do I need to take more and more in order to get the same effect?

Do I think about wanting this drug so much that it has become very important in my life?

Do I experience uncomfortable withdrawal symptoms such as weakness, anxiety, muscle twitching, nausea, sleeplessness, tremors, dizziness, hallucinations, convulsions, delirium, and delusions?

were intended for other uses. Paint thinner, gasoline, nail-polish remover, glue, spray paint, kerosene, aerosol sprays, and lighter fluid are commonly abused inhalants. Young people between the ages of seven and seventeen are the most common users. Amyl nitrate, known as "poppers," is another commonly abused substance. Used legitimately to treat heart patients, it dilates the blood vessels and speeds up the heart rate to produce a high that lasts a few minutes. Butyl nitrate, also called "locker room" or "rush," produces a similar high.

The immediate effects of inhalants include nausea, nosebleeds, sneezing, coughing, tiredness, headache, breathing problems, lack of coordination, and loss of appetite. Solvents and aerosols also decrease heart and breathing rates and affect judgment. Inhalants can also cause cardiac arrest, which is more common among Blacks than whites. Some inhaled materials coat the lung tissue and may cause severe or even fatal pneumonia. Sniffing solvents has been associated with kidney failure, among other problems. Users can also become dependent on inhalants and experience withdrawal symptoms if use is stopped.

How to Tell Whether Someone You Love Is Addicted

According to David Grant of the Institute on Black Chemical Abuse in Minneapolis, "The person with the drug problem is always the last to know she's addicted. But everyone around her knows. The addict is in denial. She can come up with a million explanations for why her life is in chaos—and none of it has to do with her drug abuse. She's like someone who's deeply in love with an abusive partner. She'll say, 'It's really not that bad. That's why I stay.' But in reality, she's dying inside."

If you or a loved one is using and your home life is beginning to show the strains of drug abuse, here are some hard questions to ask yourself about the one you love:

Am I his cover girl? Do I tell lies for him? Do I call the office and say he's sick when he's really high?

Does she spend more money on drugs than we spent on food for the entire year?

Is he secretive? Does he hide his drug use from me?

Do I hide her drugs?

Do I use drugs in an attempt to keep his drug use within limits?

Do I make apologies for her embarrassing behavior that is a result of drug abuse?

Do I cancel social engagements that might result in excessive drug use?

Do I cover his bad checks, unpaid bills, and assume his debts?

Do I support her rationalizations for drug abuse? Am I codependent?

Getting Help

If you think you've got a drug problem, get some kind of help. Don't wait until things are dire. You've lost your job. You've lost your lover. Your finances are in a shambles. Your family won't lend you money anymore. Your friends are gone. You hurt all the time, but still, you can't seem to stop using. It seems like you never get high anymore. But you're using more and more just to feel normal. You're dying inside.

If you or a loved one is using and your home life is starting to unravel, there is help out there. But all too often, we let shame stand in the way of getting help until it's almost too late. As a people, we tend not to go for treatment until we've been arrested and ordered to go by a judge. By that time, we may have lost everything—family, jobs, homes, money.

But before you reach the end of your rope, take action into your own hands. If you are addicted, contact your local state-run substance-abuse department. If a family member is in trouble, you can enlist the aid of family and friends to do an "intervention" to get the one you love to admit she's addicted. Intervention is a no-holds-barred effort usually done with the aid of a trained substance-abuse counselor. Family and friends sit the addict down for a serious heart-to-heart. One after another, they tell the addict how her problem has affected their lives, using specific details. The idea is to break through the addict's denial by telling her again and again—lovingly—that she has a serious problem and it has to stop. Experts say that an addict confronted with an intervention will usually agree to get help.

Once you've gone through the intervention process, you should contact your state's human-services department for a free assessment. During an assessment, a trained counselor will ask the addict specific questions about her drug habits: How often do you use drugs? And what are the consequences of your abuse? The person doing the assessment will recommend the appropriate type of treatment, such as a thirty-day outpatient program or a long-term inpatient rehabilitation program.

Ideally, you should try to find a rehabilitation program tailored for people of color. Historically, substance-abuse treatment programs have been tailored for white middle-class men who are alcoholics. And as a result, many treatment programs don't address the issues of class and race that may have gotten you there in the first place. Often, we get frustrated and drop out of the programs, soon lapsing back into old ways. Also, slots for women are few. If a woman has children, it's even more difficult to get help. Still, be insistent.

Recovering takes a lifetime commitment to staying straight. And to do so, you have to understand what drove you to drugs in the first place. Black women, experts say, tend to thrive in all-women groups that address the issues of being female in a male-dominated society. Programs that are specifically tailored to African-Americans are best. These days, there are a few residential programs that allow children to live on-site while their mothers get treatment. Obviously, such programs are ideal.

One of the biggest criticisms leveled against the "War on Drugs" is that it pumped billions of taxpayer dollars into fighting crime and left precious little for treatment. Today, finding—and paying for—help is no easy task. Still, it can be done. Your job may have free drug-rehabilitation programs that you can enroll in. Your insurance most likely will cover the cost of treatment; Medicaid usually only picks up the tab for detox programs. If you don't have insurance, there are some programs, such as the Minneapolis-based Institute on Black Chemical Abuse, that provide service free of charge.

If at all possible, find a long-term program that will walk you through all of the steps to recovery. First, you will need to detox from your drug. If you are a heroin addict, that may mean enrolling in a methadone program. Once you've detoxed, you'll need to go about the daunting task of learning to live drug-free. A good program is a culturally specific one that teaches the addict to control her impulses while focusing on job readiness and basic education if needed. Black-oriented support groups and African-American female therapists are invaluable for the recovering black woman. The idea is to get as much help as possible to deal with feelings of shame and disappointment.

To stay straight, you need to surround yourself with people on the outside who support your recovery. You've got to learn to live sober in every way; building a good support system is essential. Many women find comfort talking to others who are trying to stay straight, so they join a self-help support group. (For more information, see chapter 22, "The Self-Help Revolution.") Other groups to look into are twelve-step recovery groups such as Cocaine and Narcotics Anonymous.

Getting Drugs Out of Your Community

When someone stuffed a doll with a noose around its neck in Dorothy Harrell's door, the nearly sixty-year-old great-grandmother knew that she was making headway in her goal to wipe drugs out of her Philadelphia housing development.

As Harrell says, you don't make friends when you're trying to put drug dealers out of business. Her office has been firebombed twice. But

Harrell is determined to fight the good fight. "Everyone has a right to live in a healthy, decent environment," she says.

Since 1989, Harrell, along with a handful of her neighbors, has patrolled her streets, armed with a bullhorn and a lot of nerve. Her goal: to put drug dealers and their customers on notice; "We're tired and we're not going to take it anymore."

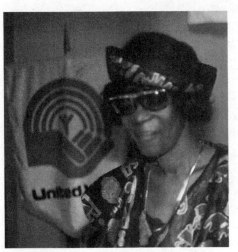

Dorothy Harrell receiving an award for her antidrug activism.
(Courtesy: Dorothy Harrell)

Within a year, Harrell's neighborhood began to change. Break-ins, muggings, and gunfights are a thing of the past. Speakeasies have been shut down. Drug dealers are out of business. Troublesome neighbors have been evicted.

"People are afraid," Harrell says. "But there's a big difference between being afraid and being a prisoner in your own home and being afraid and changing your neighborhood to clean it up. I get a high like the junkies do when I see things being done for the good of all people. But my family thinks I'm crazy."

Like Harrell, there are things you can do to take back your neighborhood. And you don't need a degree in urban policy to do it; housing experts say that citizen-run efforts go a long way to reduce crime. In Los Angeles, kids take to the streets on skateboards and bikes, reporting back to adults any drug activity they find in the 'hood. And in some parts of Washington, D.C., residents don orange hats as they patrol their streets to let drug traffickers know they're part of the antidrug gang.

If you are intent on wiping out your local drug trade, here are a few tips to keep in mind:

Clean up your act. Rundown neighborhoods send a message that people don't care about what happens there. Organize block cleanups to spruce up your environment. Once you do that, you'll have organized a task force ready to take on the dealers. And police will see that you are serious about turning your neighborhood around.

Set up a communication network among your neighbors to report drug-related activity. Some people rely on whistles; others use walkie-talkies.

Establish good relations with the local police. It's a good idea to contact them after you've organized your neighbors. That way, you will be taken more seriously by police. Ask them for training in how to spot drug activity and how to report it.

Work in groups. Use a uniform, such as T-shirts or hats, to identify that you are part of a team. Don't attempt direct confrontation with known drug dealers; it's best not to be combative.

Take away their business. Dealers may be omnipresent, but their customers don't have to be. The key is to embarrass them or make it hard for them to do business. Let them know you know what you're there for. Set up a video camera to record their comings and goings. Write down their license-plate numbers.

If possible, work with landlords, property owners, and community leaders to change the landscaping of your neighborhood. Often, drug traffic flourishes in one neighborhood because it provides easy access. One idea is to obstruct one entrance to your block so that your street doesn't become a drug drive-in.

Make sure the garbage is picked up frequently. Dealers often stash their goods in garbage Dumpsters.

If you live in an apartment development, post No Trespassing signs around the grounds. Work with housing authorities to set up security patrols to stop dealers from setting up shop outside your door.

If your landlord is indifferent or part of the problem, find out where he lives or works and picket him. Report him for any housing code violations.

Don't be discouraged if only a few show up at neighborhood meetings. Not everyone is going to get involved. But it only takes a handful of folks to make a change.

For More Information

ORGANIZATIONS

ALCOHOL AND DRUG HELPLINE, 4578 Highland Dr., Salt Lake City, UT 84117; (800) 821-4356. Referral number for drug-detox centers and rehabilitation programs across the nation. Also refers those without medical insurance to human and social services for assistance.

AMERICAN COUNCIL FOR DRUG EDUCATION, 204 Monroe St., suite 110, Rockville, MD 20850; (800) 488-DRUG or (301) 294-0600. Provides information about drug and alcohol abuse, including publications and videos.

AMERICAN SOCIETY OF ADDICTION MEDICINE, 5225 Wisconsin Ave. NW, suite 409, Washington, DC 20015; (202) 244-8948. Distributes publications and information about conferences on addiction and specific alcohol- and drug-related problems.

BLACK ALCOHOL/DRUG SERVICE INFORMATION CENTER, 1501 Locust St., suite 1100, Saint Louis, MO 63103; (314) 621-9009. Offers an outpatient treatment program and a support program for the Black community.

CENTER FOR SUBSTANCE ABUSE PREVENTION, National Clearinghouse for Alcohol and Drug Information, P.O. Box 2345, Rockville, MD 20847-2345; (800) 729-6686. A national distribution center for free information, including a catalogue of publications and other written material. Video materials are also available for a fee.

THE CENTER FOR SUBSTANCE ABUSE TREATMENT NATIONAL DRUG HOTLINE, 11426-28 Rockville Pike, suite 410, Rockville, MD 20852; (800) 662-4357. Provides drug-treatment referrals, including self-help programs. Will also answer any questions about drugs and drug abuse.

DEPARTMENT OF HOUSING AND URBAN DEVELOPMENT DRUG INFORMATION AND STRATEGY CLEARINGHOUSE, P.O. Box 6424, Rockville, MD 20850; (800) 578-3472. Provides information on drug prevention, enforcement, and treatment in public housing. Its database provides information on more than 800 national and state programs.

INSTITUTE ON BLACK CHEMICAL ABUSE, 2616 Nicollet Ave. S., Minneapolis, MN 55408; (612) 871-7878. Directs callers to inpatient services in the area and provides outpatient care for chemical dependency, including assessments and access to an on-site resource center.

NATIONAL COUNCIL ON ALCOHOL AND DRUG DEPENDENCE, 12 W. 21st St., New York, NY 10010; (800)475-HOPE or (212) 206-6770. Provides information and publications on alcoholism and drug abuse.

PROJECT INROADS, 799 South Main St., Lima, OH 45804; (419) 222-1168. This center uses an approach to substance abuse and recovery that is sensitive to the needs of people of color.

PUBLIC HEALTH SERVICE, ALCOHOL, DRUG ABUSE AND MENTAL HEALTH ADMINISTRATION, Rockville, MD 20857; (301) 656-9161. This group acts as a referral service for those in need of help with addictions. Its services include a 24-hour help line and an adult crisis center.

WOMEN'S ALCOHOL AND DRUG EDUCATION PROJECT, WOMEN'S ACTION ALLIANCE, 370 Lexington Ave., suite 603, New York, NY 10017; (212) 532-8330. Offers a resource library and holds several workshops for recovering addicts.

7

We Are at Risk: Diseases That Strike Us

Heart disease, cancer, stroke, and diabetes—these are the country's top killers, and they're more deadly among Blacks. Still, this fact remains: To a large extent, these problems are preventable. If everyone would stop smoking, switch to healthier diets, and get out and exercise several times a week, the death rates from these diseases would drop dramatically.

For Black folks, another part of the problem is the "quicker and sicker" syndrome: We Black women tend to overlook preventive care because we're too busy or too busy taking care of everyone but ourselves. Then, when we do need medical treatment, we come in sicker and die more quickly than we should. To avoid this problem, we must visit a doctor regularly for checkups and tests. Even if illness has set in, it's better to find out earlier rather than later, when treatment will be less effective.

The first step toward a healthy community is education. All of us must understand how to prevent and treat serious illness of all kinds so that we may live long and healthy lives.

Diseases That Affect Black Women

We don't have to be victims. Some of us, because of family history, may be at risk for some diseases. However, we often have the power to stay well by learning about diseases that strike us and understanding how to keep our bodies free of them.

Some healers believe that illness can occur in people who have emotional problems or are lacking spiritual grounding. The link between stress and high blood pressure, for example, is accepted even by conservative scientists. So here we must stress the importance of staying emotionally healthy and spiritually centered in order to avoid and fight disease. (For more information see chapter 21, "Emotional Pain, Stress, and Healing with Therapy," and chapter 23, "The Healing Power of Spirituality.")

For information on illnesses that are not covered here but are mentioned in other parts of this book, refer to the index. For general information on disease prevention, contact the Office of Minority Health Resource Center, P.O. Box 37337, Washington, DC 20013-7337; (800) 444-6472 or (301) 587-1938. This office responds to questions about health concerns that relate to people of color, distributes materials, and offers referrals.

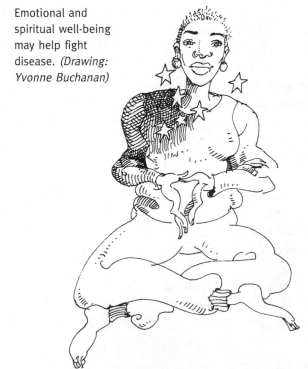

Emotional and spiritual well-being may help fight disease. *(Drawing: Yvonne Buchanan)*

Hypertension and Heart Disease

For years and years, most people didn't think that Blacks, especially Black women, had heart disease. Only overweight, overworked middle-aged white men suffered heart attacks. But that myth is dead wrong. Heart disease is the number-one killer of all Americans, including Black men and women. For Black women, heart disease is especially deadly: We are more likely to die from it than are white women. The majority of cases of heart disease in Black folks can be blamed on our high rates of hypertension, another name for high blood pressure. It is more than twice as common in Blacks than in whites, affecting one in three African-Americans.

What Is Heart Disease?

A heart attack occurs when the supply of blood to part of the heart is reduced or cut off. It happens because one or more of the arteries that supply blood to the heart is suddenly and completely blocked. Women are more at risk after menopause.

High blood pressure can lead to a heart attack. Hypertension can also be blamed for other serious diseases that strike Blacks disproportionately. For example, stroke, the interruption of blood flow to a specific area of the brain, which causes temporary or permanent paralysis of parts of the body, can be triggered by high blood pressure. Kidney damage, diabetes, and blindness or impaired vision are also associated with hypertension. The blood pressure can increase when the arteries become narrowed or the blood volume rises and the heart must pump harder and harder to force the blood to flow through the blood vessels. When this happens, the heart can become strained and the arteries can be damaged.

Inherited factors also contribute. Blacks have higher rates of hypertension than do whites for many reasons. For one, our rates of obesity are higher, and being overweight contributes to high blood pressure. Many of the foods we love are salty and fatty, and eating foods high in salt and fat also leads to hypertension. Stress, which so many African-American women have to put up with day in and day out, and smoking raise the blood pressure.

Some scientists believe that our slave past has contributed to today's high rates of hypertension. When our African ancestors were brought across the Atlantic on slave ships, many contracted diarrhea. Dehydrated and depleted of salt, these Africans died. But others who were able to retain salt survived; salt causes the body to retain water and combat dehydration. Though we no longer need it, the ability to retain salt may have been passed from generation to generation. That may have made us more "salt-sensitive," which means that our blood pressure is more likely to be affected by the amount of salt we eat.

Detecting High Blood Pressure and Heart Disease

High blood pressure is a silent killer; for many, it has no symptoms at all. That's why we must all have our blood pressure checked regularly— at least every year and more often if you know your pressure is high or have a family history of hypertension. A normal reading is 120/80. If your blood pressure is 140/90 or more, you must take steps to lower it. Many churches, health fairs, and shopping malls offer blood-pressure screenings. If your reading is high, be sure to get it *rechecked* by a physician.

Unlike hypertension, a heart attack has clear symptoms. But studies show that too often Blacks don't recognize the signs of a heart attack—or we ignore them. If you or someone you love is showing the following signs, get medical help immediately:

- Pain in the chest that radiates to the shoulders or arms—usually on the left side—or to the neck, back or jaw
- Pressure or burning sensation in the chest
- Shortness of breath
- Nausea
- Dizziness or fainting
- Indigestion that is not relieved with antacids
- Fatigue
- Excessive sweating

(For more on what to do in case of an emergency, see chapter 19, "Dealing with Doctors and Hospitals.")

Treating Hypertension and Heart Disease

Anyone with hypertension must follow the prevention strategies below. Those with more severe hypertension may need medication. Compared with whites, Blacks are less likely to take prescribed medication consistently and correctly and more likely to stop taking it without talking to the doctor. Whatever medication your doctor prescribes, don't discontinue it before checking with him or her.

As for heart disease, new research indicates that we are less likely to receive certain medical procedures, such as bypass operations, that can save a heart patient's life. This may be racism and sexism. If you or a loved one has heart disease, you must find out specific information about the best treatment and demand the care you deserve. For more information, contact the organizations listed below.

Preventing Hypertension and Heart Disease

Though hypertension and heart disease are deadly, they are also highly preventable. Follow this advice:

Cut the fat from your diet. This means you must eat less meat, switching to poultry and fish. If you do eat meat, eat it in moderation (not every day) and choose lean cuts. Trim off any visible fat and skin. Don't eat fried foods; bake, broil, or steam instead. Cut down on all oils (especially butter and bacon grease), whole milk, and other fatty foods.

Put away the salt shaker. Eating salty food can raise blood pressure. Avoid canned and processed foods, and find other ways to season your meals.

Lower cholesterol. Cholesterol is a soft, fatty substance that can build up in the arteries and impede or stop the blood flow. Have your blood cholesterol checked: It should be below 200 mg./dl. To keep blood cholesterol low, eat fewer animal fats such as meat, egg yolks, and dairy products, and cut down or eliminate coconut and palm oils.

Don't smoke. If you don't smoke, don't start, and if you do, quit. Also avoid the cigarette smoke of others.

Exercise regularly. Numerous studies have shown that lack of physical activity adds to the risk of heart disease. You must do an activity that gets your heart pumping for at least twenty to thirty minutes, three times a week. Exercise also speeds weight loss, and losing weight can help obese people lower blood pressure and help prevent heart disease.

Drink in moderation only—if it all. Studies show that more than two alcoholic drinks per day can raise blood pressure.

Keep stress in check. One study showed that when Black subjects saw racist scenes in a movie, their blood pressure shot up. To harness stress, don't bottle up your emotions; share them with sympathetic friends or family members, join a support group, or talk to a therapist. Exercise, meditation, and yoga also help reduce stress.

If you've gone through menopause, find out about estrogen. Estrogen-replacement therapy may decrease the risk of heart disease. For more information see chapter 17, "Menopause: Going Through the Change."

Cancer

Behind heart disease, cancer—the uncontrolled growth and spread of abnormal cells—is the second most frequent cause of death in Black women. Although cancer can strike many parts of the body, three cancers are particularly common and lethal in our population: lung, breast, and cervical cancer.

Lung cancer. Next to breast cancer, lung cancer is the leading cause of cancer death among African-American women. Cigarette smoking is almost entirely to blame. Blacks folks smoke more than whites, and although many sisters have quit, the decline in smoking is substantially slower among Black women than men. Nonsmokers are also at risk, especially those who have mates who smoke. Air pollution also contributes to the risk.

"To survive the
cancer, I built a
wellness support
system."

—ELAYNE M. WHITE,
SECRETARY AND
JOURNALISM STUDENT,
DECATUR, GEORGIA

When I was diagnosed with breast cancer in January of 1987, I had what could be called a disassociative experience. I, in essence, left my body. I could not handle it. I watched my life as though it were a movie starring someone else. I felt betrayed by my body. I had exercised it, fed it "healthy" food, gotten my proper rest, and checked my breasts once a month. How could this have happened to me? I was only thirty-eight years old.

When I decided to "come back to earth," I knew that I needed love, help, and support. At the bottom line, I knew that the ultimate responsibility for my health rested in my own hands, mind, and heart. However, if it had not been for the hands, minds, and hearts of others, I might not have made it to that bottom line of self-responsibility. To survive the cancer, I built a wellness support system, which included family, friends, doctors, support/self-help groups, books and tapes, spirituality, employers and coworkers, therapists, and counselors. It also included Maurice, who was my significant other for more than two years.

I was dating Maurice when I became ill. I chose to end the relationship on an intimate level, but he remains a close friend. When I found the lump in my left breast, he was the first person I told, and he immediately came to my aid. He went with me to my general practitioner and then to the surgeon's office. He also went with me to the hospital when I had the biopsy.

Maurice played a major role in my acceptance of my body after surgery. After the heavy bandages had been removed, I still had staples in my chest that were covered with surgical tape. He asked to see my chest. At first I adamantly refused. He assured me that his love for me had nothing to do with how many breasts I had. Together we looked at the scar for the first time.

During radiation therapy, after three and a half weeks of burning, itching skin that I could not touch and almost constant nausea, I refused to go for my treatment. He came from work, held me until my hysterics passed, dressed me, and drove me to the hospital for the treatment.

Be thankful to whomever is there for you. I have heard too many stories of women whose husbands or lovers, for whatever reason, chose not to deal with the disease. They left them alone in either a physical or emotional way. I know that Maurice will always have a special place in my heart, no matter what the nature of our relationship. It's okay to lean on someone when you feel that you can't make it. Things do get better.

My family—especially two of my sisters who lived in Atlanta, a number of nieces and nephews, and my two children—came forward with gifts, cards, money, transportation, prepared food, housecleaning, hugs, words of encouragement, and daily phone calls. My daughter spent the night on a cot *in my room when I was in the hospital having a modified radical mastectomy. My son held my hand while I had chemotherapy injections. He also told me that he knew I would not die because he had faith, not in God, but in me. That statement was a guiding light to me when I thought I couldn't make it.*

—Adapted from a booklet called "Building a Wellness Support System." For a copy of the booklet, contact the author, Elayne M. White, P.O. Box 37-0142, Decatur, GA 30037-0142.

Breast cancer. One in eight American women will develop breast cancer, and it is the leading cause of cancer death for African-American women. Compared with white women, breast cancer strikes Black women at earlier ages, and we are less likely to discover the cancer early on, which leads to more deaths.

Cervical cancer. African-American women are roughly three times more likely to develop cancer of the cervix and more than twice as likely to die from it than are white women. All women who are eighteen or over or are sexually active risk getting cervical cancer, and the risk increases with age.

Cancer has taken the lives of many of our best and brightest sisters, including poet, essayist, and activist Audre Lorde, who died in 1992. Still, it isn't a death sentence, and many sufferers have lived through it. In the midst of her fourteen-year struggle with breast cancer, Lorde wrote *The Cancer Journals,* a collection of journal entries and essays published in 1980 after her mastectomy. Though at times haunted by the terror of death, she discusses the need to put fear aside and continue her work as a writer and activist:

Sometimes fear stalks me like another malignancy, sapping energy and power and attention from my work. A cold becomes sinister; a cough, lung cancer; a bruise, leukemia. Those fears are most powerful when they are not given voice, and close upon their heels comes the fury that I cannot shake them. I am learning to live beyond fear by living through it, and in the process learning to turn fury at my own limitations into some more creative energy. I realize that if I wait until I am no longer afraid to act, write, speak, be, I'll be sending messages on a Ouija board, cryptic complaints from the other side. When I dare to be powerful, to use my strength in the service of my vision, then it becomes less important whether or not I am unafraid.

What Is Cancer?

Cancer is still not well understood. Scientists cannot pinpoint exactly why abnormal cells grow and spread and why some people get cancer and others don't. Cancer can be caused by many factors, both external and internal. For example, exposure to chemicals, radiation, and viruses can lead to cancer, and immune-system conditions can also trigger it. Cancer also sometimes runs in families.

Detecting Cancer

The reason Blacks are less likely than whites to survive cancer probably has nothing to do with race. It's that we are less likely to visit a doctor and have the tests that can detect cancer early. The sooner the cancer is found, the better the chance of fighting it successfully. Here are the tests and checkups you *must* have:

Routine physical examination. You must have one at least every two years and yearly after age fifty or if you have any chronic illnesses. (During this visit, your health-care provider should examine your breasts.) With many cancers, such as lung and ovarian cancer, symptoms don't appear until the disease is in advanced stages—and that's too late. It's important to listen to your body and tell your doctor every little thing that you notice.

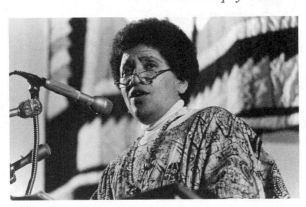

The late poet/essayist/activist Audre Lorde battled breast cancer for fourteen years.
(Photo: Marilyn Humphries)

Breast self-exam and mammogram. Together these two exams are the best way to detect breast cancer. Every woman should examine her breasts once a month. It's best to do it the week after the menstrual period or on the first day of the month for postmenopausal women. Between ages thirty-five and forty, a woman should get her first mammogram. Once you turn forty, you'll need a mammogram every one to two years, and then yearly after age fifty. If you have a family history of breast cancer, you will need mammograms more frequently. (To learn how to do a breast self-exam, see chapter 18, "Checkups and Tests We Can't Live Without.")

Pap smear and gynecological examination. All women eighteen years or older and younger women who are sexually active should have a gynecological exam once a year. This is a way to catch cervical cancer in its early stages, when it's highly curable. During your yearly checkup, a breast examination should be included.

Skin self-examination. Though our melanin provides protection against skin cancer (the rate is ten times higher in whites), we are not immune. You should examine your skin monthly and report any of these signs to a doctor:

- A change in the size, texture, or color of a mole or other darkly pigmented growth or spot
- Scaliness, oozing, bleeding, or change in the appearance of a bump or nodule
- Itchiness, tenderness, or pain in the skin
- A nonhealing sore

Watch for signs of lung cancer. If you have a chronic cough, are coughing up blood or blood-tinged mucous, or have progressive shortage of breath, see a doctor. If you haven't quit smoking yet, it's imperative that you seek treatment if you have any of the above symptoms.

(For a more in-depth discussion of these tests, see chapter 18, "Checkups and Tests We Can't Live Without.")

Treating Cancer

Treatment options include removing the cancerous tissue through surgery, killing the cancerous cells with X rays (radiation therapy) or chemicals (chemotherapy), or boosting the immune system to fight off the cancer (immunotherapy). Bone-marrow transplantation is another option. Although it can cost hundreds of thousands of dollars, it is generally covered by health insurance.

Some women suffering from breast cancer have found success with a synthetic hormone called tamoxifen, which has an "antiestrogen" quality. It fights breast cancers, many of which are fueled by the presence of estrogen, one of the body's natural hormones. Tamoxifen has also been effective in preventing cancer in the unaffected breast of women with breast malignancies and is being studied as a cancer-*prevention* treatment. (Ask your doctor about this option, or call 800-4CANCER for more information.)

Getting a cancer diagnosis is always a shock, and sorting through the treatments can be confusing and frightening. Cancer patients should seek out an oncologist (a cancer specialist) and rely on the support of friends and organizations. A positive attitude and the love of friends and relatives has helped improve the outcome of many cancer patients. You can also look into alternative therapies used for cancer treatment.

Preventing Cancer

No one knows exactly how to prevent cancer. But there are things you can do to lessen your risk of contracting it.

If you smoke, quit. If you don't, don't start, and try to avoid the smoke of others. Smoking is associated with a number of cancers, especially lung cancer.

Eat at least five servings of fruits and vegetables per day. Vegetables such as collard greens, kale, spinach, cabbage, turnips, carrots, squash, sweet potatoes, and brussels sprouts; and apples, oranges, strawberries, watermelon, and other fruits help protect against cancers of all kinds. It's best to eat them steamed or raw and to drink fresh vegetable juices. Five servings (one serving is half a cup) aren't difficult to eat in a day; you'll see once you try it.

Try to avoid foods that contain chemicals and additives. Keep the diet as fresh and natural as possible. Read labels: If the ingredients include long words you've never heard of or can't pronounce, avoid the product.

Cut down on fatty foods. Eat less meat, especially fatty cuts. If you do eat meat, trim off all visible fat. Use less oil (especially butter, oil, and lard), and avoid fried foods. Eat low-fat dairy products.

Add fiber to your diet. Whole-grain foods such as cereals, pasta, grains, and bread, as well as beans, vegetables, and fruit, help reduce the risk of cancer of the colon.

Limit alcohol use. Heavy drinking, especially in conjunction with smoking, may increase the risk of cancers of the mouth, throat, liver, and esophagus.

Limit salt-cured, smoked, and nitrite-cured foods. Bacon and even barbecued foods have been linked to cancer of the esophagus and stomach.

Avoid overexposure to the sun. To prevent skin cancer, use sunscreen of at least 15 SPF year-round, or wear protective clothing when you're going to be out in the sun. This advice applies to everyone—regardless of skin tone.

Keep your weight in check. Folks who are 20 percent or more overweight have a higher risk of cancers of the uterus, gallbladder, kidney, stomach, colon, and breast.

Exercise at least three times a week for twenty to thirty minutes per session. Consistent, moderate physical activity helps the body stay healthy and boosts the immune system to fight off all types of disease. Exercise also reduces stress, and some experts speculate on a link between negative emotions and cancer. Walking is a simple, convenient way to exercise.

Avoid exposure to radiation and chemicals. Find out whether you are being exposed to cancer-causing substances, including asbestos, at your job. If so, take steps to reduce exposure. Check your home for radon, a substance that is present in many homes and increases the risk of lung cancer. (For more information, see chapter 32, "Our Work, Our World.")

Consider supplementing your diet with vitamins. Antioxidant vitamins—A, C, and E—may reduce the risk of cancer. Keep in mind, though, that vitamins should be an addition to your diet, not a substitute for healthful eating.

Diabetes

An estimated 3 million African-Americans have diabetes, which adds up to one in every ten of us. We are 55 percent more likely than whites to have diabetes, and the disease is especially prevalent in older Black women. According to many experts, half of all patients don't even know they have it.

What Is Diabetes?

Diabetes is a disease in which the body doesn't produce or properly use insulin, the hormone needed to convert sugar, starches, and other foods into energy for the body to use. There are two major kinds of diabetes: Type I and Type II. In Type I, the body doesn't produce any insulin: This type most often strikes children, adolescents, or young adults. Type II is much more common—90 to 95 percent of all cases of diabetes are Type II—especially among Blacks. In Type II, the body is unable to make enough insulin or is unable to utilize it effectively.

Diabetes can lead to serious complications including blindness, amputation of limbs, kidney failure, and death, and Blacks are more likely than whites to experience these life-threatening side effects. Complications are more common—and worse—in people who also have hypertension and/or heart disease.

Being overweight raises the risk of contracting diabetes; in fact, 80 percent of diabetics are obese, or weigh 20 percent more than what is

Organ Donation

We take our kidneys for granted. These two small organs, located just behind the rib cage, clean and filter the blood and help regulate blood pressure. When they give out, we have serious problems. Blacks are four times more likely than whites to suffer from kidney failure, and all too often this failure requires a kidney transplant. Often a Black patient requires a Black donor organ, and we are much less likely than whites to donate kidneys or any organs. That has left thousands of African-Americans on waiting lists for new organs.

The wait for a Black person who needs a bone-marrow transplant and can't find a donor in the family is even longer. Because many of us have unusual tissue types, in most cases only another Black person will be a match for a Black person in need of a transplant. But the vast majority—80 percent—of bone-marrow donors are white.

Physicians can transplant hearts, livers, lungs, kidneys, bone, skin, corneas, and pancreases with high success rates. Donating organs can save the lives of our brothers and sisters, so we must agree to be donors. In most states you can indicate your willingness to donate on your driver's license. Otherwise, contact the organizations listed below to sign up for a donor card.

The above donations occur after death, but you can also be a living donor by donating blood and bone marrow. You can donate blood during drives in your community or workplace (you can't get AIDS by donating blood, and your donation will be screened for HIV and other diseases) or through the Red Cross or a blood center in your area. Bone-marrow donors are urgently needed. The first step is to take a blood test. Your tissue type is then entered into a national registry. If your tissue matches that of a patient in need, about 5 percent of your marrow will be removed, and you'll have to stay overnight at the hospital. Your lost marrow replaces itself in weeks, and no donor has ever suffered a serious complication. But it can save a life.

For more information and to become a donor, contact:

American Kidney Fund, 6110 Executive Blvd., suite 1010, Rockville, MD 20852; (301) 881-3052.

American Red Cross, 431 18th St. NW, Washington, DC 20006; (202) 737-8300.

Black Transplants Action Committee, 3241 Newport St., Denver, CO 80207; (303) 322-0863.

Judie Davis Marrow Donor Recruitment Program, 7700 Edgewater Dr., suite 700, Oakland, CA 94621; (510) 430-9249.

Living Bank, P.O. Box 6725, Houston, TX 77265; (800) 528-2971. Operates registry and referral service.

National Kidney Foundation, 30 E. 33rd St., New York, NY 10016; (800) 622-9010. Provides referrals and educational materials about kidney diseases.

National Marrow Donor Program, 3433 Broadway NE, suite 400, Minneapolis, MN 55413; (800) MARROW-2. Provides information and bone-marrow donor registry.

considered ideal weight. Because so many Black women weigh far more than they should, diabetes is common and serious among our ranks. (See chapter 1, "Body Weight and Image.")

Symptoms of Diabetes

Some symptoms are subtle, which is why so many people don't know they have diabetes. It's imperative to pay close attention to your body and to visit a physician once a year for a checkup. Symptoms are as follows:

- Frequent urination
- Extreme thirst
- Extreme hunger
- Dramatic weight loss with increased food intake. This generally occurs at the onset of the disease even in those who are extremely overweight.
- Weakness, fatigue, irritability, and drowsiness
- Blurred vision or changes in eyesight
- Tingling or numbness in the fingers, arms, legs, or feet.
- Frequent infections and slow healing of cuts and bruises.
- Itching of the skin or genitals. The itching may be caused by yeast infections, which are common in diabetic women.

Treating Diabetes

Although some patients must closely monitor their blood sugar and may require medication, many others will improve and keep the disease in check by following the prevention strategies below.

Preventing Diabetes

Eat right. Keeping a tight control on your blood sugar helps. Some diabetics mistakenly substitute foods that are high in fat for sugary foods. But that can make problems worse. Instead, stick to a diet that is low in fat, salt, and sugar and high in fresh vegetables and fruit, whole-grain breads, pasta, and cereals. You can also eat lean meats and poultry (nothing fatty or greasy), fish, and low-fat dairy products. It also helps to eat meals at approximately the same time every day. (For more on nutrition, see chapter 4, "Eating Right.") For a list of cookbooks designed for diabetics, contact the organizations listed below.

Lose weight if you need to, or keep weight under control. Many Black women have lost weight by following a low-fat, low-sugar diet that

"Until the day I leave this world, I will share this body with a wolf called lupus."

—ERICA K. BRIDGEMAN,
COLLEGE STUDENT,
MADISON, WISCONSIN

One morning in late March of 1992, I woke up feeling very tired, cold, and extremely ill. This was the last thing I needed. After a hellish six months of trying to adjust to the University of Wisconsin from a small Minnesota college, my life had actually started to come together. By the end of the school year, I was elected to a student-government position, and I was in a new, satisfying romantic relationship.

But as time went on, I found myself wanting to sleep more than usual, and staying up for late-night rap sessions no longer appealed to me. I began to have high fevers, and it took practically all my strength to walk from class to class. Finally I couldn't take it anymore and went to the local clinic to find some kind of explanation. Thinking it was strep throat, the doctor gave me a throat culture, but I ended up vomiting all over myself, the nurse, and the floor. My temperature registered at 104 degrees, while sweat poured from my brow. The following week I was sent to the university hospital for an IV to prevent any further dehydration.

Not in all my wildest dreams was I prepared to hear that a disease was slowly attacking my body. After three weeks in the hospital strung out on high doses of all kinds of medications, I was diagnosed as having lupus, a rare disease that in Latin means "wolf." To wake up one morning from being a healthy young woman and have "the wolf" wagging its tongue at me was completely devastating.

Because the disease attacked my body so severely, the doctor recommended that I be taken out of school to be sent home. It was all quite sudden; I barely had time to pack my clothes and say good-bye to my friends and my new boyfriend. The situation was so surreal and I was so distressed that I started to abuse my medication. This landed me back in the hospital for a third time.

This time, however, the consequences of my actions were quite severe. The lupus attacked my brain and spinal cord, and I spent three days with my legs and arms strapped down to a hospital bed while I literally acted like a wolf with rabies yelling, screaming, cursing, and hallucinating. I can still remember lying in the hospital back in Minneapolis scared to even move for fear that I would lunge back into a state of lunacy.

I was extremely sick or in the hospital from March until May. Today I am back in school entering my last year as an undergraduate. For the most part I am back to "normal," but each day through my active arthritis or my tension headaches I am reminded that until the day I leave this world, I will share this body with a wolf called lupus. Having a disability isn't the end of the world, but through many tears and much frustration, I have come to see the world in a different, more fragile light.

includes lots of fruit and vegetables, whole-grain cereals, pasta, breads, and water, and adding exercise such as walking, running, or cycling to their schedules.

Drink alcohol in moderation only or not at all. Alcohol can raise or lower blood sugar, plus it's high in calories and low in nutritional value.

Exercise. Riding a bike, roller-skating, walking, running, swimming, playing tennis, or participating in any other fitness activities at least three times a week for twenty to thirty minutes speeds weight loss and can help control blood sugar.

Lupus

Unfortunately, lupus most often affects Black women. Of the more than 500,000 people stricken with it, 9 out of 10 are women ages fifteen to forty-five, and 3 out of 5 are Black. No one knows what causes it, and there is no cure. As described by women who have it, lupus makes you feel lousy all of the time.

What Is Lupus?

Lupus is a chronic disease that affects immunity. When someone has lupus, the immune system, which generally protects the body against infection, attacks healthy tissues and organs. It's as though the body turns on itself. There are several types of lupus. Drug-induced lupus is triggered by medication, and when the medication is stopped, the lupus usually goes away. Another kind of lupus mainly affects the skin. The most serious type, systemic lupus erythematosus or SLE, may harm the skin, joints, kidneys, brain, lungs, and heart. Lupus is not contagious.

Detecting Lupus

Lupus is mild in some women and debilitating in others, and often the symptoms come and go. The signs of lupus also differ from one person to another, and the symptoms are also common signs of other diseases. For these reasons, lupus is difficult to diagnose. Common symptoms are:

- Red rash or color change on the face, often in the shape of a butterfly across the bridge of the nose
- Painful or swollen joints, usually accompanied by redness
- Unexplained, chronic fever
- Chest pain with breathing
- Unusual loss of hair

- Purple or pale fingers or toes from cold or stress
- Sensitivity to the sun
- Low blood count
- Nausea, vomiting, and abdominal pain

Treating Lupus

There is no cure for lupus, but medication and proper care can help relieve the symptoms. Lupus patients should eat right, get plenty of rest, exercise consistently, and avoid cigarettes and alcohol in order to keep the body strong and healthy. Staying out of the sun and wearing sunscreen helps. Lupus sufferers should also keep stress at a minimum by doing yoga, meditating, and seeing a psychotherapist or joining a support group. The Lupus Foundation of America (contact information below) sponsors support groups in many cities.

Sarcoidosis

In 1984 at the age of thirty-eight, Sandra Conroy was diagnosed with sarcoidosis ("sar-coy-doe-sis"). At first she was relieved to have a name for the weakness in her arms and legs and the partial paralysis that had forced her to leave her job on Wall Street. But her relief turned to dismay when she discovered that sarcoidosis has no known cause or cure and that none of the doctors she visited could give her more than sketchy information about this mysterious disease of the immune system. But instead of getting mad, Conroy got busy. She founded the National Sarcoidosis Resource Center (contact information below), which provides free literature, doctor referrals, and a quarterly newsletter and directs patients toward support groups in cities across the country. She also published *Sarcoidosis: Medical Mystery Uncovered,* a resource guide and directory, in 1991.

What Is Sarcoidosis?

No one knows exactly how many people have sarcoidosis, but it most commonly strikes African-American women ages twenty to forty. Like lupus, it is a chronic disease in which the immune system, which generally protects the body against infection, attacks healthy tissues and organs. It is not contagious.

Detecting Sarcoidosis

Sarcoidosis is mild in some women and debilitating in others, and often the symptoms come and go. The signs of the disease also differ from

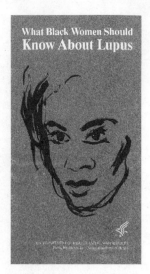

What Black Women Should **Know About Lupus**

Never hesitate to call or write for information, like this brochure on lupus, from the many organizations set up to serve you.

one person to another, and the symptoms are also common signs of other diseases. For these reasons, it is difficult to diagnose. Plus, many health-care practitioners don't know what it is. Most sufferers recover completely in about two years, with or without treatment, while about 10 percent suffer from chronic sarcoidosis. Common symptoms are:

- Sinus problems and/or a dry cough
- Unexplained tiredness or weakness
- Bruising of the skin
- Headache
- Mild pain in the center of the chest
- Shortness of breath
- Enlarged lymph nodes
- Painful, swollen, or numb joints
- Purple rash on the face
- Unexplained weight loss

Treating Sarcoidosis

There is no cure for sarcoidosis, but medication and proper care can help relieve the symptoms. Sarcoidosis patients should eat right, get plenty of rest, exercise consistently, and avoid cigarettes and alcohol in order to keep the body strong and healthy. Sarcoidosis sufferers should also keep stress at a minimum by practicing yoga, meditating, and seeing a psychotherapist or joining a support group. Conroy's organization and her book can direct you toward support groups in your area and help you find an informed physician.

Sickle Cell Disease

Having sickle-shaped, rather than round, blood cells may have helped our ancestors survive malaria. But for African-Americans, sickle cell disease can be deadly. While it also affects people in the Caribbean and those of Southeast Asian, East Indian, Latin-American, and Mediterranean descent, sickle cell disease is primarily a disease of African-Americans; it strikes one out of twelve of us.

What Is Sickle Cell Disease?

Red blood cells, which carry oxygen throughout the body, are generally donut shaped. But in people with sickle cell disease (also called sickle cell anemia), the red blood cells are curved or shaped like sickles. Because of their odd shape, the cells can pile up, stick together, and clog blood vessels, causing drastically reduced circulation. It can lead to death.

Sickle cell disease is inherited; it is not contagious and cannot be passed through a blood transfusion. About 8 percent of Blacks carry the sickle cell trait. These people are healthy, but when a man and a woman who both carry the trait have a child, that child has a one-in-four chance of having sickle cell disease.

Detecting Sickle Cell Disease

A blood test can detect sickle cell disease, and all newborns should be tested. In hospitals in many states mandatory screening programs are already in place, and babies are tested within a few days of birth. Be aware of these signs in children:

- Leg ulcers. These are sores that don't heal because of poor circulation.
- Hand-foot syndrome. Plugging of small blood vessels causes the hands and feet to swell and become hot, red, and painful.
- Slow growth. Small size, poor health, frequent colds and sore throats are characteristic of the disease.
- Jaundice. Look for a yellowish tinge on the whites of the eyes.
- Painful joints. Poor blood supply causes painful bones, especially the hips and shoulders.
- Sickle cell crisis. This is characterized by severe chest, abdominal, arm, and leg pain.

Sickle cell trait generally has no signs. To find out whether or not you carry the trait, ask your doctor for a blood test.

Treating Sickle Cell Disease

If your child has sickle cell disease, she or he will need medication and constant medical monitoring. A new treatment using butyrate, a fatty acid found in the body and in some foods, has proven promising in clinical trials.

Preventing Sickle Cell Disease

There is no way to prevent sickle cell disease. But you and your mate should get tested for traits of sickle cell and other hemoglobin disorders before you decide to have a child together. If both you and your mate have the trait, the chances are one in four that your child will have the disease. In other words, with each pregnancy the chance is:

One in four that the baby will have normal blood cells;
Two in four that the baby will also have sickle cell trait;
One in four that the baby will have sickle-shaped blood cells.

To help you determine the risk that your child will have sickle cell disease, talk to a genetic counselor. For a referral, call your local March of Dimes.

Asthma

Nearly 10 million Americans have asthma, including a disproportionate number of Blacks. Although the disease is controllable with preventive steps and proper medication, too many Black people die of it. In fact, the asthma death rate is three times higher for Blacks than for whites.

Most sadly, asthma strikes and kills far too many of our children. The number-one chronic illness among all children, asthma is more common among Black children compared with white, and it is especially dangerous and damaging to youngsters living in poverty.

What Is Asthma?

Asthma is a chronic reversible inflammatory disease of the lungs that causes recurrent breathing problems. During an attack, the bronchial tubes or air pipes become inflamed, the muscles surrounding the airways tighten, mucous clogs the smaller tubes, and air gets trapped. This leads to coughing, wheezing, and breathing difficulty.

Symptoms of an Asthma Attack

Most asthma attacks start slowly, and you can often stop an attack when you catch it early, take medication, and avoid irritating stimulants. The warning signs of an asthma episode are:

- Coughing
- Shortness of breath
- Tightness in chest
- Wheezing
- Faster breathing
- Itchy or sore throat

Treating Asthma

Asthma can range from mild to severe. Some folks manage fine without medication and keep attacks from coming by avoiding substances that

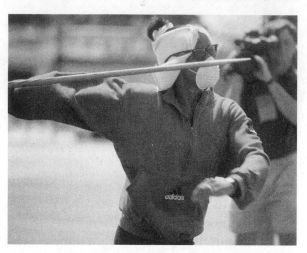

World-class athlete Jackie Joyner-Kersee suffers from asthma and sometimes wears a breathing mask to filter the air. *(Photo: Victah, New York)*

trigger them. But more serious cases require the patient to monitor her breathing and take medication every day.

In the past, physicians based treatment on the presumption that each attack of asthma was an isolated incident. Patients used medications called bronchodilators in the form of hand-held inhalers, which offer immediate relief. However, these inhalers are often misused or overused, especially the over-the-counter brands.

In 1991, the National Asthma Education Program released new treatment guidelines based on the newer theory that asthma is a chronic swelling of the respiratory system, rather than a series of isolated attacks. With that in mind, doctors now prescribe medication to reduce the inflammation along with bronchodilators. Be sure your doctor has prescribed this latest form of treatment to you.

Preventing Attacks

Though no one knows exactly what causes asthma, experts do know that certain irritants can trigger an attack. People who suffer asthma—whether mild or severe—should avoid these frequent triggers:

Airborne pollutants. We tend to live in areas with high levels of air pollution, which may be leading to our high asthma death rate. It's difficult to avoid air pollution, especially if you live in an urban area, but you can avoid another airborne irritant: cigarette smoke. Don't smoke, and everyone should avoid the smoke of others. Secondhand smoke has proven to be dangerous to those who don't smoke, especially children.

Allergens. Stay away from dust, mold, animal hair, feathers, and pollen.

Stress. Emotional upset often brings on an attack or makes it worse.

Exercise. Physical activity keeps you healthy but cannot help you prevent asthma. It can aggravate it. However, this hasn't stopped track star Jackie Joyner-Kersee from competing, and it shouldn't prevent regular people from participating in physical activities either. But asthmatic athletes must monitor the disease carefully. Many take medication before exercising. Exercising in cold weather or during pollen season can often trigger attacks in asthmatics who work out.

Respiratory infections. Cold and flu symptoms such as coughing can trigger an attack or make one worse.

Cockroaches. Surprisingly, millions of people are allergic to roaches, and 80 percent of all asthmatic children are sensitive to them.

Medication. Some prescription drugs, such as medication used to treat high blood pressure or glaucoma, can trigger an attack. But never alter a prescription without consulting a physician.

Dairy products. Dairy products create mucous in the respiratory system, and some people who suffer from asthma and allergies have curbed symptoms by cutting down on or eliminating milk products from the diet. Substitutes such as soy milk and cheese and nut milk are available at health-food stores.

Chronic Fatigue Syndrome

Everyone feels tired and drained from time to time, but imagine feeling achy, feverish, and exhausted all the time. That's what chronic fatigue immune dysfunction syndrome feels like. Commonly known as chronic fatigue syndrome or CFS, it is a relatively new, mysterious disease with no clear cause or cure. Very little is understood about it. Though it most often strikes young white women, it is mentioned here because it may be an unrecognized problem among Black women. We tend to ignore symptoms because we're too busy to deal with them or assume that "feeling poorly" is just another part of life.

What Is CFS?

No one can precisely explain CFS. It has been called the yuppie flu, because many people who sought help were well-educated, reasonably affluent women in their thirties and forties, and because so little is known about what causes the disease, even some doctors thought sufferers were simply whining or depressed.

But people who have it know that CFS is serious and debilitating. It may start after a bout with such illnesses as the flu, bronchitis, or hepatitis, it may begin gradually for no reason, or it may strike someone who is highly stressed. The sufferer experiences headache, sore throat, low-grade fever, fatigue, weakness, tender lymph glands, prolonged fatigue after exercise, sleep disturbance, muscle and joint aches, and an inability to concentrate. It's like having the flu, but the symptoms won't go away.

Experts believe CFS is caused by a virus or a breakdown of the immune system, and it has been linked with herpes, candidiasis, environmental illness, and even HIV. But no one knows for sure.

Detecting CFS

There is no sure way to diagnose CFS. A doctor will suspect CFS if the symptoms described above have persisted for at least six months and all other illnesses have been ruled out. Because so many other illnesses—diabetes, cancer, lupus, and depression, for example—also cause fatigue, these must be considered first.

Treating CFS

So far, no one knows how to get rid of CFS, so sufferers can only treat the symptoms. The most practical advice is to get plenty of rest; exercise regularly yet moderately (very vigorous exercise can make the feeling of fatigue worse); and eat a balanced diet that contains plenty of fruits, vegetables, and fiber and is low in fat and sugar. Emotional stress may make the symptoms worse, so keep it under control with moderate exercise, meditation, and other forms of relaxation.

Many sufferers have found relief with holistic treatments such as herbs, acupuncture, vitamin supplements, or very strict diets. Check with a holistic health practitioner about these options.

With so little information and research available, it may be best to talk to other CFS sufferers and see what's worked for them. The organizations below may be able to put you in touch with a support group in your area.

Disabled

Some people are born with disabilities, while others lose their sight, hearing, or use of limbs as a result of disease. Accidents, one of the leading causes of death, can also cause people to become disabled. That's what happened to Janice Jackson.

In 1984 at the age of twenty-four, Janice was hit by a car while standing around having a conversation near her home in Prince Georges

County in Maryland. She was sent flying forty-five feet in the air and landed on her neck. Doctors assumed she would be completely paralyzed until a few months later they noticed a toe move. Soon, to the amazement of her doctors, her left side regained movement.

Janice spent two years in rehab working to gain back her strength and retrain her body. Her determination, faith, and the support of her family—especially her brother, who is also disabled—helped her push on. She now lives in Baltimore and, although she is confined to a wheelchair, has a job with the IRS and is an outspoken health activist. Janice founded two support groups for other people who are physically challenged and in 1992 was elected Ms. Wheelchair Maryland. Says Janice, "Society makes us handicapped worse than our bodies make us handicapped. I want to prove to people that you can live a fulfilling life from the chair."

Having a disability of any kind can be difficult, especially in a world that generally ignores the physically and mentally challenged. In fact, says one paraplegic to people who can't face her, "You don't have to deal with my disability. I've already dealt with it. Deal with *me,* the person."

Ignorance of the differently abled extends beyond personal interactions: The rights of the blind, deaf, those who use wheelchairs, who speak differently or are mentally challenged are too often disregarded. And the situation is worse for Blacks who are physically challenged: A recent congressional study reported that for the past thirty years, African-Americans have been much more likely than whites to be rejected for benefits under Social Security disability programs. But many folks like Janice are forming support groups and fighting back against the insensitivity and discrimination so common in the "abled" world. (Some of that activism has paid off: In 1993 a national law went into effect that bans discrimination against the 14 million working-age people who have physical or mental impairments.)

For More Information

ORGANIZATIONS: Hypertension and Heart Disease

AMERICAN HEART ASSOCIATION, 7270 Greenville Ave., Dallas, TX 75235; (800) 242-8721; or contact your local office.

NATIONAL HEART, LUNG AND BLOOD INSTITUTE, P.O. Box 30105, Bethesda, MD 20824-0105; (301) 251-1222.

Books

The Black Health Library Guide to Heart Disease and Hypertension, Paul Jones, M.D., with Angela Mitchell, Henry Holt & Co., 1993.

The Black Health Library Guide to Stroke, Lafayette Singleton, M.D., with Kirk A. Johnson, Henry Holt & Co., 1993.

ORGANIZATIONS: Cancer

AMERICAN CANCER SOCIETY, 1599 Clifton Rd. NE, Atlanta, GA 30329; (800) ACS-2345; or check your phone book for a local office.

BREAST CANCER ACTION, 1280 Columbus Ave., San Francisco, CA 94133; (415) 922-8279.

CANCERVIVE, INC., 6500 Wilshire Blvd., suite 500, Los Angeles, CA 90048; (310) 655-3758.

LIVINGSTON FOUNDATION MEDICAL CENTER, 3232 Duke St., San Diego, CA 92110; (619) 224-3515.

MINORITY WOMEN'S BREAST CANCER NETWORK, P.O. Box 6444, Albany, NY 12206; (518) 385-2540.

NATIONAL CANCER INSTITUTE'S (NCI) CANCER INFORMATION SERVICE, (800) 4-CANCER. NCI also sponsors the Black Cancer Initiative and distributes literature that addresses Black patients.

NATIONAL ALLIANCE OF BREAST CANCER ORGANIZATIONS, 1180 Ave. of the Americas, 2nd floor, New York, NY 10036; (212) 221-3300.

NATIONAL COALITION FOR CANCER SURVIVORSHIP, 1010 Wayne Ave., 5th floor, Silver Spring, MD 20910; (301) 650-8868.

PEOPLE AGAINST CANCER, (800) NO-CANCER. Studies the relationship between environmental pollution and cancer and provides information about alternative methods of prevention, detection, and treatment.

SUSAN G. KOMEN BREAST CANCER FOUNDATION, 5005 LBJ Freeway, suite 370, Dallas, TX 75244; (800) I'M-AWARE.

Y-ME NATIONAL BREAST CANCER ORGANIZATION, 18220 Harwood Ave., Homewood, IL 60430; (800) 221-2141.

WOMEN OF COLOR BREAST CANCER SURVIVORS SUPPORT PROJECT, 8610 S. Sepulveda, suite 200, Los Angeles, CA 90045; (213) 418-0627.

WOMEN'S COMMUNITY CANCER PROJECT, c/o Women's Center, 46 Pleasant St., Cambridge, MA 02139; (617) 354-9888.

BOOKS

The Cancer Journals, Audre Lorde, Spinsters/Aunt Lute (San Francisco), 1980.

The Power Within: True Stories of Exceptional Patients Who Fought Back with Hope, Wendy Williams, Harper & Row, 1990.

Dr. Susan Love's Breast Book, Susan Love, M.D., Addison-Wesley, 1990.

1 in 3: Women with Cancer Confront an Epidemic, ed. Judy Brady, Cleis Press (Pittsburgh), 1991.

Revolution in Cancer Therapy: The Complete Guide to Alternative Treatments, Ross Pelton and Lee Overholser, Simon & Schuster, 1994.

ORGANIZATIONS: Diabetes

AMERICAN DIABETES ASSOCIATION, National Service Center, 1660 Duke St., Alexandria, VA 22314; (800) ADA-DISC or (703) 549-1500.

JOSLIN DIABETES FOUNDATION, 1 Joslin Pl., Boston, MA 02215; (617) 732-2400.

JUVENILE DIABETES FOUNDATION, 432 Park Ave. S., New York, NY 10010; (212) 889-7575. For information about Type I diabetes.

NATIONAL DIABETES INFORMATION CLEARINGHOUSE, Box NDIC, 9000 Rockville Pike, Bethesda, MD 20892; (301) 468-2162.

BOOKS

The Black Health Library Guide to Diabetes, Lester Henry, Jr., M.D., with Kirk Johnson, Henry Holt & Co., 1993.

ORGANIZATIONS: Lupus

AMERICAN LUPUS SOCIETY, 3914 Del Amo Blvd., suite 922, Torrance, CA 90503; (800) 331-1802 or (310) 542-8891.

LUPUS FOUNDATION OF AMERICA, Inc., 4 Research Pl., suite 180, Rockville, MD 20850-3226; (800) 558-0121.

NATIONAL ARTHRITIS AND MUSCULOSKELETAL AND SKIN DISEASES INSTITUTE, Box AMS, 9000 Rockville Pike, Bethesda, MD 20892; (301) 495-4484. (Ask for the pamphlet "What Black Women Should Know About Lupus.")

BOOKS

Living with Lupus: All the Knowledge You Need to Help Yourself, Sheldon Blau, M.D., and Dodi Schultz, Doubleday, 1993.

ORGANIZATIONS: Sarcoidosis

NATIONAL SARCOIDOSIS RESOURCE CENTER, P.O. Box 1593, Piscataway, NJ 08855-1593; (908) 699-0733.

NATIONAL SARCOIDOSIS FAMILY AID AND RESEARCH FOUNDATION, P.O. Box 22868, Newark, NJ 07101; (800) 223-6429.

ORGANIZATIONS: Sickle Cell Disease

AGENCY FOR HEALTH CARE POLICY AND RESEARCH, Publications Clearinghouse, Sickle Cell Disease, P.O. Box 8547, Silver Spring, MD 20907; (800) 358-9295. Ask for the pamphlet "Sickle Cell Disease: Screening, Diagnosis, Management, and Counseling in Newborns and Infants."

SICKLE CELL DISEASE RESEARCH FOUNDATION, 4401 S. Crenshaw Blvd., suite 208, Los Angeles, CA 90043; (213) 299-3600.

NATIONAL ASSOCIATION FOR SICKLE CELL DISEASE, 3345 Wilshire Blvd., suite 1106, Los Angeles, CA 90010-1880; (800) 421-8453.

ORGANIZATIONS: Asthma

AMERICAN ACADEMY OF ALLERGY AND IMMUNOLOGY, 611 E. Wells St., Milwaukee, WI 53202; (800) 822-2762.

AMERICAN COLLEGE OF ALLERGY AND IMMUNOLOGY, 85 W. Algonquin St., suite 550, Arlington Heights, IL 60005; (800) 842-7777.

AMERICAN LUNG ASSOCIATION, 1740 Broadway, New York, NY 10019-4374; (212) 315-8802; or find a local office in your telephone directory.

ASTHMA AND ALLERGY FOUNDATION OF AMERICA, 1125 15th St. NW, suite 502, Washington, DC 20005; (800) 727-8462.

NATIONAL ALLERGY AND ASTHMA NETWORK/MOTHERS OF ASTHMATICS, 3554 Chain Bridge Rd., Fairfax, VA 22030; (800) 878-4403.

NATIONAL ASTHMA EDUCATION PROGRAM, NHLBI Information Center, P.O. Box 30105, Bethesda, MD 20824-0105; (301) 251-1222.

ORGANIZATIONS: Chronic Fatigue Syndrome

CHRONIC FATIGUE IMMUNE DYSFUNCTION SYNDROME ACTIVATION NETWORK, P.O. Box 345, Larchmont, NY 10538; (800) 234-0037 or (212) 627-5631.

CFIDS ASSOCIATION OF AMERICA, P.O. Box 220398, Charlotte, NC 28222; (800) 44-CFIDS.

CFIDS FOUNDATION, 965 Mission St., suite 425, San Francisco, CA 94103; (415) 882-9986.

NATIONAL CFS ASSOCIATION, 3521 Broadway, suite 222, Kansas City, MO 64111; (816) 931-4777.

BOOKS

Chronic Fatigue & Tiredness: A Self-Help Program, Susan M. Lark, M.D., Westchester Publishing Co., 1993.

Curing Fatigue: A Step-by-Step Plan to Uncover and Eliminate the Causes of Chronic Fatigue, David S. Bell, M.D., Rodale Press, 1993.

Recovering from Chronic Fatigue Syndrome: A Guide to Self-Empowerment, William Collinge, The Body Press/Perigee Books, 1993.

ORGANIZATIONS: Disabled

AMERICAN COUNCIL OF THE BLIND, 1155 15th St. NW, suite 720, Washington, DC 20005; (800) 424-8666 or (202) 467-5081. Provides information and referrals.

AMERICAN FOUNDATION FOR THE BLIND, 15 W. 16th St., New York, NY 10011; (800) 232-5463 or (212) 620-2000. Provides information on visual impairments and blindness.

AMERICAN SPEECH-LANGUAGE-HEARING ASSOCIATION, 10801 Rockville Pike, Rockville, MD; (800) 638-TALK or (301) 897-5700. For information on hearing aids and certified pathologists and audiologists.

BLACK WOMEN WITH DISABILITIES ALLIANCE, c/o Deloris Costello, 45 W. 139 St., New York, NY 10027; (212) 862-2592.

CLEARINGHOUSE ON DISABILITY INFORMATION, Office of Special Education and Rehabilitative Services, Department of Education, 330 C St. SW, Switzer Bldg., room 3132, Washington, DC 20202-2524; (202) 205-8241 or (202) 205-98723. Responds to queries and provides referrals.

DEAF COUNSELING ADVOCACY AND REFERRAL AGENCY, 1539 Webster St., Oakland, CA 94612; (510) 251-6400 (has telecommunications device for the deaf, hereafter referred to as TDD). Provides information and referrals for the hearing-impaired.

HIGHER EDUCATION AND ADULT TRAINING FOR PEOPLE WITH HANDICAPS (HEALTH) RESOURCE CENTER, 1 Dupont Circle, suite 800, Washington, DC, 20036-1193; (800) 544-3284 or (202) 939-9320. Provides information on postsecondary education for the handicapped and on learning disabilities.

HEAR NOW, 9745 E. Hampden Ave., room 300, Denver, CO 80231; (800) 648-4327 (TDD). Provides hearing aids and related services for the hearing-impaired who need financial assistance.

IBM SPECIAL NEEDS SYSTEMS, P.O. Box 1328, Boca Raton, FL 33429-1328; (800) 426-2968. Provides information on how computers can help people with vision, hearing, speech impairments, learning disabilities, mobility concerns, and mental retardation.

JOB ACCOMMODATION NETWORK, West Virginia University, P.O. Box 6080, Morgantown, WV 26506-6080; (800) ADA-WORK. Provides information on accommodating workers with disabilities.

NATIONAL EASTER SEAL SOCIETY, 230 W. Monroe St., 18th floor, Chicago, IL 60606-6200; (800) 221-6827, (312) 726-6200, or (312) 726-4258 (TDD). Support services for children and adults with disabilities.

NATIONAL FEDERATION OF THE BLIND: Job Opportunities for the Blind, 1800 Johnson St., Baltimore, MD 21230; (800) 638-7518. Answers questions from blind individuals seeking jobs, parents, employers, and teachers.

NATIONAL INFORMATION CENTER FOR CHILDREN AND YOUTH WITH DISABILITIES, P.O. Box 1492, Washington, DC 20013; (703) 893-6061. Responds to questions, referrals, and technical assistance to parents, caregivers, and educators. Distributes fact sheets and provides information on parent support groups.

NATIONAL INFORMATION CLEARINGHOUSE FOR INFANTS WITH DISABILITIES AND LIFE-THREATENING CONDITIONS, Center for Developmental Disabilities, Benson Bldg., University of South Carolina, Columbia, SC 29208; (800) 922-9234 (TDD). Makes referrals for support groups and sources of financial, medical, and educational assistance for families with disabled infants up to age three.

NATIONAL INSTITUTE ON DEAFNESS AND OTHER COMMUNICATION DISORDERS CLEARINGHOUSE, P.O. Box 37777, Washington, DC 20013; (800) 241-1044 or (800) 241-1055 (TDD). Disseminates information on hearing, balance, smell, taste, voice, speech, and language.

NATIONAL LIBRARY SERVICE FOR THE BLIND AND PHYSICALLY HANDICAPPED, Library of Congress, 1291 Taylor St. NW, Washington, DC 20542; (800) 424-8567 or (202) 707-5100. Provides free library service to anyone who is visually or physically impaired. Delivers recorded and braille books and magazines.

NATIONAL REHABILITATION INFORMATION, 8455 Colesville Rd., suite 935, Silver Spring, MD 20910; (800) 346-2742 or (301) 588-9284 (TDD). Supplies publications and answers consumer questions. Center is also open to the public.

TELE-CONSUMER HOTLINE, (800) 332-1124 or (202) 223-4371 (TDD). Provides information about relay services between people with hearing or speech impairments and those without. Provides guidance on telephone issues.

TRIPOD GRAPEVINE, 2901 N. Keystone St., Burbank, CA 91504; (800) 352-8888 or (800) 287-4763 (TDD). Information on deafness including how to raise and educate a deaf child.

8

Our Bodies Growing Older

Black women age beautifully. Depending on our genes, our hair either turns silvery gray, in marked contrast to our brown complexions, or stays its natural color, even into old age. Thanks to our abundance of melanin and the thickness of our skin, we often have few wrinkles; it's not unusual to see a Black woman on the far side of sixty with a clear, smooth face. And when we do wrinkle, the lines don't mar our beauty but are the blueprint of a life lived.

And, of course, we Black women are full of personality and attitude and often get sexier and spunkier with age. Many sisters are late bloomers, coming into their own in their fifties or sixties, while others get a second wind and change careers, find a new hobby, or take up a sport at just about the same time they officially become senior citizens. Others, like our elder stateswoman Maya Angelou, who at the ripe age of sixty-four served as the "first poet" for the 1993 presidential inauguration, live amazing lives, and age does nothing to change that.

Part of the reason we age well lies in our community's collective attitude toward older folks. As our ancestors did in Africa, we love and respect the elders among us, benefiting from their wisdom and experience. The reverence and regard we offer them helps keep elders vital and thriving.

But also with age come changes in the body that can be difficult and painful. The years can take a toll, especially on Black women. Although we live longer than our men, Black women are expected to live fewer years than white women. Still, despite the changes our bodies undergo with age, we don't have to shrivel up and start looking toward the grave once we reach our fifties and sixties. Age is truly relative, and how well you age depends partly on heredity but mostly on how well you take care of your body. By exercising, eating healthy foods, keeping stress to a minimum, and avoiding bad habits such as smoking, drug use, and heavy drinking, you can feel youthful regardless of the year on your birth certificate.

Staying Healthy

As the body gets older, the immune system declines, making it harder to fight off all kinds of illnesses—from cancer and heart disease to colds and flu. On top of that, many organs in the body become less efficient as the years go by. The heart becomes less elastic and pumps less blood with each beat. The arteries stiffen and narrow, which leads to an increase in blood pressure. The lungs and airways become more rigid, leading to a less efficient respiratory system. These and other changes, combined with lowered immunity, explain why serious illnesses are more likely to strike older than younger folks.

Still, most of the health problems that plague older folks are preventable. Though the body does change with age, the effects of those changes can be lessened if you're willing to take extra care of your health. It's that simple.

Here's how.

Follow healthy habits. Age doesn't make illnesses like heart disease, stroke, diabetes, and cancer inevitable. Age is one of many risk factors, but it is one that cannot be changed. Which means that to keep your risk of getting serious illness lowered, you have to pay attention to factors you can control. So, stick to a healthy low-fat, low-salt diet; learn to avoid or handle stress; don't smoke; keep your weight in check; exercise consistently; and get a medical checkup at least once a year.

Have your blood pressure checked. Because blood pressure rises with age, it's imperative to keep yours under control. High blood pressure is much more common among Blacks than whites and leads to heart disease—the nation's number-one cause of death. Get a yearly blood-pressure reading; a reading of 120/80 or lower is normal. (You may need to get checked more often if you have hypertension or other health problems.) To keep your blood pressure within the normal range, avoid high-fat foods and salt, make sure to exercise consistently, and learn to control stress.

Take care of your breasts. A woman's risk of breast cancer increases with age, so older women must get their breasts checked frequently and properly. Women over forty should have mammograms every one or two years, and women over fifty should have yearly mammograms. You should also have your breasts checked as part of your yearly health exam, and you should check your own breasts once a month. (For specific information see chapter 18, "Checkups and Tests We Can't Live Without.")

Pay attention to your gynecological needs. The risk of cancers of the female reproductive organs increases as a woman ages. So even if you have gone through "the change," you still need yearly Pap smears and pelvic exams.

Talk to your doctor about taking vitamin supplements. Zinc and vitamins C, E, A, and the B's are all immune boosters, and research has shown that vitamins help older folks stay healthy.

Get a flu shot. People over sixty-five should do this once a year.

Think positive. A State University of New York at Buffalo study concludes that although older Blacks and older whites report similar health-related behaviors, Black folks are more likely to *perceive* that their health is poor. Say the researchers: "The subjective sense of feeling bad, even above and beyond actual health-related behaviors, still may have costs in terms of longevity and more objective health further down the road." The message here: Try not to allow stress and negativity to lead to poor health.

Understanding and Preventing Problems

Alzheimer's Disease

Alzheimer's disease is a confusing and frightening illness that strikes approximately one person in twenty over the age of sixty-five. It is a progressive disorder that slowly kills nerve cells in the brain and is particularly difficult for friends and relatives who watch a cherished person lose touch with the world. The first sign is generally a slight personality change and memory loss. Your loved one may feel more easily tired, upset, or anxious. As Alzheimer's progresses, the memory worsens, and decision making becomes difficult. In later stages, many Alzheimer's patients develop dementia, a syndrome characterized by deterioration of reasoning, judgment, and impulse control as well as changes in memory and personality. Dementia may be of particular concern to Black women: A Duke University study found that although white males and females had similar rates of dementia, Black women had twice the rate of Black men.

In its later stages, the Alzheimer's patient loses physical coordination and has increasing trouble identifying family and friends. Eventually the patient loses touch with reality and requires constant care.

No one is sure what causes the disorder, though researchers are focusing on a number of leads.

It may be extremely frightening for you if you notice that an older relative starts to lose her or his memory. Is it the first signs of Alzheimer's, or is it just normal memory loss that occurs with aging? The American Psychiatric Association offers these comparisons:

AVERAGE PERSON	OLDER PERSON	ALZHEIMER'S PATIENT
Is seldom forgetful	Forgets parts of an experience (can remember eating but doesn't remember what fruit was served)	Often forgets entire experiences (may not remember eating a meal)
Remembers later		
Acknowledges memory lapses lightly		Rarely remembers later
Maintains skills such as reading	Often remembers later	Acknowledges lapses grudgingly after initial denial and attempts to compensate for lapse
Follows written or spoken directions readily	Acknowledges lapses readily, often with a request for help in recalling information	
Can use notes or reminders	Skills usually remain intact	Skills deteriorate
Can care for self	Usually able to follow directions	Increasingly unable to follow directions
	Usually able to use notes or reminders	Increasingly unable to use notes or reminders
	Usually able to care for self	Increasingly unable to care for self

Although Alzheimer's can be very frightening, books and organizations can provide help, hope, and resources. For more information, see the list at the end of the chapter.

Arthritis

Many older folks know arthritis as aching, stiffness, and "cricks." Arthritis is characterized by joint swelling, pain, and loss of motion and can be caused by more than one hundred different problems. However, the most common type, osteoarthritis, affects more than 30 million Americans and most often strikes older people, especially women. In fact, according to the American College of Rheumatology, virtually everyone over the age of seventy-five complains of some degree of arthritis in the joints of the fingers, neck, lower back, or legs.

Though some forms of osteoarthritis have a hereditary link, it is most often due to the deterioration of the cartilage (the tissue that pads and cushions the joints) that can occur due to age-related wear and tear.

If you have problems with arthritis, here are some things you can do to find relief.

Exercise. Some arthritis sufferers avoid exercise, thinking it'll make the problem worse. But being sedentary may be what makes the pain worse: When you don't exercise your body, ligaments, muscles, and tendons become stiff and tight. That can make you feel achy and worsen any joint pain you may have. Instead try a workout that's easy on the joints, such as walking (be sure to wear well-cushioned shoes), biking, or swimming. A stretch or yoga class can also be a great way to get your joints moving and increase flexibility and range of motion. It's important, too, to stretch thoroughly before and after your exercise session.

Watch your weight. Extra weight puts stress on the hip and knee joints.

Keep your spirits up. Emotional factors, such as stress, can intensify the pain, and some experts suspect that stress may even increase inflammation of the joints.

Don't overuse painkilling medication. At least 13 million people take nonsteroidal anti-inflammatory drugs (NSAID's) every day for arthritis.

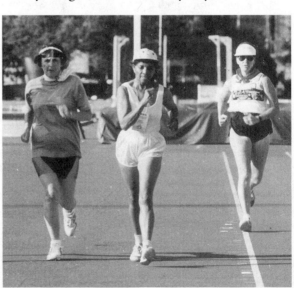

Competitors participating in the Senior Sports Classic. *(Photo: USNSO, Robin Fellows)*

Medications such as aspirin, ibuprofen (Advil and others), and prescription drugs reduce pain and swelling, but they can also cause stomach irritation, indigestion, and heartburn and may lead to stomach ulcers. If you do use them regularly, take them after meals, and spread them out throughout the day.

Incontinence

Incontinence, the involuntary loss of urine, is a problem many women suffer as they get older. It generally starts with a little bit of leakage and then gets worse. Though it's not a disease and is not necessarily caused by aging, it can be extremely stressful and embarrassing for the millions of older women who suffer from it. To make matters worse, in this country, public rest rooms for women are scarce, and this can lead to "accidents."

Several factors can lead to incontinence. As the body ages, the muscles grow weaker, including the pelvic muscles that are vital for bladder control. Childbirth may cause temporary or permanent incontinence, although some health activists suspect that the problem is sometimes triggered by obstetrics practices rather than the natural phenomenon of having a baby. After menopause, bladder control may lessen, because the reduction of estrogen affects the urethra through which urine flows. Stress, some medications (such as hypertension drugs), some medical procedures (such as hysterectomy), and specific health problems (such as Alzheimer's disease and strokes) can all trigger incontinence.

If you have bladder-control problems, discuss it with your doctor to rule out a serious medical problem. You may not look forward to this conversation, and with good reason: Male doctors can be unsympathetic about urinary incontinence, which is perceived as an "old-lady problem." But do it anyway. Remember, loss of bladder control isn't something to be

Caring for Your Elders

Census data reports that compared with older white people, our elders are more than twice as likely to live with a relative other than a spouse. And our older folks are half as likely to be living in a nursing home or with a nonrelative. That means that many Black women in their twenties, thirties, forties, and fifties are responsible for the care of an older relative. And this makes sense given the communal culture of African-descended people and our respect for our elders.

But caring for an older loved one can be extremely difficult, especially for women who are working and raising children as well. There are plenty of resources that can help you as a caregiver and can also help older folks who are managing on their own but could use a little help. Check out the lists of organizations at the end of this chapter for information and help.

ashamed of but something that needs to be taken care of. Insist that your doctor take the problem seriously.

You can also try these self-help tips:

Drink at least six glasses of water a day. Even though drinking less can ease the problem temporarily, it can also lead to dehydration and urinary-tract infections.

Cut down on alcohol, soft drinks, and caffeine. These are all diuretics, which will make you have to urinate more often.

Plan trips to the bathroom, and go frequently. If you walk around with a full bladder, a cough, sneeze, or laugh may trigger leakage.

Make sure your weight is in check. When large women lose weight, bladder-control problems tend to lessen. Do this by exercising and sticking to a diet full of vegetables, fruit, fish, and lean meat—not fat and sugar.

Keep a "bladder schedule." Figure out when the problem started: after surgery? When you started taking a certain medication? Jot down how often you go to the bathroom and when: When you feel stressed? After you drink coffee or soda? This will help you get a grip on the problem.

Strengthen your pelvic muscles—even if you're not incontinent—to prevent the problem. Do this with Kegel exercises. Start by sitting on the toilet and urinating. Try to halt the flow, and notice which muscles you use to stop it. These are the muscles you need to build. Now, when you have a moment, clench the muscle for a count of three, then relax it. Do this at least one hundred times per day. You can do it anywhere; no one needs to know.

Osteoporosis

Black women have strong, thick bones that are 10 percent denser than white women's. That makes us less prone to osteoporosis, the excessive loss of bone that strikes 20 million mostly older women and leads to hunched backs and broken bones. But that doesn't mean we're immune to the disease: Black women, especially thin, small-boned women, those who don't exercise or eat right, and smokers are still at risk for osteoporosis. What's more, for Black women who do have osteoporosis, the outcome is worse: Our survival rate is lower than that of our white counterparts.

Osteoporosis most often strikes women after menopause. Bone density peaks at about age thirty-five, then begins to decrease. It declines rapidly during the first few years after menopause because of decreasing levels of estrogen, which protects bone.

The easiest way to protect against osteoporosis is to keep your skeleton strong by doing the following:

Exercising. Bones are living tissue, and they can be built up with exercise. Weight-bearing exercise, such as walking and running, are the best bone builders.

Taking care of yourself. Smoking, drinking large amounts of coffee (several cups a day), and poor eating habits have been linked to osteoporosis.

Getting adequate calcium. Consuming high levels of calcium-rich foods can help build bones or even retard bone loss. Older women need at least 1,000 to 1,200 milligrams per day, and low-fat dairy products, fish, and leafy green vegetables are all calcium-rich. You can also try hijiki, a black sea vegetable that looks like spaghetti and has fourteen times more calcium than milk. You can find it in health-food stores. You may also need to take calcium supplements if you can't get enough from food.

Asking your doctor about hormone-replacement therapy (HRT) or estrogen-replacement therapy (ERT). Many menopausal women swear by replacement therapy because it not only slows or even stops bone loss, it also relieves menopausal symptoms. But studies have also linked replacement therapy to serious illness, including some kinds of cancer. Read up on this before you and your doctor decide. (See chapter 17, "Menopause: Going Through the Change.")

Emotional Health of Older Women

The later years can be a joyful time for women, but aging can also be a scary, lonely experience, especially for sisters in poor physical health. Aging also signals loss, as friends and family members die. We live longer than our men, so many sisters over sixty-five are widowed. And compared with older white women, we are three times more likely to be separated or divorced. Money can be a large worry for older folks, and Black women have the lowest incomes of any group of elderly in America today.

These kinds of worries take their toll: The suicide rate for folks over sixty-five is 50 percent higher than for the general population, making them the group at most risk for suicide. Alcoholism and the abuse of prescription drugs are particularly problematic for older folks.

For many women, however, the later years are a time of really living. Many sisters manage to do their best, most creative work in later life, and many are happiest and most content in their sixties or seventies.

These women are the ones who know how to live—surrounding themselves with good friends, taking care of their bodies, using their minds to their fullest, and staying busy with work, hobbies, and classes.

Being happy as an older woman means:

Looking at the positive. Don't let yourself slip into sad, negative thoughts. Think about all the things you *do* have.

Surrounding yourself with family and friends. You can never have too many friends, so make and keep lots of them.

Hanging around with children. We have so much to teach and tell our children, and they need us more than ever. Plus, kids are lots of fun.

Getting a pet. A dog or cat can make a nice companion, providing a way to give and receive affection. Some research shows that older folks who have pets live longer than those who don't.

Cultivating hobbies and interests. As you grow older, you may have more time to learn something new or to dive into an activity you love. So take an adult education class, perfect your fishing skills, read books, expand your garden, take pictures, get involved in your community's theater, learn to roller-skate, start a political action group, or teach Sunday school.

Asking for help if you need it. There's no shame in knowing when you need assistance and reaching out for it. You've probably spent many years caring for others, so let them help you out for a change.

Taking care of your body. There's no reason to be tired or in pain. Why waste the time? Get the checkups and tests you need, and talk to your health-care provider if something feels wrong. And if you feel good physically, your emotional self will also improve.

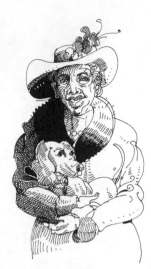

Studies show that having a loving pet can help combat the psychological problems associated with aging. *(Drawing: Yvonne Buchanan)*

Older Women and Sex

Sex can get better and better as you get older. For one, you will have had plenty of time to learn and perfect your skills and to understand and communicate what gives you pleasure. Studies also show that older folks enjoy sex. A 1992 University of Chicago report found that nearly 40 percent of married people over sixty have sex at least once a week, and 16 percent have sex several times a week. A 1984 Consumers Union survey of more than four thousand people fifty and older noted that "the panorama of love, sex, and aging is far richer and more diverse than the stereotype of life after fifty. Both the quality and quantity of sexual activity reported can be properly defined as astonishing." (For heterosexual sisters, finding a partner may prove challenging. Black men die earlier than women, making nearly three out of every five older Blacks a woman.)

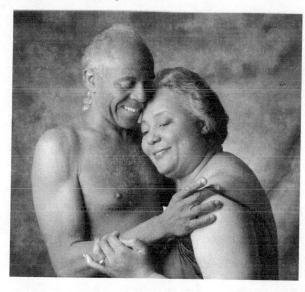

Age is no obstacle to love, affection, and sex.
(*Photo: Dwight Carter Photography, New York*)

Though sex can be wonderful after sixty, you should also be aware of the changes in your body that may affect your sexuality. According to a February 1993 supplement to the *Mayo Clinic Health Letter* on sexuality and aging, here's what to expect:

A Change in Your Desire

This varies greatly from woman to woman, but hormones such as estrogen and testosterone (the male hormone, which is also present in women) play a role. At menopause the ovaries stop producing estrogen, and this may affect your sex drive. Of course, it may not.

What to do: There are many ways to get turned on, especially if you're open and creative. For ideas, see chapter 27, "Sexuality and Having Sex Safely." You may want to discuss estrogen-replacement therapy (ERT) with your doctor. For more information on this option, read chapter 17, "Menopause: Going Through the Change."

Vaginal Changes

After menopause, estrogen deficiency causes the folds of skin that cover your genital region to shrink and become thinner. This causes more of the clitoris to be exposed, and may lead to an increased sensitivity. For some women, stimulation to the clitoris feels unpleasantly tingly or even prickly. The opening of the vagina may also become more narrow, particularly if you aren't very active sexually. This can lead to painful sexual intercourse.

What to do: Talk to your partner about how you feel during sex. You may need to adjust the way the two of you make love. Remember, sex isn't just about the genitals; if clitoral stimulation or vaginal penetration aren't comfortable, remind your partner about the many other sexy spots on your body. Estrogen-replacement therapy is also an option.

Lack of Lubrication

Because of decreased estrogen, lubrication of the vagina may occur more slowly with age. (Diabetes can also trigger this problem.) And even when you're excited, your vagina may feel less moist than when you were younger.

What to do: Use a lubricant. You can buy it at the drugstore, and it's best to get a water-based type. One note: In some cases you may not be excited by your partner or you may have been pressured to have sex, and that may be what's slowing down your ability to get wet.

One more important thing to remember: When you have sex, do it safely. The risk of contracting sexually transmitted infections, including the AIDS virus, doesn't decrease with age. If you need more information on safer sex, see chapter 27, "Sexuality and Having Sex Safely."

For More Information

ORGANIZATIONS: Alzheimer's Disease

ALZHEIMER'S DISEASE AND RELATED DISORDERS ASSOCIATION, INC., 919 N. Michigan Ave., suite 1000, Chicago, IL 60611-1676; (800) 272-3900. You can get free information or inquire about its very helpful kit for Alzheimer's caregivers and families, "Just the Facts and More" ($8).

AMERICAN PSYCHIATRIC ASSOCIATION, 1400 K St. NW, Washington, DC 20005; (202) 682-6000. Ask for its pamphlet on Alzheimer's.

THE ALZHEIMER'S DISEASE EDUCATION AND REFERRAL CENTER (ADEAR), P.O. Box 8250, Silver Spring, MD 20907-8250; (800) 438-4380 or (301) 495-3311.

BOOKS

The Alzheimer's Cope Book: The Complete Care Manual for Patients and Their Families, R. E. Markin, Citadel Press, 1992.

Alzheimer's Disease: A Guide for Families, Lenore S. Powell and Katie Courtice, Addison-Wesley, 1992.

Caring for the Alzheimer Patient: A Practical Guide, Raye Lynne Dippel and J. Thomas Hutton, M.D., Golden Age Books, 1991.

The 36-Hour Day, Nancy L. Mace and Peter V. Rabins, Warner Books, 1992.

ORGANIZATIONS: Arthritis

AMERICAN COLLEGE OF RHEUMATOLOGY, 60 Executive Park S., suite 150, Atlanta, GA 30329; (404) 633-3777.

ARTHRITIS FOUNDATION INFORMATION HOTLINE, (800) 283-7800.

NATIONAL ARTHRITIS AND MUSCULOSKELETAL AND SKIN DISEASES INFORMATION CLEARINGHOUSE, P.O. Box AMS, 9000 Rockville Pike, Bethesda, MD 20892; (301) 495-4484.

BOOKS

All About Arthritis: Past, Present and Future, Derrick Brewerton, M.D., Harvard University Press, 1992.

Arthritis: A Comprehensive Guide, James F. Fries, M.D., Addison-Wesley, 1990.

Arthritis: A Guide to Controlling Your Illness and Working with Your Doctor, Mike Samuels, M.D., and Nancy Harrison Samuels, Summit Books, 1991.

Arthritis: What Works, Dava Sobel and Arthur C. Klein, St. Martin's Press, 1991.

The Duke University Medical Center Book of Arthritis, David S. Pisetsky, M.D., Fawcett Books, 1992.

ORGANIZATIONS: Incontinence

HELP FOR INCONTINENT PEOPLE, P.O. Box 544, Union, SC 29379; (800) BLADDER or (803) 579-7900.

BOOKS

Overcoming Bladder Disorders, Rebecca Chalker and Kristene E. Whitmore, M.D., HarperCollins, 1991.

Staying Dry: A Practical Guide to Bladder Control, Kathryn L. Burgio,

K. Lynette Pearce, and Angelo J. Lucco, M.D., Johns Hopkins
University Press, 1989.

ORGANIZATIONS: Osteoporosis

NATIONAL OSTEOPOROSIS FOUNDATION, 1150 17th Street NW, suite
500, Washington, DC 20036; (800) 223-9994 or (202) 223-2226.

BOOKS

Preventing and Reversing Osteoporosis: Every Woman's Essential Guide,
Alan Gaby, M.D., Prima Publications (Roseville, Calif.), 1993.

ORGANIZATIONS: Aging

ADMINISTRATION ON AGING, U.S. Department of Health and
Human Services, 330 Independence Ave. SW, Washington, DC 20201;
(202) 619-0556. Call (800) 677-1116 for elder-care locator information
and assistance. Call (202) 619-0011 for the AoA's Office of State and
Community Programs.

AMERICAN ASSOCIATION OF RETIRED PERSONS, 601 E St. NW,
Washington, DC 20049; (800) 424-2277 or (202) 434-2277. AARP
offers a variety of services including information about and help obtaining group health insurance, auto and homeowner's insurance, and phar-
maceuticals. Brochures and pamphlets are available.

AMERICAN GERIATRICS ASSOCIATION, 770 Lexington Ave., suite 300,
New York, NY 10021; (212) 308-1414. Provides some information for
the public.

ELDERHOSTEL, 75 Federal St., Boston, MA 02110; (617) 426-8056.
Information on college-campus–based educational experiences for older
adults.

GERONTOLOGICAL SOCIETY OF AMERICA, 1275 K Street NW, suite
350, Washington, DC 20005-4006; (212) 842-1275. GSA has an information service for referrals to various specialists in the field.

GRAY PANTHERS, 2025 Pennsylvania Ave. NW, suite 821, Washington, DC 20006; (202) 466-3132. The Gray Panthers is an advocacy
group "dedicated to fighting the 'isms' of society." With 60 local networks nationwide, the Panthers confront issues of education, economic
and tax justice, and affordable housing, among others.

NATIONAL ASSOCIATION OF AREA AGENCIES ON AGING, 1112 16th

St. NW, suite 100, Washington, DC 20036; (202) 296-8130. For information or referrals to services in your area, or call (800) 677-1116 for elder-care locator information and assistance.

NATIONAL COUNCIL OF SENIOR CITIZENS, 1331 F St. NW, Washington, DC 20004; (202) 347-8800. For referrals and assistance with Social Security and Medicare concerns, help in choosing a nursing home, and long-term care.

NATIONAL COUNCIL ON THE AGING, 409 3rd St. SW, 2nd floor, Washington, DC 20024; (800) 424-9046 or (202) 479-1200. Write or call for resources, information, and referrals.

NATIONAL ELDERCARE INSTITUTE ON OLDER WOMEN, c/o National Council of Negro Women, Inc., 1667 K Street NW, suite 700, Washington, DC 20006; (202) 659-0006. The Institute has taken on a leadership role on important issues concerning aging and people of color, particularly those who are at special risk because they are low-income or live in rural areas.

OLDER WOMEN'S LEAGUE, 666 11th St. NW, suite 700, Washington, DC 20001; (800) TAKE-OWL or (202) 783-6686. OWL is an advocacy organization that deals with women's issues from midlife on.

ORGANIZATIONS: Support and Advice for Caring for Elders

AMERICAN ASSOCIATION OF HOMES FOR THE AGING, 901 E St. NW, suite 500, Washington, DC 20004; (202) 783-2242. Ask for the free brochure "Choosing a Nursing Home: A Guide to Quality Care." Other consumer literature is available.

CHILDREN OF AGING PARENTS, 1609 Woodbourne Rd., suite 302A, Levittown, PA 19057; (215) 945-6900. Information and support for caregivers.

FAMILY SERVICE AMERICA, Headquarters, 11700 W. Lake Park Dr., Milwaukee, WI 53224; (800) 221-2681. Call or write for a referral to a member agency in your area and for information on the counseling and support services.

FOUNDATION FOR HOSPICE AND HOMECARE, 519 C St. NE, Washington, DC, 20002; (202) 547-6586. The Foundation runs education, certification, and accreditation programs for providers in the field of home health care.

NATIONAL ASSOCIATION FOR INDEPENDENT LIVING, c/o National Rehabilitation Association, 633 S. Washington St., Alexandria, VA 22314, or NATIONAL COUNCIL ON INDEPENDENT LIVING, 2539

Telegraph Ave., Berkeley, CA 94704. Write for information on centers that provide services for disabled folks who live at home.

NATIONAL INSTITUTE ON ADULT DAYCARE, c/o National Council on the Aging, 600 Maryland Ave. SW, West Wing 100, Washington, DC 20024; (202) 479-1200. For information on centers that provide activities, meals, and medical services during the day for older folks.

SHARED HOUSING RESOURCE CENTER, 6344 Greene St., Philadelphia, PA 19144; (215) 848-1220. For information on housing arrangements between elderly friends, elders with younger people, or help finding an arrangement for five to fifteen older folks to live together.

BOOKS: Aging

Growing Old Together: A Couples' Guide to Understanding and Coping with Late Life Crises, Barbara Silverston and Helen Kandel Hyman, Pantheon, 1993.

Having Our Say: The Delany Sisters' First 100 Years, Sarah and A. Elizabeth Delany with Amy Hill Hearth, Kodansha America, Inc., 1993.

How a Woman Ages, Robin Marantz Henig, Ballantine, 1985.

Longevity: The Science of Staying Young, Kathy Keeton, Viking/Penguin, 1992.

Ourselves, Growing Older: Women Aging with Knowledge and Power, Paula Brown Doress, Diana Laskin Siegal, and the Midlife and Older Women Book Project, Simon & Schuster/Touchstone, 1987. An excellent book by the women who produced *Our Bodies, Ourselves.*

Reverse the Aging Process Naturally: How to Build the Immune System with Antioxidants—the Super-Nutrients of the Nineties, Gary Null, Villard Books, 1993.

Staying Young: The Whole Truth About Aging and What You Can Do to Slow Its Progress, Thomas Hager and Lauren Kessler, Facts on File Publications, 1987.

We Live Too Short, We Die Too Long: How to Achieve and Enjoy Your Natural 120-Year-Plus Life Span, Walter M. Bortz, II, M.D., Bantam Books, 1992.

BOOKS: Caring for Elders

The Caregiver's Guide: Helping Older Friends and Relatives with Health and Safety Concerns, Caroline Rob and Janet Reynolds, Houghton Mifflin, 1992.

Caring for Your Aging Parents: A Sourcebook of Timesaving Techniques and Tips, Kerri S. Smith, American Source Books (Lakewood, Colo.), 1992.

How to Care for Your Parents: A Handbook for Adult Children, Nora Jean Levin, Storm King Press (Friday Harbor, Wash.), 1993.

When Parents Age: What Children Can Do, Tom Adams and Kathryn Armstrong, Berkley Books, 1993.

Where Can Mom Live? A Family Guide to Living Arrangements for Elderly Parents, Vivian F. Carlin and Ruth Mansberg, Free Press, 1987.

You and Your Aging Parent: A Family Guide to Emotional, Physical, and Financial Problems, Barbara Silverston and Helen Kandel Hyman, Pantheon, 1993.

terrifyingly terrific teens! that year when mama sent me down south like she did every summer my aunt said i couldn't be running around the fields naked all day like me & my cousins did cuz i was getting titties. titties meant clothes all the time no matter how hot it was. i still haven't quite recovered.

teen time was dreaming about doin it, listening to big girls tell about doin it & looking up words about doin it in the dictionary. in those early 1950s segregation days in a central jersey factorytown my longings were fueled by innuendoes overheard in the girls bathroom or gleaned from r&b sides like "work with me annie" by the midnighters or "fever" by little willie john & by non-stop food cravings—candy! cookies! potato chips! soda! hoagies! hair was growing on my legs under my arms & between my legs. boys & men noticed me in a new way that made mama nervous & that excited & scared me. men in cars followed me yelling dumb stuff. older boys tried to train-gang me. i felt real grown when i first inserted a tampon into my virginal vagina. i did the grind & made out til finally i experienced the thrill of a finger a tongue—gasp!—a penis. pregnancy & a kitchen table abortion followed.

free at last! in the early 60s black-power-free-sex anti-war days i moved my 19-year-old self to the lower east side in new york city & said goodbye to pressed hair & other forms of repression. shedding my countrified underwear—panties, girdle, stockings, longline bra, whole slip—for skimpy briefs & pantyhose. i draped my black is beautiful self in revolutionary pants suits

"The terrifyingly terrific teens to the fiercely 40s & 50s!"

HATTIE GOSSETT,
AUTHOR OF *PRESENTING SISTER NOBLUES*,
NEW YORK CITY

or african clothing. freedom! when i had sex in bed—no more car backseat action—my new afro meant no worries about my hair going back. freedom!

my body was an engine of endless energy. i regularly hung out all night at political meetings, experimental theaters, smoky jazz clubs & after hours spots. i got 3 hours sleep & was at work almost on time the next morning. friends called me the secret weapon cuz i could hang longer than anybody. when the revolution came all counter-revolutionaries would be sentenced to hang out night after night with me til they dropped dead or repented. in my hi heels i ran for subways & cabs & up & down the steps of the 5-floor walk-ups everyone lived in on the lower east side. exercise? in my artist/social activist set we were too busy reading; thinking; doing dope; debating integration, nationalism, pan africanism & marxism; eating spareribs; making art; fucking; going to rallies, demonstrations & poetry readings. birth control pills & legal abortions inspired us to throw open our legs even wider.

where're my toenails? *that night i was gonna wear my hi heeled suede sandals so i had to polish my toenails. by then i had been married & annulled & was loving being a single diva in demand. i put my foot up on the bed & bent over but couldn't make the nail polish brush reach my toenails. so i tried it from another position. no matter how i twisted & turned i couldn't reach my toenails. what?! my mid-30s body was rebelling. byebye natural muscletone, hello african dance class—stretch, twist, bend, push, breathe, breathe, breathe—oh the pain. slowly, slowly the power of my body was restored—just in time for accelerated p.m.s. & membership in that circle of women who only have 4 or 5 good days per month what with pre-period stress followed by period stress followed by post-period stress. tirelessly euphoric one minute wearily evil the next. a new concept: rest? uh huh rest.*

enter womanism & the understanding of how race, class, gender & patriarchy intersect. i started therapy, joined a sisters support group then put 2plus2 together about my dick happiness & learned to sublimate excess sexual energy toward creative ends: writing & performing instead of worrying why some man wouldn't romance me right. the scary thing about my bout with fibroid tumors was the near impossibility of finding a doctor to surgically remove them without removing all my reproductive organs too. though i didn't want no babies, i didn't want no hysterectomy or surgically induced early menopause either.

fiercely free 40s & 50s! *mama suffered a totally incapacitating stroke while i was in my late 20s. one day i found her asleep with her gown wide open & her genitals exposed. i was shocked at how thin & grey her pubic hair was! mama died soon after but when i discovered my own first gray pubic hair 20 years later i was ready. yes* all *hair can get gray & fall out too.*

*when my dreads started falling out i spent a year meditating on baldness &
woman-ness & sanity. conclusion? no wigs, hair pieces or magic hair restoration formulas (herbal or chemical) for me. on my 50th birthday i discovered
the joys of baldheadedness.*

*menopause manifested in the late 80s just when the post world war 2
american dreamland hologram—with its promise of endless socioeconomic
expansion—was exhibiting alarmingly finite limitations. menopause
brought joy over the approaching end of my period & the promise of another
era of freedom. my mind was eager. on the other hand there were powerful
mood swings & diminished physical energy along with broadening hips &
breasts pointing toward the earth not the sky. talk about ironic timing! my
body & the world were changing in scary ways. renewed racial ethnic sexist
homophobic & economic violence were deepening global realities. a.i.d.s.
was the final straw.*

*just the time to re-program my life: to figure how to make a living doing
what i wanna do instead of wasting away in some brain-eroding day gig; to
adjust to safe sex & menopause & touches of arthritis; to appreciate less as
more. vitamins, lots of walking, acupuncture, increased attention to my attitude & what i eat & more rest are very helpful. books, experimental theater,
political discussions, jazz, cocktails, talking on the phone, making art, hanging out & bonding with my sisters continue to promote affirming power.
here i am standing at the crossroads on the shoulders of my ancestors looking
for a share of the sweetness of life & struggling for a brighter day by all
means necessary.*

© 1993 hattie gossett

PART II

OUR REPRODUCTIVE HEALTH

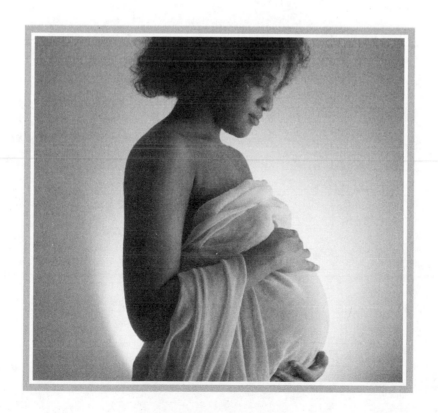

9

The Reproductive System and Menstruation

Most of us have been taught to be ashamed or embarrassed about our reproductive organs—don't look at them, don't talk about them, and for goodness sake, don't touch them. But in order to understand our bodies and keep them healthy, this is exactly what we must do: look at, talk about, and touch all of the parts of our bodies.

Find a well-lit private spot that is quiet and warm, such as your bathroom after bathing or your bedroom as you're undressing for bed, and take a look at the parts of your body that you always hurry to cover up. Though every woman's body is slightly different, this is what you'll see.

Our Breasts

The breasts come in all shapes and sizes—much to the frustration of some women who may feel that theirs are too large, too small, or too saggy, thanks to this society's preoccupation with breast size. Actually every woman has about the same amount of glandular tissue, and it is that tissue that produces milk when a woman is nursing. Fat supports the glandular tissue, and the more fat a woman has, the larger her breasts will be. The size of the breasts are determined by heredity, hormones, and weight, and size has absolutely nothing to do with sexual responsiveness or the amount of milk a woman produces after she gives birth. You can't increase breast size by doing exercises, although you can strengthen the muscles that support the breasts. If you gain or lose weight, the size of your breasts may change.

In the middle of the breast you can see a circle of darker skin called the areola, and on the tip is your nipple. The areola ranges from being pinkish in white women and light-skinned Black women to nearly black in darker sisters. (During pregnancy, this area generally grows larger and darker.) You may notice small bumps on your areola (these are oil glands, which are normal) and hairs growing around it, especially if you're on the Pill. Your nipples may be large, they may stick out, they may be flat, or may even turn inward—all of these kinds of nipples are normal. When you are sexually aroused or cold, your nipples become more erect. You may also notice milky fluid coming out of them, even if you're not pregnant or nursing. If so, talk to your health-care provider, especially if the fluid is greenish or yellowish, it comes out without you touching your nipple, or it is accompanied by breast tenderness, fever, or swollen glands.

This shouldn't be the last time you look at your breasts: You should be examining them every month. See chapter 18, "Checkups and Tests We Can't Live Without," for more on breast self-examination.

To examine your genitals, you'll need a mirror. You can either squat over it or sit down and hold a hand mirror between your legs.

The Vulva, or Outer Genitals

We usually refer to the reproductive organs in the pelvic area as the vagina, but actually the vagina is located behind the vulva, the outer genitals. As you can see, the sum of those parts is shaped like the delicate bud of a flower, and some women artists have used the flower as a metaphor for the female genitals.

Looking at the vulva, you first see the *mons pubis,* round, plump outer folds that are covered with pubic hair. Moving down, you'll notice the outer lips, known as the *labia majora.* Also covered with hair, these dark flaps of skin protect the opening of the vagina against infection. If you pull back that skin, you'll see the inner lips or *labia minora.* These soft and sensitive flaps of hairless skin fold over the vagina as the last line of defense against infection.

You can find the hood of the *clitoris* just below the *mons pubis* at the

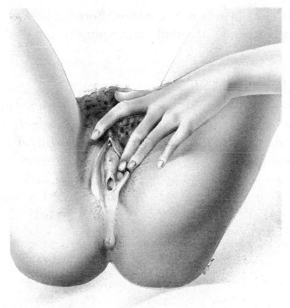

External view of the female
reproductive organs.
(Drawing: Keelin Murphy)

top of the inner lips. If you pull back the hood, you'll encounter the highly sensitive clitoris, which tenses, swells, becomes erect, and produces orgasm during sexual excitement. In the past it was thought of as a shrunken or underdeveloped penis (others preferred to think of the penis as an oversized clitoris!), but it is actually a much more complex structure with several parts. For more on the clitoris and orgasm, see chapter 27, "Sexuality and Having Sex Safely."

Gently pull apart the inner lips, and you'll encounter the entrance to the urethra, the opening through which you urinate. It leads directly to the bladder and shouldn't be confused with the larger vaginal opening. (Menstrual blood and vaginal secretions come through the vagina, not the urethra, and penises are inserted in and babies pass through the vagina, not the urethra.)

The entrance to the vagina lies behind the urinary opening. If you insert your finger inside it, it feels damp, thanks to the *Bartholin's glands,* situated alongside the vaginal opening. These glands provide moisture, especially during sexual arousal. The *hymen,* a thin membrane of skin, separates the vaginal opening from the internal reproductive organs. The myth is that the hymen can only be torn through sexual activity. But these days, most girls tear their hymens because of activities like soccer, bike riding, ballet, and gymnastics.

To the rear of the vaginal opening is the *perineum,* which separates the vagina from the anus, the opening to the *rectum*. Bowel movements pass from the bowel (large intestine), through the rectum and out of the anus.

The Internal Reproductive Organs

The internal reproductive organs lie in the pelvic area. Though they are more difficult to see than the external organs, you can use a speculum (an instrument gynecologists use to open the vagina), a flashlight, and a hand mirror to get a good look at some of your organs. (For complete instructions on how to do a gynecological self-exam and to order an inexpensive plastic speculum, contact the Federation of Feminist Women's Health Centers, 633 E. 11th Ave., Eugene, OR 97401; 800-995-2286 or 503-344-0966.)

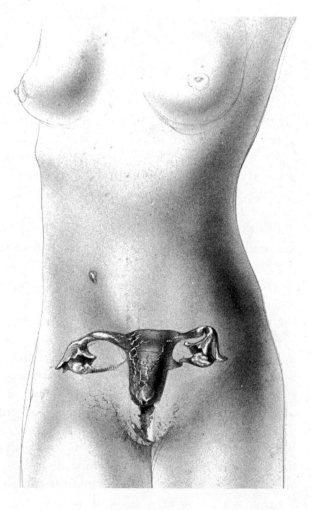

Internal view of the female reproductive organs.
(Drawing: Keelin Murphy)

The Vagina

The vagina is an extremely flexible organ, stretching to accommodate a tampon or a penis, and eventually allowing a baby to pass through. It measures about three to five inches and connects the uterus to the outside of your body. Though we've been led to believe that the vagina is dirty or nasty, actually it's a clean, efficient organ. It constantly sheds its cells along with secretions, which you know as discharge. This clear discharge thins and turns whitish during the ovulation stage of the cycle; this is normal. If your discharge has a foul odor, is greenish, yellowish, or thick and lumpy, see a doctor because you may have an infection. (For more on reproductive-tract infections, see chapter 12, "Reproductive-Tract Infections.")

The Cervix

The cervix sits at the top of the vagina; it is the lower part of the uterus. It feels like a small bump with a dimple in the middle, which is actually the os, a tiny hole through which the sperm enter the uterus. Though the opening is very small, it expands greatly during childbirth. A plug of mucous covers the os to prevent bacteria from infecting the uterus and other internal organs.

The Uterus

Located behind the bladder, the tough but extremely flexible uterus stretches to the size of a large melon to house the fetus when a woman is pregnant. All other times, it is about the size of a fist and only large enough to hold a teaspoon of fluid. The inside of the uterus is lined with the endometrium, which sheds unless conception takes place. Mixed with blood and fluid, this lining is what we know as menstrual blood.

The Fallopian Tubes

Branching out from the top of the uterus are the two fallopian tubes, which are also known as oviducts or egg tubes. When the microscopic egg is released from the ovary, the strands of tissue on the end of the tube scoop it up, and it is propelled through the tube by microscopic hairs. Once in the fallopian tubes, the egg may meet up with a sperm and get fertilized; if so, it will travel to the uterus, where it attaches to the uterine wall. Otherwise, it disintegrates or is flushed out of the body with vaginal secretions.

The Ovaries

A woman's main reproductive organs, the two ovaries are suspended by ligaments on either side of the uterus. They contain hundreds of thousands of follicles, and each month one of the ovaries produces a mature egg. The ovaries also manufacture hormones that regulate the menstrual cycle and prepare the body for pregnancy.

Menstruation

Our menstrual period, the monthly expelling of blood and tissue, is a natural body process that will be with most of us for some forty years—from puberty until menopause. Yet for something so natural, menstruation (though it's frequently pronounced wrong, the correct pronunciation is "men-strew-ay-shun") has been shrouded in secrecy, myth, and taboo. Too many of us feel ashamed or embarrassed about our period, calling it "the curse," something women must endure as punishment for the biblical Eve's sins.

Since the beginning of time, men have approached our bodies and our ability to reproduce with a mix of envy, awe, and terror. Write Janice Delaney, Mary Jane Lupton, and Emily Toth, the authors of *The Curse: A Cultural History of Menstruation*: "Greater than his fear of death, dishonor, or dismemberment has been primitive man's respect for menstrual blood."

In Hebrew tradition, a menstruating woman is seen as spiritually unclean and must be avoided, and some orthodox and conservative Jewish women are still forbidden contact with their husbands during menstruation. In Muslim cultures a menstruating woman cannot visit a shrine or mosque, and she is forbidden to have sexual intercourse.

Not all cultures abide by these kinds of paranoid taboos. In a series of interviews with !Kung women, a contemporary hunting/gathering tribe in Africa, anthropologist Marjorie Shostak found that "because [women] held positions in their society almost equal to men, sharing decision making as well as labor, their menstruations were not objects of fear or taboo." (Interestingly, these !Kung sisters reported no PMS symptoms and were surprised to learn they even existed!)

Despite what the larger society thinks about menstruation, like the !Kung women, we must look at our periods as something natural and healthy. The more we understand about menstruation—why it occurs, how it works—the more we can appreciate the monthly cycle as a normal bodily function.

The Menstrual Cycle

Your reproductive cycle is an ongoing process that your body goes through. Slight changes in vaginal discharge, premenstrual symptoms, and, of course, your monthly "bleeding" or period are the only signs of this complex, continuous process. From start to finish the cycle lasts approximately twenty-eight days, though it varies from as many as thirty-five to as few as twenty days depending on the woman. To learn more about your own cycle, keep a menstrual chart. Use a calendar to jot down the start of your cycle. Keep track of your period, and record any cramps, breast tenderness, mood changes, and fluctuations in vaginal discharge. Soon you'll be able to pinpoint when your period is to arrive, and you'll be aware of your body's monthly changes.

Assuming your period is twenty-eight days, here's how it works:

Days 1 through 14. Though the monthly bleeding seems like the end result of the reproductive cycle, the first day of your menstrual period actually marks the first day of the cycle. At this point, your levels of the hormones estrogen and progesterone have decreased, causing the lining of the uterus (the endometrium) to shed. This lining is mixed with blood, vaginal secretions, and cervical mucus to become your menstrual blood. You'll probably expel about four to six tablespoons of brownish fluid, though it may feel like more. (If your period is extremely heavy, see a doctor; heavy menstrual bleeding may be a sign of fibroid tumors or other gynecological problems.) You may notice cramping (due to contractions of the uterus) during the first day or two of your period.

The average woman's period lasts five days, though it can be as long as eight and as short as two. Your period may fall at the same time every month, but if it doesn't, that shouldn't be cause for alarm and doesn't mean that you're irregular. If your cycle is about thirty days long, you'll be better able to predict when your period will appear. But if it's longer or shorter, your period will fall at a different time each month.

During this time, the hormones are at work. The pituitary gland (located at the base of the brain) releases the follicle-stimulating hormone (FSH), which triggers some of the immature follicles (egg cells) to grow. Eventually one follicle, destined for ovulation, will grow larger while the others die off. At this point, the developing eggs also produce estrogen and the endometrium thickens.

During days 15 and 16, one egg, stimulated by the luteinizing hormone (LH), emerges from one of the ovaries and is swept into the fallopian tube. This period of about forty-eight hours is known as ovulation and is the easiest time of the month to conceive. The mucous that blocks the cervix has become watery, making it easy for sperm to travel through the uterus and into the fallopian tube where the egg is resting.

What to Say to Your Daughters

Your daughter is about to reach adolescence, and you know it's time to have that "little talk" with her. You may find yourself excited to tell her about her growing body and her period. Or you may put it off, afraid that you won't be able to explain it right, ashamed and embarrassed to talk to her about her body and her period and eventually about s-e-x. You try to avoid facing the inevitable: that your baby is growing up.

But we must have these talks with our daughters. In a study of 120 African-American women, researcher Beryl Jackson, Ph. D., found that 67 percent of respondents were not adequately prepared for the onset of menstruation. She cites author and researcher Joyce Ladner's findings that compared with white women, "twice as many black women had no premenarcheal preparation, a factor that might have influenced their poor adjustment to menarcheal experiences."

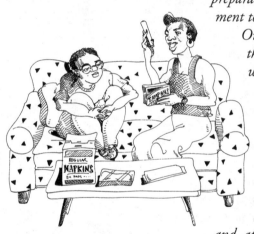

On the other hand, Jackson notes, ". . . literature suggest[s] that when prepubertal girls were prepared for menstruation within a loving, caring, and accepting relationship by the mothering person, their response to the first menstruation experience was not traumatic or anxiety-ridden."

We can't allow our own feelings of shame, anxiety, and embarrassment about our bodies and our periods to get in the way, leaving our daughters dangling with no one to explain menstruation and the reproductive system. Our children shouldn't have to rely on piecemeal information or misinformation and end up, at best, confused or afraid and, at worst, pregnant.

It's important for mothers and daughters to have that "little talk." (Drawing: Yvonne Buchanan)

Just before your daughter reaches puberty (about age eight or nine or before she reaches fifth grade), sit down with her and explain to her about the changes that will soon be taking place in her body. Using simple language and correct terms, explain the menstrual cycle. (A University of Miami School of Medicine study of adolescent Black girls notes that vague comments like "you will bleed every month" or "you will become a woman" aren't enough.) Have books, diagrams, and samples of napkins and tampons on hand. Let her know that every woman menstruates—it's as natural as a heartbeat—and that her monthly period will be a sign of good health, not a curse or disease. You can discuss sex and reproduction now, or you can do that at another time. Try not to rush or feel embarrassed; our sensitive youngsters will be able to pick up on those subtle cues.

On Becoming a Woman: Mothers and Daughters Talking Together *can help. This 104-minute video features a group of sisters and their teenage daughters talking together about menstruation, sex, birth control, and love, and why it is so hard for mothers and daughters to talk. A twenty-four-minute animation covers male and female anatomy, reproduction, birth control methods, and the risks and responsibilities of sex, including safer sex. For more information contact the National Black Women's Health Project, 1237 Ralph David Abernathy Blvd. SW, Atlanta, GA 30310; (800) ASK-BWHP.*

There are also books that will help you explain things. With your daughter read books such as Changing Bodies, Changing Lives: A Book for Teens on Sex and Relationships, *by Ruth Bell et al.;* Period, *by J. Gardner-Loulan, B. Lopez, and M. Quackenbush;* The What's Happening to My Body Book for Girls *by Lynda Madaras with Area Madaras; and* You're in Charge: A Teenage Girl's Guide to Sex and Her Body *by Niels H. Lauersen and Eileen Stukane.*

During ovulation your discharge is thinner, your temperature drops and then rises slightly, and you may experience slight cramping as the follicle bursts to release the microscopic egg.

After the egg follicle bursts, during days 17 though 28, it turns yellow and is now known as the corpus luteum or "yellow body." Stimulated by LH, it produces increasing amounts of hormones, especially progesterone. This new stock of progesterone changes the mucus covering the cervix back to its thick consistency and plugs the entrance to the uterus. The hormone also enriches the endometrium, causing it to thicken even more.

At this point, the egg makes its way to the uterus. If it has been fertilized, it will attach itself to the newly enriched endometrium, and the yellow body will continue to pump out progesterone. If the egg hasn't been fertilized, it is flushed out of the body, the corpus luteum disintegrates, and progesterone levels fall. With no hormones to support it, the endometrium breaks down and the uterus is filled with blood and tissue. Soon the uterine walls contract, sending the contents of the uterus out of the body as menstrual blood. That marks day one of the next cycle.

During the final part of your cycle, you may notice physical and emotional changes. Many women feel their breasts swelling and becoming tender and their bodies bloating. This is the hormones preparing the body for pregnancy by conserving fluid. (This fluid leaves the body once you start menstruating.) Hormonal changes also cause some women to feel depressed, moody, hungry, tense, and sexually aroused. They also stimulate oil glands in the skin, which can lead to acne flare-ups.

Toxic Shock Syndrome

In the late seventies women received a huge scare: Tampons became deadly. That was when cases of toxic shock syndrome (TSS), a rare but sometimes deadly infection, were first reported. The disease coincided with the introduction of superabsorbent tampons, designed to "absorb your worry."

In the next few years scientists recognized the link between these superabsorbent tampons and TSS, which causes sudden fever (102 degrees or more), vomiting, diarrhea, flulike symptoms, fainting, dizziness, or a red rash. Experts believe that the synthetic materials used to make the superabsorbent tampons enhanced the production of the bacterial toxin that causes TSS. Plus, women tend to leave in superabsorbent tampons for longer periods of time, allowing bacterial organisms more time to grow.

Manufacturers have yanked superabsorbent products such as Procter & Gamble's Rely (which was known as the "killer tampon") off the market, and other makers have changed the contents of tampons. Tampons are now safe as long as they're used correctly. Be sure to change your tampon every four to six hours, and never use a product with more absorbency than you really need. (Don't use super if regular or "junior" will do.) Some women prefer to alternate tampons and napkins.

Napkins and Tampons

Women in Borneo and other cultures prefer to allow their menstrual fluids to flow, while our ancestors used plants, rags, or gauze to catch them. Now we can choose from several different kinds of "sanitary products" during our periods. Whichever you choose, be sure to read and follow all instructions carefully.

Sanitary napkins are rectangles made of highly absorbent fibers that catch the menstrual fluid. You can still buy the old-fashioned kind that fit tightly between your legs, held in place with an elastic belt. Most women prefer pads with an adhesive backing that attach to the panties. Shorter and thinner than regular napkins, minipads are used with a tampon or alone when your flow is light. Perfumed pads and those with artificial fibers may be itchy and irritating; if so, switch brands.

A *tampon* is a small, white cylinder of cotton that fits into the vagina to absorb menstrual fluid before it leaves the body. A string is attached at the bottom for removal. Tampons come in different sizes and absorbencies, with or without scent and applicators.

Here are some tips to follow when using tampons:

Follow instructions carefully. These instructions, which often have drawings, can be very helpful if you're inserting a tampon for the first time. Some companies offer toll-free numbers to call with any questions.

Never choose a tampon with more absorbency

than you need. High-absorbency tampons raise the risk of toxic shock syndrome, a bacterial illness that can be fatal (see box). Rather than using a "super" tampon, choose a lower absorbency and change it more often (tampons should be changed every four to six hours). If your flow is very heavy, wear a tampon and a pad.

Make a decision about applicators. Applicators make tampons easier to insert, but some women don't need them and prefer applicatorless tampons which are smaller, easier to carry, and better for the environment. If you like applicators, be sure they're made of cardboard (not plastic), which is biodegradable.

Understand that scented products are unnecessary. Many women find that scented tampons are irritating to the vulva and vagina. Menstrual fluid doesn't have any odor until it hits the air, so you don't need to use perfumed tampons anyway.

Toward the end of the period, use a pad or smaller-size tampon to avoid pain and vaginal abrasions.

Choose alternative products. The Keeper, for example, is a reusable rubber cup inserted into the vagina to collect menstrual blood. For more information, contact The Keeper, P.O. Box 20023, Cincinnati, OH 45220; (513) 221-1464. You can also find reusable cloth sanitary pads in health food stores. Both of these products save money and the environment.

How We Feel About Our Periods
When some of us saw that first brownish stain in our panties, we were shocked and scared. Because no one had explained how the menstrual cycle worked, many of us simply thought we were sick and bleeding to death. Others were embarrassed, sure that everybody in the world could see huge, bloody stains or worse, could smell the odor of menstrual fluid.

To sell their products, companies that produce tampons, sanitary napkins, and other "feminine hygiene products" play on these fears. In a study of imagery associated with menstruation in advertising targeted to adolescent women, researchers noted that, "The ads depict menstruation as a 'hygienic crisis' that is best managed by an effective 'security system' affording protection and peace of mind." In one magazine ad, a teenage girl was "worried that he (her date) would know I had my period," presumably because of the smell. (Actually the odor isn't so strong—unless the pad isn't changed frequently enough—but has been exaggerated by men who are afraid of menstrual fluid and companies trying to hawk their products.)

Some of us were taught to think of our "time of the month" as an illness. We weren't supposed to exercise, swim, take showers, or have sexual intercourse, and many of us used the monthly excuse to get out of gym class or unwanted sex. (These are, of course, myths; we can participate in all of these activities during menstruation—if we want to.) This idea of menstruation as illness has been used against us by men who say that our periods make us unfit for certain jobs, especially the prized ones, such as the heads of companies or countries. (Who hasn't heard a man say: "How could we have a woman president? What would happen if the country were in a crisis and she got her period?")

Menstrual Problems

Some women skate through their menstrual periods pain-free. They see the bit of breast tenderness they have right before their periods as sexy, and they notice that they feel more creative and sexually aroused several days before the onset of menstruation. These sisters may look at their periods as a bodily cleansing ritual and feel closer to other women during this time. (This could be attributed to menstrual synchrony, the tendency of women in a group to menstruate at the same time.)

Many of us don't feel that way. We have varying degrees and types of menstrual problems from premenstrual symptoms such as bloating and moodiness to cramps or irregular periods. To ease these problems, it's best to understand the facts about your period and what menstrual pain means and come up with solutions that are right for you. Use a calendar to keep track of your menstrual cycle. Jot down when symptoms occur, the remedies you used, and whether or not they worked.

Dysmenorrhea.

This literally means "painful flow," and symptoms can range from mild cramping to incapacitating cramps accompanied by vomiting and diarrhea. There are two types: primary and secondary dysmenorrhea.

Primary dysmenorrhea is menstrual pain that cannot be blamed on another disorder; it is triggered by menstrual-cycle changes that cause contractions in the uterus. It is fairly common in young girls who have just started to menstruate, and many women notice it the first day or two after bleeding begins. No one knows exactly why some women have horrible cramps while others are pain-free, but it may be due to the amount of prostaglandin (a fatty acid similar to a hormone) that is released into the uterus when the lining breaks down every month.

Without definitive answers, you can't stop the pain from coming, you can only relieve it. Here are some of the ways to try.

Ibuprofen. This is a painkiller that works as an antiprostaglandin medication, which you probably know by the over-the-counter brand names Motrin, Advil, Nuprin, and so on. Stronger formulas such as prescription Motrin, Anaprox, and Naproxen are available from a doctor. Remember that all of these medications may cause stomach distress.

Exercise. Yoga, stretching, and aerobic exercise can relieve menstrual cramps by relaxing the muscles and increasing circulation. It certainly can't hurt, and there's absolutely no reason *not* to exercise during your period.

Orgasm. This seems like a wonderful way to get rid of cramps, with or without a partner. The strong orgasmic contractions of the uterus may be followed by relaxation of the organ that provides relief from pain. Some women swear by it as a temporary measure.

Massage. Try massaging your pelvic region while lying on your back with your knees bent. Or ask someone else to massage your lower back. Women with severe cramps may want to try acupuncture.

Heat. This can relax the muscles temporarily, so try a hot water bottle, heating pad, or hot bath.

Eat right. You should be doing this all the time, but it's especially important during your period. Be sure to eat plenty of whole grains and fresh fruit to avoid constipation, which can exacerbate cramping.

Herbal teas. Raspberry leaf, yarrow, chamomile, and black-currant teas are helpful to some women. Other herbs such as lady's mantle may also relieve the pain, but it's best to check with an herbalist or naturopath before experimenting with herbal remedies.

The Pill. Oral contraceptives eliminate ovulation and, in turn, get rid of cramps. Though doctors may immediately recommend the Pill as a solution to dysmenorrhea, it should be used only as a last resort. It's best left to women who have severe problems and need contraception and isn't recommended for young girls.

Menstrual pain that has an underlying cause is referred to as *secondary dysmenorrhea.* It occurs mostly in women over thirty and is generally the result of a disorder such as fibroids, endometriosis, or pelvic inflammatory disease. It is imperative that you have yearly gynecological examinations to make sure that none of these problems is causing your painful periods.

Amenorrhea.
This term refers to the absence of menstruation and occurs in two forms: primary and secondary amenorrhea.

In primary amenorrhea a girl has reached age eighteen and hasn't begun menstruating. But even a sixteen-year-old who hasn't started her period should be seen by a doctor to make sure she doesn't have any reproductive-system abnormalities. Amenorrhea can be embarrassing to young girls who don't want to be "late bloomers," the last girl among her friends to get her period.

Secondary amenorrhea describes menstruation that has started, but then stops. Many women miss their periods occasionally, but several missed periods signal a problem. The most obvious reason is pregnancy, so if you're sexually active with men and your period has ceased, get tested right away. If you're older, stopped periods may be a sign of menopause. Amenorrhea also occurs frequently in young girls whose menstrual cycles haven't yet begun regulating properly. It isn't highly unusual for a girl to have one or two periods and then not see another sign of menstruation for six months or longer.

Other explanations for amenorrhea:

Fluctuations in weight. Losing or gaining as little as five pounds can throw off your period and cause it to cease. Amenorrhea is common in women who have anorexia nervosa, which occurs when a woman has a distorted image of her body and diets, exercises excessively, and/or uses laxatives to become sickly thin. (For more on anorexia, see chapter 1, "Body Image and Weight.") Generally, once your body settles into your new weight or you bring your weight back to healthy levels, your period will return.

Serious illness. Health problems such as diabetes, thyroid disease, anemia, hormonal imbalance, drug abuse, and ovarian cysts or tumors can cause amenorrhea. You must be treated for these medical concerns.

Very strenuous athletic training. It is common for high-level athletes, especially long-distance runners, to lose their periods during times when they are training heavily. Once workout levels are lowered, most women start menstruating again.

Emotional problems. Stress and depression can cause you to miss your period. To find your way out of emotional pain, find a therapist or self-help group.

Birth control pills. Some women skip a period while taking the Pill or when they stop taking it. Talk to your doctor; you may need to switch to a different oral contraceptive. The strength and flow of the period are also greatly reduced when you're on the Pill. If you've just stopped taking the Pill, several months without a period isn't unusual as your ovary reregulates itself. However, if you aren't menstruating after about three months, see your doctor.

Endometriosis.

This is a condition in which cells that make up the lining of the uterus—the endometrium—break away and grow outside of the uterine cavity. They implant themselves in many locations within the pelvic area, including the ovaries, ligaments of the uterus, cervix, appendix, bowel, and bladder. Acting as though they were still in the uterus, these "lost" endometrial cells respond every month to the same hormones produced during the menstrual cycle. In other words, they thicken, enlarge, and bleed as though they were still in the uterus. However, unlike normal bleeding, when these implants bleed they can't be expelled from the body through the vagina. Instead, blood from the refugee cells remains trapped in the pelvis, where it can cause inflammation, cysts, scar tissue, and other structural damage.

Endometriosis affects 7 to 15 percent of women and is more common in white than Black women. The cause has not yet been pinpointed. Some scientists have speculated that it may be an autoimmune condition similar to lupus that is caused by a backup of the menstrual flow, or that it is inherited.

Common symptoms are premenstrual pain and pain during menstruation. Other symptoms depend on where the stray cells land.

Understanding Symptoms of Endometriosis

SITE	SYMPTOM
Vagina	Painful intercourse
Bowel wall	Rectal bleeding, constipation, painful defecation
Ovaries, fallopian tubes	Infertility
Bladder, urethra	Frequent urination, pain in the groin, blood in the urine
Small intestine	Vomiting, abdominal pain, and swelling
Appendix	Pain before menstruation, acute symptoms that mimic appendicitis

In some cases, the endometrial cells travel as far as the thighs, forearms, armpits, and lungs.

Endometriosis is sometimes confused with other conditions such as pelvic inflammatory disease or ectopic pregnancy (pregnancy outside of the uterus). It can be diagnosed preliminarily through a pelvic exam, but a laparoscopy (the insertion of a lighted, tubelike instrument through an incision at the navel) is necessary for a conclusive diagnosis.

Pregnancy offers temporary relief from the disease, although women with endometriosis sometimes can't conceive. However, no one should get pregnant only to get rid of a medical condition. Hormonal treatments and surgery are also used to treat endometriosis.

Taking care of yourself by eating foods high in fiber and B vitamins, getting plenty of rest, exercising, and keeping stress to a minimum may also help. Some women use acupuncture and herbs for relief.

Other Menstrual Problems

Lighter, Shorter Periods. The Pill could cause a change in your period. Lighter, shorter periods may also be the result of menopause.

Heavier, Longer Periods. This may be a sign of fibroid tumors (which are much more common in Black than in white women) or another reproductive-system illness. Women who use the IUD as birth control may also have long, heavy periods because the IUD irritates the lining of the womb. If you notice that you're using more sanitary napkins and tampons or your period is lasting longer, see your doctor.

Bleeding or Spotting Between Periods. This could be a sign of pregnancy or fibroids or another reproductive-system disorder. Sexually transmitted infections such as chlamydia and gonorrhea can cause spotting, and stress can also throw off your hormones and cause spotting as well. New Pill users may notice spotting as the body adjusts to the contraceptive or because they aren't using it correctly. In IUD users, spotting may be a sign that the body is rejecting the IUD and should be removed. In any of these instances, you'll need to see a physician.

Premenstrual Syndrome (PMS)

The front of a greeting card has a drawing of a scary creature with tears running down her cheeks, a hot-water bottle on her head, and fangs coming out of her mouth where her two front teeth should be. Inside the card reads: "Beware—PMS victim." For many women, however, premenstrual syndrome (PMS) is no joke but a set of confusing, sometimes debilitating symptoms experienced each month.

While many women have premenstrual symptoms, PMS is much more distressing. Scientists do not agree on exactly what causes PMS, and some 150 symptoms have been identified with it. And there seem to be just as many remedies. What is clear is that PMS occurs between ovulation and the onset of menstruation, sometime during the two weeks before bleeding begins. The most common symptoms will probably be familiar to you: breast tenderness, fatigue, bloating and weight gain, headache, food craving (generally for chocolate, sugar, and salt), clumsiness, changes in sex drive, acne, mood swings, difficulty concentrating, and crying jags.

Nsenga Warfield-Coppock, Ph.D., a psychologist and president of

Boabab Associates, Inc., in Washington, D.C., has studied PMS in Black women and notes that our symptoms sometimes differ from those experienced by white women. White women tend to report more physical symptoms, while Black women are more likely to complain of emotional problems such as mood swings and irritability, notes Dr. Warfield-Coppock, who began studying PMS because of her own symptoms, which left her "moody, snappy, and with a lack of self-confidence that gave me only about one good week a month."

Dr. Warfield-Coppock speculates that PMS may be more severe in Black women. "Women who have more stress, worse diets, lack exercise, and have a lower ability to take care of themselves will have more PMS. We're talking African-American women," she says.

Though experts and women alike are comfortable discussing symptoms, treatment isn't so easy to pinpoint. With no definitive word on what to do about PMS, you'll have to go through a period of trial and error to determine what works best for you and your particular set of symptoms. Keep an accurate record of your periods, symptoms, and successful treatments, and don't forget to talk to your gynecologist about the problem. Here are some suggested treatments for you to consider:

Dietary Changes. Many women have found success by altering their diets during premenstrual times. Sticking to a diet that is high in carbohydrates and low in fat, sugar, salt, processed foods, caffeine, and alcohol has helped many—but of course, you should be eating that way anyway. Though you may crave salty foods, salt will only exacerbate bloating, and studies have shown that cutting down on or eliminating caffeine has lessened the severity of PMS for many women.

For nutritional advice, read *Premenstrual Syndrome Special Diet Cookbook* by Jill Davies. In her book, Davies discusses the link between PMS symptoms and low blood sugar. To help stave off PMS by keeping blood-sugar levels normal, she recommends eating six small meals that are high in complex carbohydrates (rice, pasta, and whole-wheat bread), rather than the traditional two or three large meals.

Healthy Lifestyle. Exercise, adequate amounts of sleep, sound nutrition, avoiding excessive amounts of alcohol and caffeine, and avoiding smoking at all should already be part of your life. If not, healthy lifestyle changes can help abate PMS symptoms. Exercise proves especially helpful to premenstrual women, perhaps partly because it also helps combat depression.

Progesterone. British doctor Katharina Dalton is the main advocate of treating PMS with supplements of progesterone, the hormone that is

"PMS now means Pamper My Self."

—DANELLA CARTER, WRITER, NEW YORK CITY

Much like a pushy parent, PMS ruled my life for years. I hid my bloated body in a dark room where I indulged in crying jags and bouts of hysteria; fatty food that held my blood cells hostage; more intense sex, but not really because I was so bitchy that no one wanted to be around me. I'd begun to hate my period, an odd concept for someone who bought her first box of napkins two years before I had ever started to bleed.

It was time for a change.

I began by reading as much as I could about premenstrual syndrome and learned that many women control their symptoms by changing their diet. I read that in the ten days prior to my period—at the onset of PMS—the body requires more protein, calcium, and magnesium. I started keeping a daily journal of my moods and a log of the foods I ate, and I noted that my diet was poorest at that time. I would succumb to cravings for salty snacks, chocolate, and sugar.

Though my body buzzed with confusion and rebellion, I replaced the junk food with lentils, white beans, broccoli, and fresh apple juice. I ate bulky foods like brown rice and grains and washed it down with three quarts of liquids daily, mostly water, but also freshly squeezed juices, lemonade, and herbal tea. Cucumber juice was my main tonic, persuading my pimples to camp out elsewhere. Now nutritionally correct with some of my physical symptoms abated, I was better able to deal with my emotional state.

Knowing that I felt like committing murder on the days before my period, I decided that I needed to take care of myself, really take care of myself. Now I treat myself to a facial, foot massage, or body wrap instead of breathing fire. On days I want to pick fights, I peace out with a hot candlelit bath, meditation, or a favorite CD. By day five, I'm ready to deal, so I meet a friend to have afternoon tea or maybe buy myself a gift. During these ten days I pop six capsules per day of an herb called Evening Primrose. By the time I get my period I'm feeling, well, great.

This wasn't an overnight discipline, nor was it a cheap investment. But PMS had dictated my well-being for so long that I was willing to do whatever was necessary to take back my life. I seem to have succeeded because the letters PMS now mean only one thing: Pamper My Self.

secreted during the second half of the menstrual cycle and the time PMS occurs. After making lifestyle changes (cutting down on sugar, processed foods, caffeine, and salt, exercising, and controlling stress), Dr. Warfield-

Coppock went on progesterone therapy, and she swears by it. After a symptom-free two years, she took herself off progesterone but still eats right, exercises, and tries to keep stress under control, and PMS is no longer a problem.

However, many health advocates are wary of women taking hormones—synthetic or natural—because their long-term effect is not known. If your symptoms are very severe, read Dr. Dalton's book *Once a Month: The Original Premenstrual Syndrome Handbook,* and talk about this option with your doctor.

Other Remedies. As one women's health activist noted about PMS treatment: "Everything works for somebody, but nothing works for everybody." See the list of resources at the end of the chapter.

Emotional Help. If you know other women who suffer from PMS, you may want to form a support group to talk about how you feel and what to do about it. If you have emotional problems, hormonal changes that happen before your period may make you feel even worse. If that's the case, find a therapist and get help.

For More Information

ORGANIZATIONS

THE ENDOMETRIOSIS ASSOCIATION, 8585 N. 76th Pl., Milwaukee, WI 53223; (800) 992-3636.

PMS ACCESS, P. O. Box 9326, Madison, WI 53715; (608) 833-4767. Provides free information and resources.

BOOKS

Blood Magic: The Anthropology of Menstruation, Thomas Buckley and Alma Gottlieb, eds., University of California Press, 1988.

The Curse: A Cultural History of Menstruation, Janice Delaney, Mary Jane Lupton, and Emily Toth, University of Illinois Press, 1988.

Endometriosis, Julia Older, Macmillan, 1985.

Fibroid Tumors and Endometriosis: A Self-Help Program, Susan M. Lark, M.D.

Menstrual Health in Women's Lives, Alice Dan and Linda L. Lewis, eds., University of Illinois Press, 1992 (see chapter 16, "Black Women's Responses to Menarche and Menopause" by Beryl Jackson).

Menstruation, Health, and Illness, Diana Taylor and Nancy Woods, Hemisphere Publishing Co., 1991.

Premenstrual Syndrome Self-Help Book: A Woman's Guide to Feeling Good All Month, Susan M. Lark, M.D., Celestial Arts, 1989.

Red Flower: Rethinking Menstruation, Dena Taylor, The Crossing Press (Freedom, Calif.), 1988.

Self-Help for Premenstrual Syndrome, Michelle Harrison, Random House, 1985.

What Women Can Do About Chronic Endometriosis, Judith Sachs, Dell 1991.

Wise Wound: The Myths, Realities and Meanings of Menstruation, Penelope Shuttle and Peter Redgrove, Bantam Books, 1990.

10

Birth Control

As Black women, we must be free to decide whether and when to get pregnant. However, controlling our fertility has never been easy, and it's still plagued with problems. All forms of birth control—from the Pill, which has side effects and has been linked to serious illness such as breast cancer, to condoms, which we don't control because it's men who have to wear them—have some drawback. Nonetheless, birth control is absolutely necessary. The majority of women who are sexually active do not want to conceive and do use some form of birth control. We deserve to be able to make love without the threat of pregnancy, and we must have that right.

Birth Control and You

As individuals we must decide which method to use to prevent pregnancy. It's a complex choice, and one that a woman must decide with her sexual partner. It's also a joint venture. But the final decision lies with the woman, because the responsibility and the consequences are ultimately hers. You should start thinking about birth control early, at the same time you're thinking about having a first sexual encounter. Parents should discuss birth control with their children at the time they first explain pregnancy.

Follow this guide as you choose, and use the method that's right for you. The more you know about each type of contraceptive and the better you understand your own body, the easier the choice will be. The Alan Guttmacher Institute estimates that 47 percent of unplanned pregnancies occur in women who use birth control inconsistently or incorrectly. So whichever method you decide upon, use it correctly, consistently, and carefully.

Birth Control at a Glance

According to the Alan Guttmacher Institute, in the U.S. the five most common forms of birth control are:

1. Sterilization (male and female combined)
2. The Pill
3. Condoms
4. Diaphragm
5. Natural family planning (periodic abstinence)

Methods that are not recommended because failure rates are too high:
- Spermicides alone
- Withdrawal method

Methods that the National Black Women's Health Project recommends be used with caution:
- Depo-Provera (the shot)
- Norplant (implants)

Methods that provide adequate protection against sexually transmitted infections, including HIV:
- Condoms (male and female)

Cervical Cap

How it works: A small rubber device about one and a half inches long, the cap is inserted into the vagina to cover the cervix and form a barrier between the opening of the uterus and the sperm. Spermicide is placed inside the cap to kill any sperm that gets by the barrier.

Cost: The cap itself costs about $30, but the clinic fee for fitting it can be $100 or more.

Failure rate (estimated percentage of U.S. women experiencing an unintended pregnancy in one year of use): When used perfectly, 6 percent. When used by the average couple: 18 percent.

Pros

Entirely controlled by the woman. Unlike the condom, the cap can be inserted in advance to avoid disrupting sexual activity.

No systemic or long-term health problems.

Practical for women who have infrequent intercourse.

When used properly and with spermicide, may provide some protection against sexually transmitted infections. However, it should *not* be relied upon.

Small, easy to use, and can be left in longer than a few hours.

Cons

Not widely available. For a list of practitioners and clinics that fit cervical caps, contact Cervical Cap Ltd., 430 Monterey Ave., suite 1B, Los Gatos, CA 95030; (408) 395-2100.

Cap must be properly fitted by health personnel.

Users must be trained to ensure proper placement over the cervix and to recognize if it has become dislodged during intercourse.

Cannot be totally relied upon to prevent sexually transmitted diseases.

Cap may increase the risk of vaginal infections and abnormal Pap smears.

Who shouldn't use it: Any woman who has lacerations on her cervix shouldn't use the cap, nor anyone who has had toxic shock syndrome (TSS). Associated with tampon use, TSS is very rare but dangerous. The warning signs are fever, vomiting, diarrhea, muscular pain, dizziness, and rash. If you notice two or more of the symptoms, get help immediately.

Tips for using it correctly:

To better avoid pregnancy and to prevent sexually transmitted diseases, use with a condom.

If the size of the uterus changes, the cap should be refitted. It may change following full-term pregnancy, abortion, or miscarriage beyond the first four months, pelvic surgery, or weight change of ten pounds or more.

Choose a spermicide that contains nonoxynol-9.

Male Condom

How it works: A condom is made of latex (thin rubber), and is placed over an erect penis before sexual intercourse. It prevents sperm from entering the vagina.

Cost: About $1 each.

Failure rate (estimated percentage of U.S. women experiencing an unintended pregnancy in one year of use): When used perfectly, 2 percent. When used by the average couple, 16 percent.

Pros

Widely available and easy to find. You can buy them at convenience stores and drugstores.

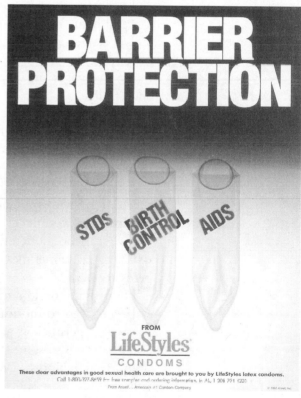

This promotional poster underlines the importance of condoms. *(Courtesy of Healthcare, Ansell Medical)*

Don't cost much.

Provide the best protection against sexually transmitted infections, including the AIDS virus, for both partners.

No systemic or long-term health effects.

Cons

Because they must be used by men, women don't control them. Some men refuse to use them.

Some people complain that they disrupt sexual activity and reduce enjoyment.

Many people use them incorrectly. The failure rate for typical use is fairly high, and breakage during use is common.

Tips for using it correctly:

Carefully take the condom out of the package. Squeeze the tip to remove excess air, which could cause the condom to break. Place it on the tip of his erect penis, and roll it all the way down.

To remove the condom after sex, he should withdraw his penis while it is still hard. You or he should hold on to the rim of the condom as he pulls it out, so nothing spills. Roll the condom off the penis, and discard it. Both of you should avoid further sexual contact until you have washed your sex organs and any other areas that came in contact with body fluids.

Never reuse a condom.

Keep condoms away from extreme heat or cold and direct sunlight. Store in a cool, dry place, but not in a wallet or glove compartment. Remember to check the expiration date.

Be sure to use a latex condom. Avoid "natural" condoms made of sheep or lamb membrane. They are porous and can allow transmission of viruses, including HIV. Some people also believe that colored condoms break more often than the regular type.

Condoms sometimes come in sizes. Make sure the condom fits his penis correctly.

Don't use a condom that feels sticky or brittle or looks damaged.

If you need to lubricate, choose a water-based lubricant such as K-Y jelly or a spermicidal gel or foam. Condoms also come prelubricated, and according to some, these tend to be less prone to breakage than the unlubricated kind. Never use oil-based lubricants such as petroleum jelly, baby oil, or shortening. They can weaken the latex and lead to breaks and tears.

If the condom breaks and semen spills or leaks out, you and your partner should wash wherever you had sexual contact right away.

For best results, use a condom with another form of birth control such as a diaphragm or the Pill. This way, you can better avoid pregnancy and protect against sexually transmitted diseases.

Female Condom

How it works: This new device consists of a thin polyurethane sheath with two flexible rings. One ring lies inside the closed end of the sheath and is used to insert the device and to hold it in place. The other ring remains outside the vagina after insertion. When the man inserts his penis into the woman's vagina, the sheath covers her labia and the tip of his penis. It is prelubricated and is over-the-counter in drugstores and convenience stores.

Cost: $2.50 each.

Failure rate (estimated percentage of U.S. women experiencing an unintended pregnancy in six months of use): When used perfectly, 3 percent. When used by the average couple, 12 percent.

Pros

Completely controlled by the woman.

Will be widely available and easy to find. You'll be able to buy them at convenience and drugstores without needing medical facilities or personnel.

Failure rate is fairly low when used correctly.

Because it is made of polyurethane, which is generally stronger than latex, it is more resistant to tears than the male condom.

Prevents the transmission of sexually transmitted infections.

No systemic or long-term health effects.

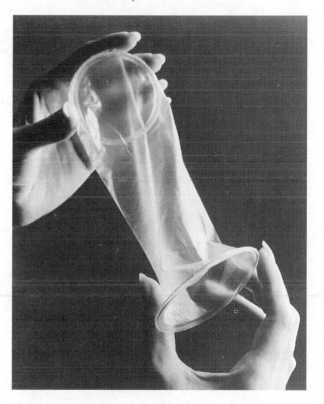

The female condom is one of the newest forms of birth control. *(Courtesy of Wisconsin Pharmacal Co.)*

Cons

Some people complain that they disrupt sexual activity and reduce enjoyment.

Some women have complained that they are unattractive, uncomfortable, somewhat awkward to use, and difficult to insert.

Expensive to use. They cost more than twice as much as the male condom.

Tips for using it correctly:

To insert, squeeze the inner ring and insert it similar to the way you'd put a tampon in. Push the inner ring up as far as it will go. The inner ring should be resting on the cervix, the sheath should fill the vaginal cavity, and the outer ring should be resting on the labia, outside of the vagina.

Each female condom must be used only once and should be discarded like a condom.

What Black women need to know:

In focus group discussions conducted by New Orleans psychiatrist Denese O. Shervington, Black women endorsed the female condom. They did not find it cumbersome or aesthetically unpleasing. Noted Shervington: "Many [women] took ownership of Reality, referring to it as a 'safe shield.'"

Depo-Provera ("The Shot")

How it works: Depo-Provera, an injectable synthetic hormone, which was approved for use in the United States in 1992, is controversial (see "What Black Women Need to Know" below). It has been available in other countries for many years. A synthetic form of the female hormone progesterone, it is shot into a woman's arm or buttock to suppress ovulation. It also thickens the cervical mucus to block sperm and makes the uterine lining unsuitable for implantation. A woman must receive the shot once every three months.

Cost: $25 to $30 per shot plus doctor or clinic fees.

Failure rate (estimated percentage of U.S. women experiencing an unintended pregnancy in one year of use): When used perfectly, .3 percent. When used by the average couple, .4 percent.

Pros

Highly effective and long-acting.

Good for women who want to practice birth control discreetly but have little privacy.

Easy to use. You don't have to take a Pill or insert a device.

May reduce anemia, which is a possible benefit to women with sickle-cell trait.

Cons

Requires regular visits to a physician or clinic for injections.

Return to fertility is often delayed for several months or longer.

Some women experience side effects such as weight gain, menstrual irregularities, headaches, irritability, dizziness, and mood swings. Other reported side effects: depression, hair loss, diminished sex drive, and breast discharge.

Not immediately reversible if side effects occur; it takes three or more months for effects to wear off.

Studies show that Depo-Provera slightly increases the risk of breast cancer in women under thirty-five, and it may also increase the risk of developing cervical cancer. One study suggests that it may temporarily lower bone density, a factor in osteoporosis.

Does not protect against HIV or other sexually transmitted infections.

Who shouldn't use it: Women with acute liver disease, unexplained vaginal bleeding, breast cancer, or blood clots in the legs, lungs, or eye. A woman who suspects she's pregnant should not get the injection, which may cause low birth weight in babies.

What Black women need to know: The National Black Women's Health Project (NBWHP) and other groups such as the National Women's Health Network oppose Depo-Provera. The possible increased risk of breast cancer in women under age thirty-five may be an especially dangerous problem for Black women, who are more likely than other women to develop breast cancer at younger ages.

For Black women, whose health status as a group is poor, Depo-Provera's side effects can be extremely risky. Weight gain caused by the drug can be as high as 20 to 50 pounds in some women. Nearly half of us are obese, and many suffer from problems such as high blood pressure and diabetes, which are worse for overweight women, so we can't afford to take a drug that will exacerbate the problem. Depression is another side effect of Depo-Provera, and given the high levels of stress so many Black women already endure, we can't risk compounding the problem.

Because Depo-Provera must be dispensed through the health-care system, like Norplant, it can easily be administered inappropriately and coercively to poor women and women of color. Incidents of coercive use of the shot have been reported among Black women in South Africa and in Zimbabwe before independence. In the early 1980s, African-American women were part of the Depo-Provera trials in Atlanta. NBWHP believes that many women who signed consent forms and received the shot may not have understood what they were signing or what they were getting.

Diaphragm

How it works: A woman inserts a round soft-rubber device with a flexible rim into her vagina to cover the cervix and form a barrier between the opening of the uterus and the sperm. Spermicide is placed in the diaphragm before insertion to kill any sperm that get past the barrier.

Cost: Between $15 and $35, plus doctor or clinic visit.

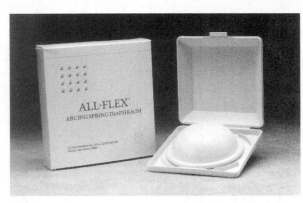

The diaphragm can be inserted before intercourse to retain the spontaneity of sexual activity.
(Photo: Ortho Pharmaceutical Corp.)

Failure rate (estimated percentage of U.S. women experiencing an unintended pregnancy in one year of use): When used perfectly, 6 percent. When used by the average couple, 18 percent.

Pros

Entirely controlled by the woman. Unlike the condom, the diaphragm can be inserted in advance to avoid disrupting sexual activity.

Doesn't cost much.

No systemic or long-term health problems.

Practical for women who have infrequent intercourse.

Can last for at least two years if cleaned and stored in a cool, dry place after each use.

When used properly and with spermicide, may provide some protection against sexually transmitted diseases. However, it should *not* be relied upon.

Cons

Diaphragm must be properly fitted by health personnel.

Users must be trained to ensure proper placement over the cervix and to recognize if the diaphragm has become dislodged during intercourse.

Lack of spontaneity and slight hassle.

Cannot be totally relied upon to prevent sexually transmitted infections.

Who shouldn't use it: Women who are prone to urinary-tract infections. The diaphragm may trigger them. Any woman who is allergic to rubber.

Tips for using it correctly:

Be sure to have your health-care practitioner explain how to insert the diaphragm. When you get home, follow instructions carefully.

Before inserting, place a teaspoonful of contraceptive cream or jelly

I like being able to say that I've never used the Pill. To me, birth control pills are just too much medicine. The idea that you could swallow something that would stop your period seemed like too strong an effect. It also seemed like overkill to take a pill every day when I wasn't having sex nearly that often.

I began using birth control at age nineteen, and I chose the diaphragm for several reasons. For one, I liked that I put it in only when I was going to have sex. Also, I liked getting to know my body—touching my cervix and knowing how to place the diaphragm just so. The experience made me feel empowered, in control of my body. Kind of like the control I feel when I'm driving a car that has a stick shift. Finally, a barrier method seems more natural than other methods like the Pill or Norplant, which are more convenient but alter the body's functions.

I've been happily wedded to the diaphragm for sixteen years, but as with many relationships, this one is under serious reevaluation. I no longer love it in the same way because my life has changed. Now that I'm married to a real live man who is in possession of a healthy sexual appetite, I have sex more often. Now, suddenly, the diaphragm may not be my best choice.

I'd like to have more spontaneous sex, but that's a big problem when you use the diaphragm. Making love in places other than the bedroom and at odd times is vital, but that's not so easy to do when you've got to worry about carrying around an oversized plastic compact.

One compromise has been that my husband takes responsibility half of the time by wearing a condom. He doesn't mind this, but we still have the problem of no spontaneity. We try to remember to keep them next to the bed, but that doesn't always work. Even when it does, we still have our foreplay interrupted, because we have to put the condom on. I have to admit that both the diaphragm and the condoms now seem like a pain. I have even entertained thoughts of getting the Pill.

Struggling with the birth control dilemma has made me realize one thing: There is no perfect method. If men were responsible for controlling births, and it was guys who had to worry about getting pregnant, I'm sure we'd have better options.

"I liked getting to know my body—touching my cervix and knowing how to place the diaphragm just so."

—BENILDE LITTLE, WRITER, SOUTH ORANGE, NEW JERSEY

into the diaphragm, and spread a small amount around the edge with your fingertip.

You can insert the diaphragm up to six hours before intercourse, and it must be left in place for at least six hours following intercourse, but not more than twenty-four hours. If sexual intercourse is repeated, insert additional spermicide into the vagina.

To better avoid pregnancy and to prevent sexually transmitted diseases, use with a condom.

If the size of the uterus changes, the diaphragm should be refitted. It may change following full-term pregnancy, abortion, miscarriage beyond the first four months, pelvic surgery, or weight change of ten pounds or more.

Intrauterine Devices (IUD's)

How it works: A physician inserts a small T-shaped plastic or metal device into the uterus; a string, which extends down into the vagina, is attached to the end of the device. An IUD can remain for up to eight years, depending on the type. How IUD's work is unclear; researchers speculate that the device inhibits the eggs from implanting on the uterine wall or by blocking fertilization by the sperm. Two types are available in the United States: the Copper T380A, also known as TCU-380A (ParaGard), which can be used for four to eight years, and the Progesterone T (Progestasert), which releases progesterone and might need to be replaced yearly. An IUD must be removed by a health professional.

Cost: About $300 plus doctor or clinic fees.

Failure rate (estimated percentage of U.S. women experiencing an unintended pregnancy in one year of use): When used perfectly, .8 percent. When used by the average couple, 4 percent.

Pros

Highly effective and easy to use.

Reversible. Very appropriate for women who want a reversible method but find other methods difficult to use.

It can be inserted right after a baby is delivered or immediately following an abortion without negative health effects.

Can be inserted after unprotected sex to prevent the implantation of the fertilized egg.

Cons

Insertion and removal require access to trained health personnel with appropriate equipment and facilities.

Insertion can sometimes be painful.

May cause irregular or heavy bleeding and occasionally severe cramping.

The device can become expelled from the uterus without the woman knowing it, and in rare cases it can perforate the uterus.

Provides no protection against sexually transmitted infections, including HIV.

IUD's may increase the risk of developing pelvic inflammatory disease. At the time of insertion, microorganisms in the cervix or vagina may enter the uterus and cause infection. However, the risk decreases as time passes.

Tips for using it correctly: Make sure you can feel the string, since it's the only way to know that your IUD is in place. Also, don't skip follow-up visits to your clinic or doctor, especially if you have side effects.

Who shouldn't use it: Women who have unprotected sex with multiple partners are at high risk of contracting sexually transmitted infections and should not choose the IUD.

What Black women need to know: Though the current types of IUD's are safe, it wasn't always that way. Between 1971 and 1974 physicians inserted over 2 million Dalkon Shields, IUD's that looked like metal insects, into American women and sent another 2 million abroad. Black women received the Shield disproportionately because it was promoted and available at health clinics, Planned Parenthood, and city hospitals. But the device turned out to be a time bomb. It brought bacteria into the uterus, causing pelvic inflammatory disease, which often went undetected. Hundreds of thousands of women suffered bleeding, pain, and eventual scarring and blocking of the fallopian tubes. Because of the Shield, many women had abnormal pregnancies or were left sterile.

Thousands of women were part of a class-action suit against Robins Company, the Shield's maker. During the 1980s, IUD usage dropped dramatically, and several models were removed from the market. If by some chance you still have a Dalkon Shield in place or you know someone who does, have it removed immediately.

Natural Family Planning (Periodic Abstinence)

How it works: This method calls for abstaining from sex during times of fertility—just before ovulation when fertility is at it's highest. Some women keep detailed written records of their menstrual cycles to calculate fertile periods, while others monitor the amount and consistency of cervical mucous to determine when they're most fertile. During ovulation, cervical fluid increases and becomes thinner, wetter, and more slippery; just after ovulation it is more sticky and rubbery. Other women take and record their waking body temperature, which dips to below normal during ovulation and then rises to slightly above normal just after it. Natural family planning works best when women keep track of body temperature, cervical mucus, and the menstrual cycle.

Cost: Free.

Failure rate (estimated percentage of U.S. women experiencing an unintended pregnancy in one year of use): When used perfectly, 9 percent. When used by the average couple, 19 percent.

Pros

It's free and can be controlled by the user.

Doesn't require medical personnel, drugs, or devices.

No systemic or long-term health effects.

Increases knowledge of the body and the reproductive cycle.

Increases the chances of conception when the woman is ready to have a child because she will understand when her fertile periods are.

Cons

Failure rates are high.

May require up to two weeks of abstinence.

Several months of practice are required to interpret symptoms correctly, and the user must be meticulous about record keeping.

Vaginal infection, stress, fever, and other health problems may alter signs of fertility and lead to inaccurate calculation of fertile period.

Doesn't protect against sexually transmitted infections.

Who shouldn't use it: This method works best for couples and is not suggested for unpartnered women who are more likely to have sex spontaneously.

Tips for using it correctly:

You must keep very good records of your menstrual cycle and the changes in your body that go with it.

You must also have the cooperation of your partner. Natural family planning doesn't work unless you abstain from sex during your fertile periods.

Most experts believe that the ovulation method is the most accurate method of natural family planning. Community organizations and religious institutions sometimes offer classes to teach this method, and charting kits are available. You can also use over-the-counter ovulation predictor kits for accurate readings.

My experiences with birth control have been frustrating, to say the least. I've tried the sponge. I've tried the diaphragm. Foam. Suppositories. Condoms. All of them required some kind of elaborate preparation process. Putting in the diaphragm was a joke. My partner would have a reaction to the spermicide. I would have reactions to the spermicide. I was worried about complications from putting those chemicals in my body, and so was my partner. And I didn't want to be on the Pill because I didn't want to interrupt the natural processes of my body.

I discovered natural family planning in 1990. I was in a health-food store one day, and I found a book, Your Fertility Signals: Using Them to Achieve or Avoid Pregnancy, Naturally by Merryl Winstein. It was exactly what I'd been looking for. I'm very much into preventive health and the natural ways of healing ourselves. Even so, I was surprised at how much I didn't know about my body. I learned that every month, the cervix secretes a slippery mucus discharge signaling that your body is fertile. You're considered to be fertile any day the mucus is present, plus four dry days after the mucus ends. I never knew that—I just assumed it was discharge. Now I know that once you understand the signals in your body, you know when you're fertile. If you are trying to get pregnant, that's helpful. If you're not, that's helpful too. But don't get me wrong: This isn't the rhythm method. This is very scientific.

Soon, using this method became very natural to me. I loved being in tune with my body and my reproductive health. And it was certainly cost-effective. And knowing when I'm fertile helps me predict when I'm going to have PMS symptoms. Of course, to do this method properly, you need the support of a stable partner. You really need someone who is cooperative and concerned about your well-being and your health. He's got to be patient, too: Your body doesn't always cooperate with anniversaries and romantic evenings or with making up after a fight. Once I was fertile on Valentines' Day! We had to be very disciplined. We learn about other ways to make love without intercourse, such as taking a bubble bath together. But there are times when we'd get frustrated, and we'd fall back on a condom and spermicide.

Discovering this method was incredibly important to me as an African-American woman. We're not educated about our bodies. Using natural family planning helped me feel less alienated from my body. This way, I took control of my body and my life.

> "Using natural family planning helped me feel less alienated from my body."
>
> —AARONETTE WHITE, SOCIAL PSYCHOLOGY PROFESSOR, ST. LOUIS

For more information on the ovulation method write to Family of the Americas Foundation, P.O. Box 1170, Dunkirk, MD, 20754-1170; (800) 443-3395 or (301) 627-3346. You can also read *Love & Fertility* by Mercedes Arzu Wilson, published by the Family of the Americas Foundation, and *Your Fertility Signals: Using Them to Achieve or Avoid Pregnancy, Naturally* by Merryl Winstein.

Norplant (Implants)

How it works: Norplant is controversial; see "What Black women need to know" below. First the upper arm is numbed with a local anesthetic. Through a small incision, the health-care practitioner inserts six thin, matchstick-size Norplant capsules under the skin in an arc formation. Each capsule contains the synthetic hormone progestin. Released at a slow, steady rate, progestin suppresses ovulation, thickens cervical mucus to block sperm, and makes the uterine lining unsuitable for implantation. The procedure takes about fifteen minutes, and protection lasts for five years.

Cost: $400 to $600 for the capsules and procedure.

Failure rate (estimated percentage of U.S. women experiencing an unintended pregnancy in one year of use): .05 percent.

Pros

Highly effective.

Good for women who are not planning to have children or who have had enough children but don't want to be sterilized. Also good for women who aren't planning children for a few years.

Easy to use. You don't have to take a pill or insert a device.

Reversible. Once the implants are removed, a woman can get pregnant. Or they can be removed if side effects occur.

Good for women who want a reversible method but find other forms of birth control difficult to use or lack a reliable source of contraceptive supplies.

May reduce anemia, which is a possible benefit to women with sickle-cell trait.

Cons

The majority of users report irregular bleeding—either spotting between periods or throughout the month. (Some women had enough bleeding to require a panty liner.) Other women report long periods, while others stop menstruating altogether. In most cases, the irregular bleeding disappears in a few months.

Other reported side effects: headaches, sore breasts, enlarged ovaries, acne, moodiness, nausea, slight weight gain or loss, gain or loss of facial hair.

Though it's inexpensive in the long run, several hundred dollars is too much for some women to pay on the front end.

Implants are less effective for large women, those weighing over 150 pounds. This is an important factor for Black women to note, since we have so many large sisters in our community.

Cannot be removed by the user, and removal is more difficult than insertion.

Scar tissue may form around the implants, especially if they are inserted improperly. This is a problem for us because of our tendency to form keloids.

Does not protect against HIV or other sexually transmitted infections.

Although five-year studies show no adverse effects on women, the long-term safety of Norplant (beyond five years) has not been determined. No one knows the effect on women and the children they bear after using Norplant.

Who shouldn't use it: Women with undiagnosed genital bleeding, known or suspected pregnancy, acute liver disease or tumors, known or suspected breast cancer. Women who smoke heavily are also advised against using Norplant. Women with health histories that include diabetes, high cholesterol, high blood pressure, cardiovascular disease, migraines, depression, epilepsy, gallbladder or kidney disorders should consider Norplant use with extreme caution.

Signs that something might be wrong: Serious problems are rare but possible. These are the warning signs:

- Vaginal bleeding that is heavier than your normal period
- Delayed menstruation after a long period of regular cycles
- Arm pain
- Severe lower abdominal pain
- Pus or bleeding at the implant site
- One of the implants seems to be coming out

What Black women need to know: While Norplant is a safe, effective option for some women, as described above, it has been used coercively. The fact that some policy makers and opinion leaders see this birth control drug as a potential tool to be used against the poor and women of color is inhumane and unconscionable. We must monitor and organize action against the offering of so-called "incentives" that limit choice of contraceptives, punitive and racially discriminatory regulations, and legislation targeting poor women.

The Pill

How it works: A woman takes a small tablet containing synthetic hormones every day for either twenty-one or twenty-eight days. There are

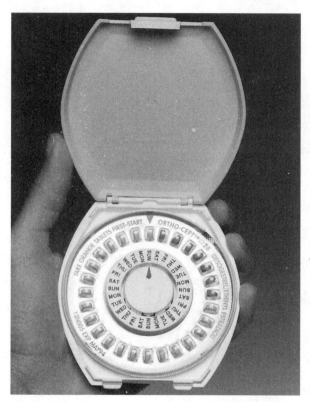

two types: combined oral contraceptives (birth control pills) and progestin-only oral contraceptives (minipills). The combined birth control pill contains estrogen and progestin, which suppress ovulation, thicken cervical mucus to block passage of sperm, and thin the endometrial lining. The minipill contains only progestin.

Cost: About $10 to $20 a month plus doctor or clinic fees.

Failure rate (estimated percentage of U.S. women experiencing an unintended pregnancy in one year of use): When used perfectly, .1 percent. When used by the average couple: 6 percent.

The Pill is the country's most common nonsurgical form of contraception. (*Photo: Ortho Pharmaceutical Corp.*)

Pros
Entirely controlled by the woman.

Highly effective and reversible.

Protects against cancer of the ovaries and uterus as well as ovarian cysts and benign breast cysts. It also reduces the risk of some pelvic infections and ectopic pregnancies.

Causes lighter, regular periods and less cramping.

Doesn't interrupt sex.

Cons
Requires strict daily pill taking.

Requires a prescription and medical personnel.

For women who smoke, it may increase the risk of blood clots.

Some women experience a slight weight gain (it generally levels off or disappears after the first month), as well as spotting between periods and tender breasts. Less frequently, women complain of nausea and mood swings.

Does not protect against sexually transmitted infections, including HIV.

Who shouldn't use it: The combined birth control pill contains estrogen, which is not recommended for women who have diabetes, high blood pressure, or are prone to headaches. Women who have problems with estrogen should not take the combined birth control pill but can take the minipill. The combined birth control pill may also reduce the quantity of breast milk, especially if used within six weeks after delivery. The combined pill may also delay fertility for several months following discontinuation. Neither of these problems is associated with the minipill. However, the minipill is slightly less effective than the combined pill. Discuss the pros and cons of each pill with your doctor to determine which one is right for you.

Tips for using it correctly: You must take the Pill regularly for it to work. It's best to take your pill at the same time each day so pill taking becomes routine.

What Black women need to know: In the 1960s and '70s, experts warned that taking the Pill increased the risk of cancer and heart disease. That led many women to stop taking it or to avoid it altogether. However, today's Pill contains much lower dosages of hormones, and new studies indicate that those health risks no longer exist. In fact, for women who don't smoke, the Pill can reduce the risk of cancer. The only exception is the relationship between the Pill and breast cancer; that remains somewhat unclear. The Pill appears to *increase* the risk of breast cancer for younger women and *decrease* the risk in older women. Older women are more likely to contract breast cancer than younger women. However, breast cancer is more common in young Black women (under age thirty-five) than in young white women.

All of this is complicated. It's best to have a detailed discussion with your doctor about the risks and benefits of the Pill for you.

Spermicides

How it works: Foam, cream, jelly, or a suppository is inserted into the vagina up to fifteen minutes before intercourse. This creates a barrier that kills sperm on contact and inhibits their movement up the vagina into the cervix.

Cost: About $4 to $12 for a tube or canister.

Failure rate (estimated percentage of U.S. women experiencing an unintended pregnancy in one year of use): When used perfectly, 3 percent. When used by the average couple, 30 percent.

Pros

Completely controlled by the woman.

Is widely available and easy to find. You can buy them at convenience and drugstores without needing medical facilities or personnel.

Provides some protection against sexually transmitted infections.

No systemic or long-term effects.

Cons

Extremely high rate of failure when used by the average person.

Sometimes causes itching and burning. Some people don't like the mess and odor.

Must wait fifteen minutes before intercourse takes place, and lasts only an hour.

Who shouldn't use it: This method is not a reliable form of birth control, nor does it provide adequate protection against sexually transmitted infections including HIV. It should be used with a condom.

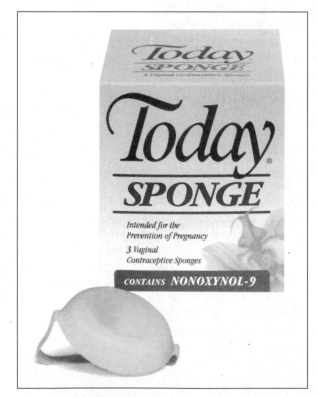

The contraceptive sponge can be purchased over the counter. (*Courtesy of Whitehall-Robins*)

The Sponge

How it works: A soft, dome-shaped sponge saturated with spermicide is inserted into the vagina prior to intercourse. It covers the cervix to block sperm from entering the vagina, and the spermicide kills any sperm that gets by the barrier. It remains effective for about an hour.

Cost: About $4 for three sponges.

Failure rate (estimated percentage of U.S. women experiencing an unintended pregnancy in one year of use): When used perfectly, 9 percent. When used by the average couple, 24 percent.

Pros

No systemic or long-term health effects.

It is controlled by the woman and does not require trained providers or medical facilities.

Can be left in place for twenty-four hours.

Good for women who have only infrequent sexual intercourse.

Provides limited protection against some sexually transmitted infections.

Cons
The failure rate when used by the average person is fairly high.

The sponge is expensive when used routinely.

Some women (and men) are allergic to the spermicide the sponge contains. This can lead to itching, irritation, and a rash.

Who shouldn't use it: Any woman who has had toxic shock syndrome (TSS) should not use the sponge. Associated with tampon use, TSS is very rare but dangerous. The warning signs are fever, vomiting, diarrhea, muscular pain, dizziness, and rash. If you notice two or more of these symptoms, get help immediately.

Tips for using it correctly: For the sponge to be effective, you must wait six hours after the last act of intercourse before removing it. Never leave the sponge in longer than about thirty hours after insertion.

Sterilization, Female (Tubal Ligation, Tubectomy)
How it works: The world's most widely used contraceptive method, voluntary female sterilization is a surgical procedure to block the fallopian tubes and prevent sperm from reaching and fertilizing eggs. Most are performed under general anesthesia (which means the patient is unconscious), but it can also be done under local anesthesia and is fairly simple. A small incision is made in the lower abdomen, and the fallopian tubes are cut and tied, clipped or cauterized.

Cost: $1,000 to $2,500.

Failure rate (estimated percentage of U.S. women experiencing an unintended pregnancy in one year of use): When used perfectly, .2 percent. When used by the average couple, .5 percent.

Pros
Highly effective.

Entirely controlled by the woman.

One-time procedure with little long-term follow-up care required.

No hassle; nothing to insert and no pill to take.

Cost is relatively low if spread out over years of effectiveness.

Good for women who do not want children or more children.

Cons
Generally not reversible. Though it can sometimes be reversed through microsurgery, that operation is more expensive and complicated.

High initial cost and requires a skilled practitioner and appropriate facilities.

The Morning-After Pill

Sometimes accidents happen: The condom breaks, the diaphragm slips out of place, a woman forgets to take the Pill or has unprotected sex. At worst, she gets raped. In these instances there is an alternative to getting pregnant and having an abortion or taking the pregnancy to term. It's called the morning-after pill, and most women don't know a thing about it.

The name "morning-after pill" is catchier, but experts prefer the term "emergency contraceptive pills (ECP's)." Most commonly, the method works this way: Within seventy-two hours after unprotected sex or birth control failure, a woman takes two combined contraceptive pills (this is the Pill that contains both estrogen and progestin), then twelve hours later takes two more. Depending on exactly when the woman takes them, the ECP's either prevent fertilization or stop the fertilized egg from implanting in the lining of the uterus.

In Canada and several European countries doctors prescribe birth control pills for morning-after use. Here, the Food and Drug Administration has not approved the Pill for morning-after use; however, ECP's are not illegal. Some Planned Parenthood clinics offer them, and emergency rooms often provide them to women who have been raped. Many doctors have never heard of this method, but you can request a prescription from your doctor. Clinics that receive federal funding cannot offer ECP's, and manufacturers of the birth control pill are not allowed to market them for morning-after use.

To read a full-scale discussion of ECP's, see "The Morning-After Pill: A Well-Kept Secret" in the January 10, 1993, issue of The New York Times Magazine.

As with any surgery, general anesthesia involves some risk.

Complaints after surgery include temporary pain or discomfort.

Does not protect against sexually transmitted infections.

Who shouldn't use it: A woman should not consider sterilization unless she is positive that her childbearing days are over. It should be thought of as a permanent method.

Tips to use it correctly: You must find a skilled surgeon. Get a referral from the Association for Voluntary Surgical Contraception, 79 Madison Ave., 7th floor, New York, NY 10016; (212) 561-8000. Be sure to ask how many operations of this type she or he has performed.

Sterilization, Male (Vasectomy)

How it works: Vasectomy is a surgical procedure that keeps sperm out of a man's semen. Sperm is made in the testicles and passes through tubes to glands where they mix with other fluids that make up semen. In a vasectomy, each tube—called vas deferens—is blocked. The newest procedure is called the "no-scalpel method," which requires a small puncture rather than cutting the tubes.

Cost: $250 to $500.

Failure rate (estimated percentage of U.S. women experiencing an unintended pregnancy in one year of use): When used perfectly, .1 percent. When used by the average couple, 0.2 percent.

Pros

Highly effective.

Safe and simple. It is simpler than female sterilization and generally performed at a doctor's office under local anesthesia.

One-time procedure with little long-term follow-up care required.

No hassle; nothing to insert and no pill to take.

Cost is low if spread out over years of effectiveness. Cheaper than female sterilization.

Good for couples who do not want children or more children.

Cons

Generally not reversible. Though it can sometimes be reversed through microsurgery, that operation is expensive and complicated.

High initial cost and requires a skilled practitioner and appropriate facilities.

Not controlled by the woman. If a man claims that he's had a vasectomy, there's no way for a woman to confirm it.

Complaints after surgery include temporary pain or discomfort, swelling, bruising, and bleeding.

Does not protect against sexually transmitted infections.

Who shouldn't use it: This procedure is best for couples who have completed childbearing. It should not be thought of as reversible. Also, two 1993 studies found that a vasectomy may increase a man's risk of developing prostate cancer. Because Black men are more likely than white men to contract this type of cancer, a Black man must discuss vasectomy carefully with his doctor before choosing it as a birth control method.

Tips for using it correctly: A man must find a skilled surgeon. Get a referral from the Association for Voluntary Surgical Contraception, 79 Madison Ave., 7th floor, New York, NY 10016; (212) 561-8000. Be sure to find out how many operations of this type she or he has performed.

What Black couples need to know: Many men shy away from vasectomy, worried that it will affect their manhood or masculinity. This is not the case. Male sterilization is not castration. No glands or organs are removed. Hormones and sperm continue to be produced. Sperm are just absorbed into the body. Vasectomy will not affect a man's ability to get or maintain an erection. It will also have little effect on ejaculation; sperm make up only about 5 percent of ejaculate.

Withdrawal (Coitus Interruptus)

How it works: The man rapidly pulls his penis out of the vagina before he is about to ejaculate.

Cost: Free.

Failure rate (estimated percentage of U.S. women experiencing an unintended pregnancy in one year of use): When used perfectly, 4 percent. When used by the average couple, 24 percent.

Pros

Requires no device or medical personnel.

Can be done on the spot.

Is free and requires no training.

Cons

Has an extremely high failure rate. Accidents are easy, and preejaculation fluid, which contains sperm and viruses, gets into the vagina.

Doesn't protect against sexually transmitted infections that can be passed, for example, through sores.

Interrupts lovemaking.

What Black women need to know: Withdrawal is not an acceptable method of birth control.

For More Information

ORGANIZATIONS

THE ALAN GUTTMACHER INSTITUTE, 120 Wall St., 21 floor, New York, NY 10003; (212) 248-1111. Provides information and statistics about contraception and women's reproductive health.

AMERICAN COLLEGE OF OBSTETRICIANS AND GYNECOLOGISTS, 409 12th St. SW, Washington, DC 20024-2188; (202) 638-5577. Provides literature about women's reproductive health.

AMERICAN SOCIAL HEALTH ASSOCIATION, P.O. Box 13827, Research Triangle Park, NC 27709; (919) 361-8400. Provides educational materials on sexually transmitted infections and contraception.

ASSOCIATION OF REPRODUCTIVE HEALTH PROFESSIONALS, 2401 Pennsylvania Ave. NW, suite 350, Washington, DC 20037; (202) 466-3825. Provides educational materials on sexual and reproductive health.

CENTERS FOR DISEASE CONTROL, 1600 Clifton Rd. NE, Atlanta, GA 30333; (404) 639-3311. Offers information on sexually transmitted infections and reproductive health.

ADVOCATES FOR YOUTH, 1025 Vermont Ave. NW, suite 200, Washington, DC 20005; (202) 347-5700. Provides information on youth sexuality and reproductive health.

FAMILY HEALTH INTERNATIONAL, P.O. Box 13950, Research Triangle Park, NC 27709; (919) 544-7040. Request printed information on contraceptive health.

PLANNED PARENTHOOD FEDERATION OF AMERICA, 810 7th Avenue, New York, NY 10019; (800) 829-7732 or (212) 541-7800. Pamphlets on health topics, contraception, and sexuality, or call (800) 230-PLAN to find a clinic.

REPRODUCTIVE HEALTH TECHNOLOGIES PROJECT, 1601 Connecticut Ave. NW, suite 801, Washington, DC, 20009; (202) 328-2200. For information about abortion, RU-486, and other forms of reproductive-health technology.

11

Abortion

In our community, the issue of abortion has produced contradictions. Though as Black women we are twice as likely as white women to have abortions, it was long assumed that we didn't support abortion rights. Because most opinion polls ignore or exclude us, the myth persisted. Supposedly we disapproved of abortion because of our strong religious roots and because we saw the procedure as genocide, a white plot to kill our babies.

In 1991, however, the Communications Consortium Media Center and the National Council of Negro Women Inc. conducted the Women of Color Reproductive Health Poll, a landmark study that refuted many previously held assumptions about our attitudes toward abortion. The study showed that 83 percent of African-American women believe that a woman should be able to make her own decision about abortion. Eighty-five percent believe that it is wrong for anti-choice demonstrators to block women from entering abortion clinics, and 76 percent reject the notion that abortion is a white-engineered genocidal plot. Sixty-two percent believe there should be federal funding for poor women's abortions.

Abortion History
During slavery, plantation owners—who relied on slave labor to keep the economy alive—forbade any kind of birth control among slaves.

They profited directly from Black babies who would grow into workers, a valuable commodity. Forced breeding and rape were the norm, so any attempt among slaves to abort was met with the wrath of the slave owners—even though abortion was actually legal in America until 1800. Nonetheless, slave narratives mention concoctions from a "root gotten from the woods" and other brews used to abort. In fact, some slave women used abortion as a way to revolt against slavery by taking control of their own fertility.

The first large antiabortion fight began around the turn of the nineteenth century as physicians and a few denominations of the Protestant church campaigned against abortion. Neither group had pure motives. The doctors used the campaign as a way to limit herbalists and midwives (who often dispensed potions that induced abortion) from practicing. The Protestants, worried that the numbers of Catholics, Blacks, and other ethnic minorities were growing too fast, opposed abortion, but *specifically* for middle-class Protestant white women. By the twentieth century, every state had some kind of criminal statute against abortion.

Between that time and the landmark 1973 *Roe* v. *Wade* decision, which legalized abortion, millions of women underwent illegal abortions, and each year thousands died or were left infertile as a result of these "back-alley" procedures. Most often, victims were women of color and poor women who couldn't afford or didn't have access to private physicians who could perform safe abortions; or they were women who couldn't travel to the few states where abortion wasn't completely outlawed. In the early seventies, just before *Roe* v. *Wade,* the death rate from illegal abortions for women of color was twelve times that of white women.

Out of desperation, women resorted to drastic means. They inserted pens, pencils, crochet hooks, umbrella ribs, knitting needles, hatpins, curtain rods, and the infamous coat hanger into the uterus to expel the fetus. Others drank or douched with quinine, turpentine, bleach, drain cleaner, hydrogen peroxide, or toxic combinations of herbs—and died from poisoning.

Following the legalization of abortion in January 1973, however, death from abortion dropped dramatically. Today the risk of death is actually lower for a woman undergoing abortion than for pregnancy and childbirth.

Despite the anti-choice view that women decide to abort frivolously and for selfish reasons, most women struggle over this very difficult

Facts About Abortion

Who has abortions and why?

Women of color have more than twice as many abortions as our white counterparts.

Young women—ages eighteen to twenty-four—have the highest abortion rate. Most turn to abortion because they cannot afford to have a baby or because they aren't ready to be a parent or don't want a child.

Most women (82 percent) are unmarried at the time of the abortion.

More than 50 percent of the pregnancies among U.S. women are unintended, and half of these are terminated by abortion.

When do women have abortions?

Though antiabortion activists would like you to think otherwise, 90 percent of women have abortions in the first trimester of pregnancy. And half of all abortions are obtained in the first eight weeks of pregnancy.

Only about .01 percent of abortions take place after twenty-four weeks.

How safe is abortion?

The risk of complication is minimal—less than 1 percent of all abortion patients experience a major complication associated with the procedure.

The risk of death associated with childbirth is about eleven times higher than that associated with abortion.

Who pays for abortion?

At last count, only 12 percent of all abortions in the U.S. were paid for with public funds, virtually all of which were state funds.

For every $1 spent by government to pay for abortions for poor women, about $4 is saved in public medical and welfare expenditures incurred as a result of unintended birth.

—from the Alan Guttmacher Institute

decision and may suffer physical and emotional consequences, though it differs for each woman.

If You Need an Abortion

Before you make the decision to get an abortion, first you'll need to make sure that you're actually pregnant and, if so, exactly how far along you are. Even if you've used a home pregnancy test and gotten a positive result, you'll still need to be tested by a health professional, since home test kits are sometimes inaccurate—especially if used incorrectly. Doctors and abortion clinics always perform their own test and internal examination, even if this has been done elsewhere, before scheduling an abortion.

Deciding to get an abortion is a straightforward choice for many women—especially those who are sure that they aren't ready to raise a child, can't afford one, or don't want to do it alone. After they've had abortions, most women are comfortable with the choice and have no regrets, positive that they did the right thing.

For others, weighing whether or not to abort can be an excruciating process. Though polls show that the majority of Americans favor a woman's right to choose, right-wing politicians and anti-choice terrorists have loudly worked to convince us that abortion is at the least selfish and at worst murder. These extremists prey on women's worst fears and the ambivalence many of us have about the control of our reproduction and our lives. But the decision to conceive or have a child belongs to each individual woman and to her alone. That choice is sanctioned by law. She is the one who will have to live with that decision long after the antiabortionists have moved on to terrorize the next pregnant woman.

Though the choice is ultimately yours, you don't have to make it alone. Talk to someone you trust, such as a close friend or partner who cares about you, a parent or family member you're comfortable with, or a teacher, social-service counselor, or therapist. Most clinics that perform abortions offer some kind of group or individual counseling.

Your decision may be difficult, but it's important not to put it off: Abortions that take place between seven and thirteen weeks of pregnancy are safer, easier, and less expensive than later abortions, which are more complex.

Barriers to Abortion

For many women, especially those who are poor and of color, a number of state restrictions hinder our ability to have an abortion. Here are some of the roadblocks to abortion, depending on where you live:

Funding. In most states a woman cannot use Medicaid to pay for an abortion unless her life is in danger. (A few states allow public funding in additional circumstances, for example, if the pregnancy resulted from rape or incest.) Only twelve states fund most or all abortions.

Minors' access. Most states prevent women under eighteen from obtaining abortions without parental consent or notice.

Informed consent/intimidation requirements. Half of all states have laws that require health care workers to give women seeking abortion intimidating or irrelevant state-prepared materials designed to dissuade them from having abortions. However, some states don't enforce the law.

"That abortion will be with me forever. But I don't regret it."

—Name withheld, unemployed, Chicago

I knew I was pregnant when my period didn't come. And when I started feeling real queasy in the morning and in the afternoon, I thought, "Woooooo—what am I going to do?"

I'm not married, my partner wasn't with me, and there was no guarantee that he'd be by my side. I already have an eight-year-old daughter and a fifteen-month-old baby. I want things out of life; I don't want to be on public aid forever. I'd like to go to college and become a nurse or maybe even a computer programmer.

But things had been hard lately. On New Year's Eve, my neighbors broke into my apartment. They stole clothes, my baby's clothes, his stroller. They ripped up my baby's books and even stole my diaphragm. I told the police, but that just made things worse, and the neighbors started threatening my life. I started sleeping with a butcher knife under my bed.

At that point, my mind was not in a state to deal with another baby. I was depressed, still am. I felt like a little bit of nobody. I was going through too many changes to be pregnant. But I knew my stomach would get bigger and bigger and my problems would get closer and closer.

I went to the doctor and asked him was there a place where he knew I could get an abortion. He refused to give me any information on it. He told me it was a sin for me to kill my baby. He went on and on about the Lord and told me his church would find someplace to take care of my baby. He gave me a bunch of religious pamphlets. He made me feel bad, and I cried.

The one good thing that doctor gave me was an ultrasound to see how far along I was. He gave me a copy of the sonogram and asked me if I wanted to see what my baby looked like. I could see where his head and feet and legs and heart would grow. I still have it. I keep it as a reminder, so that I won't put myself in that position ever again.

Eventually I found someone who would do the abortion at Planned Parenthood, and my partner came through with the money. I don't know what I would have done if he hadn't had it. I didn't want to give the baby up for adoption, because I'd always wonder if my baby was okay. If it was being abused, if it was in a nice home, if it was being taken care of.

The waiting room at the abortion clinic was packed. I was nervous and shocked to see how many young girls were going through what I was going through. But the worst thing was all the questions. Everybody was asking me questions. It was really awkward. They kept counseling me, telling me to focus on trying to forgive myself. But a lot of what they were telling me kept going in one ear and out the other. And the more they talked about it, the more nervous I got.

The pain. It's not the same type of pain that you get from having a baby. I felt like I was going through this pain—raising the money and going through all that trouble—to kill a baby. That's a hurting pain. When you're having a baby, you're sweating and hollering, but it's a happy pain. When you're done, you have something to look at. For me, the abortion was the worst kind of pain to have; you have nothing to show for it.

That abortion will be with me forever. But I don't regret it. People can tell you what to do, but they're not going to be there to help me with the baby. I made the right decision.

Facilities. A handful of states ban abortions in public facilities such as public-health clinics.

Because the laws vary state by state and are subject to change, call the National Abortion Rights Action League or the National Abortion Federation hotline for specific information and updates (numbers listed at the end of the chapter).

Choosing a Facility

Abortions are generally performed by medical or osteopathic doctors in clinics, doctors' offices, and sometimes in hospitals. In some states other practitioners such as physician's assistants can legally perform the procedure. The vast majority (83 percent) of abortions are performed at freestanding clinics, which may or may not specialize in abortion. Women who are low-income, eligible for Medicaid, or are women of color are much more likely than wealthier white women to have abortions in hospitals. Many low-income women utilize hospitals for most of their medical care; in many communities, the hospital may be the only available health-care facility. In the case of late-term abortions (in which the procedure is more complicated and, while still relatively safe, carries more risk) hospital care may be necessary. And, sad to say, many poor women are forced to resort to late abortion in hospitals because they are unable to get the fee together earlier in their pregnancies.

Costs vary depending on the location, but the average charge for a clinic abortion at ten weeks is $245, and the price may be more than double that for the same procedure performed in a hospital. The later in the pregnancy, the more the abortion will cost: The average price of a clinic abortion at sixteen weeks is $509; at twenty weeks of pregnancy the price increases to $897.

In general, when you check out any kind of facility, it's important to ask the following questions:

What kind of pre- and postabortion counseling does the facility provide? How many (if any) of the counselors are women of color?

How does payment work? Do I have to pay the fee all at once? Is any of the fee covered by Medicaid or private health insurance?

Can I get other services, such as a Pap smear, birth control counseling, breast exam, tests for sexually transmitted infections? How will I have to pay for those additional tests? What kind of follow-up services are available?

Can I bring a friend or family member with me during the procedure? Is child care provided?

In checking out facilities, the National Abortion Rights Action League warns women to beware of fake abortion clinics. These are bogus facilities set up to lure pregnant women who want abortions. They are sometimes listed in the Yellow Pages under "abortion," and they appear to provide abortion services. But once a woman gets to the bogus clinic, she is given false information by anti-choice extremists trying to frighten her out of having an abortion. Also, Operation Rescue and other right-wing groups sometimes target abortion clinics by picketing and harassing clients and personnel. If this is happening at the time you must visit the clinic, bring a friend along, and stay strong in your decision.

For help in choosing a facility in your area, the National Abortion Federation provides a confidential, toll-free hotline: (800) 772-9100, or (202) 667-5881 in Washington, D.C.

The Abortion Procedure

At the facility you've chosen, a physician should explain the procedure and tell you what to expect. She or he should answer any questions you have and explain any risks. You'll also need a pregnancy test (even if you've had one somewhere else), blood tests to check for anemia and RH factor, and a brief physical examination. After confirming how far along you are (health-care professionals call this LMP, which refers to the number of weeks since your last menstrual period), your physician will determine the type of abortion you'll need.

First-Trimester Abortion

Nearly all abortions take place during the first trimester or the first three months of pregnancy. The standard method is called vacuum aspiration

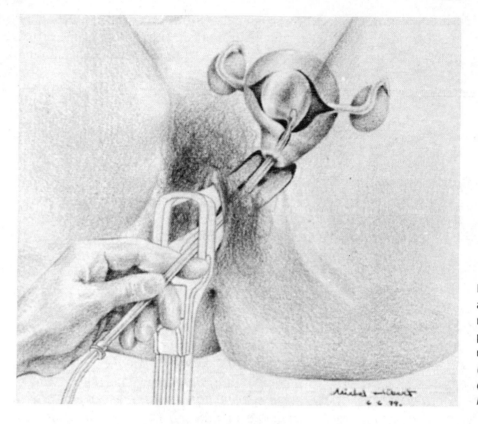

In first-trimester abortions, suction removes the fetus and placenta from the uterus.
(Drawing: Michel Hebert; courtesy of Montreal Health Press, Montreal)

or suction curettage and is performed safely on an outpatient basis with local anesthesia.

You will lie on your back on an examining table with your feet in stirrups, as you would for a pelvic examination. The doctor inserts a closed speculum (widening tool) into the vagina, then opens it to hold the vaginal walls apart. At this point, she or he will usually clean the vagina and then administer the local anesthesia.

The physician will then gradually widen (dilate) the cervix, increasing the size until the opening is about 1/2 inch or the size of a drinking straw. She or he will then insert a small tube, which is attached to an aspirator machine; it's like the small suction device dentists use to clear the mouth of saliva. The machine's suction empties the contents of the uterus. Then the doctor checks the walls of the uterus with a small, spoon-shaped instrument (curette) to make sure no placental tissue is left. The entire procedure takes about ten minutes and is usually followed by some light vaginal bleeding. (The bleeding can last for up to a week or occasionally longer. You should call the doctor if the bleeding is causing severe cramping or is soaking more than one regular-size sanitary pad per hour.) Some women will also notice pain (similar to menstrual cramps) during the procedure and for some time afterward. Cramping

Menstrual Extraction

In the early 1970s, a group of women in Los Angeles came up with a technique for "self-help" abortions. Known as menstrual extraction (ME), this method allows women to remove the contents of the uterus and avoid doctors and the medical setting. As well as being used as an abortion method in the early stages of pregnancy (up to eight weeks), menstrual extraction has also proven valuable for women who want to free themselves from their periods, for example, to get rid of severe menstrual cramps.

Though ME is controversial, it has proven to be a viable choice for some women. Carol Downer, one of the creaters of ME, notes that over the last two decades, perhaps one thousand to two thousand women have learned how to do the procedure, and it has been used to terminate pregnancy about twenty thousand times. It is generally done in groups and works best for women who are experienced with other self-help gynecological techniques (such as performing gynecological exams on other women). Notes Rebecca Chalker, coauthor with Downer of A Woman's Book of Choices: Abortion, Menstrual Extraction, RU-486 (Four Walls Eight Windows, 1992), "Over the past 20 years, ME has been practiced by women who are highly aware of self and body. These women often work in tight-knit, friendship groups. They normally consist of up to a dozen women who meet monthly or more often to discuss their feelings about ME, to study reproductive anatomy and polish their skills."

In the event that we lose our right to abortion, groups of women performing ME in their homes will become the norm. To use the method, your group will need an experienced leader (someone who has done the technique several times) and some specific equipment, most of which is available at grocery, hardware, and medical-supply stores. We aren't going to explain how to do the procedure, because you should not do it unless someone in your group is experienced in ME. One note of caution: The safety record of ME has not been studied thoroughly. Compared with surgical abortion, no national record can confirm that it is safe.

For more information, contact the Federation of Feminist Women's Health Centers, 633 E. 11th Ave., Eugene, OR 97401; (800) 995-2286 or (503) 344-0966. Ask for a reprint of the chapter on menstrual extraction from their book A New View of a Woman's Body.

can last from an hour to a week, but it shouldn't be so severe that you are doubled over in pain. Patients are given antibiotics to fight infection.

Second-Trimester Abortion

If you are more than twelve or thirteen weeks pregnant, you will probably have a procedure called dilation and evacuation or D&E. It is similar to the aspiration technique except that because the fetus is larger, it is a little more complicated. With this procedure, the dilation takes longer, sometimes overnight. On the first day, the health-care provider inserts a laminaria stick, a small compressed bundle of sterilized seaweed—about the size of a tampon—into the cervical opening to gradually stretch it in order for dilation to take place. After the laminaria is removed at the time of abortion, it may be necessary to use a dilator to further enlarge the cervical opening.

The actual procedure generally occurs the following day. A D&E takes from ten to thirty minutes and may be more painful than aspiration. If so, the doctor may prescribe pain medication. A smaller percentage of abortions are obtained by induction or instillation. Here, the physician injects a substance through the abdomen into the uterus to induce labor and expel the fetus and placenta.

After the Abortion

NAF and others strongly urge that you contact the facility that provided the abortion if you have any of the following symptoms after an abortion:

- Severe pain that makes you double over. This may feel like very violent menstrual cramps and is not alleviated by ibuprofen or other over-the-counter medication.
- Abdominal tenderness to the touch.
- Chills or fever with a temperature of 100.5 degrees F. or higher.
- Bleeding that is heavier than the heaviest day of your normal period or that saturates one sanitary pad in an hour or less.
- Foul-smelling vaginal discharge.
- Continuing symptoms of pregnancy that last for more than a week or a delay (six weeks or more) in resuming menstrual periods. Your period should reappear about a month to six weeks after the abortion.
- You should take good care of yourself after the procedure. Don't do any heavy lifting or exercise too much. Get plenty of rest, and try to

take time off work or from child-care responsibilities if you need to. To prevent infection, don't insert anything into the vagina, douche, or take baths. That means take showers, and avoid tampons and intercourse for a couple of weeks. It's imperative that you get a checkup in two or three weeks to make sure you're okay.

- Many women report feeling sad or depressed after an abortion, although this response has been greatly exaggerated by the anti-choice movement. In fact, postpartum depression is usually worse than depression after an abortion. Still, if you do feel down, talk it over with someone close to you, or discuss it with a counselor or therapist. You might also feel better if you write about your feelings.

The Politics of Abortion

Though it is often characterized more narrowly, the pro-choice movement is about much more than simply the right to choose abortion. This struggle is ultimately about the right of women to control our bodies and improve and maintain our quality of life. For us it might be better called the "pro-survival" movement.

The legalization of abortion in 1973 saved the lives of many women of color, but each of the laws that followed have whittled away at that right, and these changes have enormous effects on Black women. Yet for a variety of reasons, we have been slow to become involved in the pro-choice movement.

For one thing, during the Black Power movement of the sixties and early seventies many Black nationalists strongly disapproved of abortions (and birth control) for African-American women. In her book *When and Where I Enter: The Impact of Black Women on Race and Sex in America*, Paula Giddings recalls that the 1967 Black Power Conference in Newark, New Jersey, passed an anti–birth control resolution. The following year an *Ebony* article published the views of a physician who saw a revolutionary baby boom as a way to build Black power. He believed that if Black women kept producing babies, whites would have to either kill Blacks or grant us full citizenship.

Of course many revolutionaries such as Angela Davis and Kathleen Cleaver complained about this sexism coming from the men in the movement. Such conflicts have understandably left many African-American women ambivalent about getting involved in the pro-choice struggle.

What's more, many Black women feel left out of the mainly white pro-choice movement and are angered by the racism of white feminists. Black feminists believe that leaders of the women's movement didn't

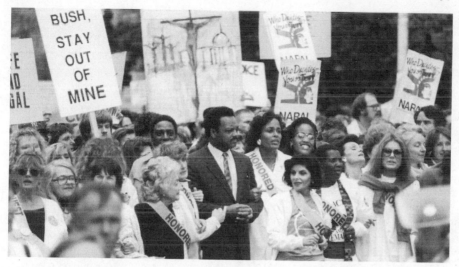

Pro-choice activist Faye Wattleton marches with the Reverend Jesse Jackson. Also shown are author Betty Friedan (black dress), actress Susan Sarandon (sunglasses, left), Gloria Steinem (sunglasses, right), and National Black Women's Health Project founder Byllye Avery (wearing kente cloth). *(Photo: Planned Parenthood)*

fight hard enough to prevent passage of the Hyde Amendment. This 1977 law prohibits the use of federal funds, primarily channeled through Medicaid, to pay for abortion and most affects poor women, who are disproportionately women of color.

In recent years, however, our involvement in the movement has become more apparent as Faye Wattleton, Byllye Avery, Dr. Dorothy I. Height, bell hooks, Marcia Ann Gillespie, Eleanor Holmes Norton, and other African-American women have stood out as vocal and visible pro-choice activists.

The reason Black faces are largely absent from the pro-choice movement may come down to practical considerations. Although we support abortion, many of us don't have the luxury that many white women have to spend time marching, protesting, and organizing. There are so many struggles to fight—racism, sexual abuse, violence, drugs in our communities, and the crumbling educational system— that sometimes the abortion issue takes a back burner. Many of us are struggling to survive, just trying to have enough energy to get through the day to day.

Nonetheless, abortion is *our* issue. You can become involved in the movement by joining a pro-choice group through NARAL, the National Organization for Women, Planned Parenthood, the National Black Women's Health Project, or by making choice an issue in an organization that you belong to. Be visible by participating in pro-choice marches, and be vocal letting those around you—including your legislative representatives—know that you support abortion rights for all women.

*"I felt like a
soldier at war."*

—Victoria Shepler-
Carter, pro-choice
activist, Cleveland

During the summer of 1991, I had watched TV reports of Operation Rescue's action in Wichita, Kansas, wishing they would come somewhere near where I live so that I could personally let them know whose life they had decided to dictate and control. I was an activist with time on my hands, so when I heard about a few white sisters who were going to drive up to Buffalo during Operation Rescue's attempted occupation of the clinics there, I knew I had to make the trip.

Saturday morning we arrived at the Main Street Clinic in Buffalo. We needed to be ready at the drop of a dime for the anti-choice thugs. Their so-called "spring of life rescue" was not due to begin until the next day (Easter Sunday), but trusting their public announcement was not wise. Small groups on each side had gathered, and Buffalo United for Choice had the front and side entrances of the clinic secured. The anti-choice protestors were directly across the street, and a few city police were in the area observing the situation. As the afternoon progressed, one of the local anti-choice ministers decided to venture to our side of the street. He knelt on the curb in front of our secured line and began to mutter his gibberish. Of course our people reacted with outrage, and some even became combative physically.

I saw that things had gotten out of hand as the police stood there and did nothing. I stated very loudly, "Let's pick him up and remove him!" As I said this I locked my arm into his and began to raise him. Immediately I felt his entire body weight and realized no one was helping me. I continued to escort him across the street back to his side. Midway across the street another woman finally came to assist me. The media converged on the scene and began to snap their cameras. I didn't care and continued to do what I had started. We reached the other side of the street and he fell to his knees as if I had knocked him down. I again attempted to lift him, but he resisted, so I left him there on the ground.

I returned to our side of the street, and immediately people gathered around to conceal me. A few whispered that the police were looking for me. Because I was the only large African-American woman, I was easily identifiable, so I quickly left the scene to change my appearance. Having to leave upset me—the white woman who assisted me halfway across the street didn't have to leave—but after changing my head wrap, I returned to the clinic-defense site as though nothing had occurred. Eventually, the day ended and the clinic remained opened and all medical procedures were completed.

The next day we returned to the clinic and by 6:00 A.M., we had the perimeter secured with at least two hundred of our people. In the wee hours of the morning, the anti-choice protestors would circle the block scoping us out, and we could usually identify them with ease. I felt like a soldier at war, which in a great sense is exactly what I was. We never knew when they would attack, how many of them would come, and if we could maintain the entrance, but we were determined to win this battle. There were no rules to this battle, and the police were no help—not that I expected anything from them. By midmorning, the anti-choice protestors were occupying the sidewalk across from the clinic and had poured over into the street; only a yellow police tape separated them from us.

We would stand in the rain literally in the same position for hours on end. Side by side, arms and legs locked to form a line that stretched about 100 yards. Each time one of the anti-choice thugs attempted to break through our secure line, our bodies would tense up with strength, and we chanted even louder to drive them away. It was a very powerful display of group participation.

RU 486

RU 486 is an innovative reproductive technology that combines a dosage of antihormone medication with the hormone prostaglandin to interrupt pregnancy. It has been called the "abortion pill," but its creator prefers the term "contragestion," somewhere in between birth control and abortion. The drug works early in pregnancy by preventing the embryo from implanting itself in the uterine wall.

American women may never have the chance to take advantage of this abortion option, thanks to groups like the National Right to Life Committee, which have fought to keep RU 486 out of the U.S. Presently the drug is being tested here on a limited basis but is banned from being imported here (the Supreme Court upheld the ban in 1992). It is legal in some European countries. In France, where the drug has been licensed since 1988, surveys show that women who have used it are satisfied with it and would take it again.

European women use RU 486 during the first seven weeks of pregnancy under the strict supervision of a physician in a controlled medical setting. The entire process takes several weeks, which includes four office or clinic visits. French women pay $240 (most of which is paid for by national health insurance) and must agree to a surgical abortion should RU 486 fail, since little is known about the possible side effects of the drug on the growing fetus.

Despite the obvious benefits of having another abortion option, even women's health activists point to its drawbacks in this country. The crumbling state of our health-care system would prevent widespread access to the procedure. The cost in time and money of repeated visits to a medical facility might be viable for middle-class French women but seems out of the question for poor women in America, especially those who live in rural areas.

The most important drawback of RU 486 may be in its safety. Though it has been studied in a limited way by U.S. researchers, the import ban prevents thorough, long-term monitoring of the drug. In the wake of the damage that the Dalkon Shield, DES, and breast implants have caused to women's bodies, we cannot risk using another poorly studied medical technology. There are also side effects to RU 486 such as cramps, vomiting, dizziness, and bleeding.

Little is known about the effect of RU 486 on future fetuses of women who have used the drug. And because most research subjects have been middle-class white women, no one knows whether the drug will work differently for women of color. For example, for reasons that remain unclear, Black women are much more likely to suffer from fibroid tumors; that being the case, no expert can be sure RU 486 will not increase the likelihood of fibroids or that the fibroids will not hamper the safety and effectiveness of the drug.

Still, until the government ban is lifted we'll never know the answers to these questions and never find out whether RU 486 is a viable abortion alternative for us. For more information read *The Case for Antiprogestins: RU 486: The First in a New Generation of Birth Control,* a report of the Reproductive Health Technologies Project, 1601 Connecticut Ave. NW, suite 801, Washington, DC, 20009; (202) 328-2200; *A Woman's Book of Choices: Abortion, Menstrual Extraction, RU-486* by Rebecca Chalker and Carol Downer; *The Abortion Pill: RU 486, A Woman's Choice* by Etienne-Emile Baulieu; *RU 486: The Pill That Could End the Abortion Wars and Why American Women Don't Have It,* by Lawrence Lader.

For More Information

ORGANIZATIONS

CATHOLICS FOR A FREE CHOICE, 1436 U Street NW, suite 301, Washington, DC 20009; (202) 986-6093. Provides a pro-choice Catholic voice.

CENTER FOR REPRODUCTIVE LAW AND POLICY, 120 Wall Street, New York, NY 10005; (212) 514-5534. Provides law-related abortion information and a free newsletter, *Reproductive Freedom News.*

FEDERATION OF FEMINIST WOMEN'S HEALTH CENTERS, 633 E. 11th Ave., Eugene, OR 97401; (800) 995-2286 or (503) 344-0966. Practical information on abortion and menstrual extraction from a feminist and self-help perspective.

INTERNATIONAL WOMEN'S HEALTH COALITION, 24 E. 21st St., New York, NY 10010; (212) 979-8500. For information on abortion and women in developing countries.

NATIONAL ABORTION FEDERATION, 1436 U St. NW, suite 103, Washington, DC 20009; (202) 667-5881. Ask for the group's free information packet, or call the toll-free hotline—(800) 772-9100—for answers to practical questions and referrals state by state.

NATIONAL ABORTION RIGHTS ACTION LEAGUE (NARAL), 1156 15th St. NW, 7th floor, Washington, DC 20005; (202) 973-3000. The political arm of the grassroots pro-choice movement.

NATIONAL ORGANIZATION FOR WOMEN (NOW), 1000 16th St., suite 700, Washington, DC 20036-5705; (202) 331-0066. For information on abortion rights and legislation.

PLANNED PARENTHOOD FEDERATION OF AMERICA, 810 7th Ave., New York, NY 10019; (800) 829-7732 or (212) 541-7800. Call for information or to find a clinic in your area.

RELIGIOUS COALITION FOR ABORTION RIGHTS, 100 Maryland Ave. NE, suite 307, Washington, DC 20002; (202)-543-7032. The Coalition's purpose is to make clear that abortion can be a moral decision that must be made by the woman, according to her own religious understanding without government interference.

REPRODUCTIVE HEALTH TECHNOLOGIES PROJECT, 1601 Connecticut Ave. NW, suite 801, Washington, DC, 20009; (202) 328-2200. For information about abortion, RU 486, and other forms of reproductive-health technology.

BOOKS

Abortion Then and Now: Creative Responses to Restricted Access, The National Women's Health Network (Washington, D.C.), 1989.

Abortion Without Apology: A Radical History for the 1990s, Ninia Baehr, South End Press (Boston), 1990.

Back Rooms: Voices from the Illegal Abortion Era, Ellen Messer and Kathryn E. May, St. Martin's Press, 1988.

The New Our Bodies, Ourselves: A Book By and For Women, *The Boston Women's Health Book Collective, Simon & Schuster, 1992.*

A Woman's Book of Choices: Abortion, Menstrual Extraction, RU-486, Rebecca Chalker and Carol Downer, Four Walls Eight Windows, 1992.

12

Reproductive-Tract Infections

Reproductive-tract infection (RTI) is a catchall term that refers to infections that originate in the external genitals, vagina, and cervix. It includes everything from bacterial vaginosis and yeast infections to serious sexually transmitted infections such as gonorrhea, syphilis, and even AIDS. With the proper screening, early diagnosis, and correct treatment, most RTI's are little more than annoying. But when they aren't taken care of, they can spread to the upper tract—the uterus, fallopian tubes, and ovaries—and lead to pelvic inflammatory disease (PID), ectopic pregnancy, infertility, cervical cancer, miscarriage, and infant death. Having some RTI's also puts women at risk for acquiring the virus that causes AIDS.

RTI's are extremely common, affecting millions of people—primarily women—every year. Health officials are alarmed by the rise in cases of sexually transmitted infections (STI's), especially now in the age of AIDS, when all of us should be practicing safer sex. In fact, according to the Alan Guttmacher Institute, more than one in five Americans, or 56 million people, are infected with an STI. Such infections will strike at least one in four Americans sometime during their lives. The Guttmacher research also points out that Blacks and teenagers are disproportionately affected by STI's.

Part of the problem is the shroud of shame that surrounds all RTI's, especially those that are transmitted sexually. Many women are embarrassed to talk openly and honestly about symptoms such as discharge and itching or to discuss their sexual practices with their physicians. Some doctors also feel uncomfortable discussing sexual health. And even though so many sisters have had RTI's, many of us find bringing up the subject with other Black women awkward.

But we must begin talking with one another and with our physicians about RTI's of all kinds. People have a wide range of sexual habits, and chances are doctors have heard it all. A good doctor will be sensitive to the awkwardness some women feel, and a smart patient will insist on getting answers to all her questions despite any discomfort. Black women must learn about both sexually and nonsexually transmitted infections, and we must share that information with our sisters so that we can all protect our reproductive health.

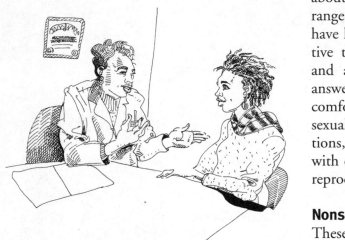

It's crucial to talk openly and frankly with your physician about your sexual practices.
(Drawing: Yvonne Buchanan)

Nonsexually Transmitted Infections

These are problems that are often referred to under the general term *vaginitis*. Vaginitis is any irritation or inflammation of the vagina that may cause pain, soreness, burning, itching, painful intercourse, abnormal vaginal discharge, and odor. These kinds of problems often occur when the normal bacteria that help keep the vagina healthy grow out of control. They can irritate the walls of the vagina and lead to infections.

Some of these kinds of RTI's, such as bacterial vaginosis and yeast infections, usually require treatment. Other kinds don't. But symptoms can be tricky, and some nonsexually transmitted RTI's are difficult to diagnose. A Pap test *does not* detect all these problems. That's why you must pay close attention to your body and learn to understand your discharge, its consistency and its odor. Be sure to report any chronic symptoms to your health-care practitioner.

Many kinds of irritations can lead to vaginitis. If you get rid of whatever is causing the irritation, sometimes symptoms go away. Some of the most common are:

- Douches that interfere with the balance of acidity in the vagina.
- Allergies to soap, deodorants, and other products used around the vagina. Sensitivity to fabric such as panty hose or the crotch of panties can also trigger the problem.
- Lowered resistance from stress, poor eating habits, and lack of sleep.
- Serious illness such as diabetes. The high sugar content of a diabetic woman's vaginal secretions can trigger infection, generally yeast.
- Medication such as birth control pills, antibiotics, and hormones.
- Sexual intercourse can sometimes cause irritation of the vagina, especially when there isn't enough lubrication. This is sometimes a problem for postmenopausal women. Tampons can also irritate the vagina in some women.

To prevent vaginal infections of all kinds, follow this advice:

Keep your genital area clean. Use a cleanser made for sensitive skin, and avoid perfumed and deodorant soaps. Pat the area dry with a clean towel, and avoid using other people's towels.

Wear clean, cotton-crotch underwear. That will help keep the genital area dry and discourage bacteria that grow in warm, moist environments. Avoid pants that are tight in the crotch, and don't sit around in a wet bathing suit for long periods of time. Bypass panty hose, or always wear it with cotton underwear.

Don't Douche

Compared with white women, we are twice as likely to douche—flush the vagina with water or other cleansing agents. Most of us do it to try to relieve symptoms such as discharge or itching or as birth control or to keep the vagina clean and odor-free. But douches aren't necessary; in fact, they can cause more problems than they solve. A recent study published in the journal Obstetrics and Gynecology found that women who douched at least once weekly were four times more likely to report having been diagnosed with pelvic inflammatory disease (PID) than women who douche less often or not at all. PID can lead to serious problems including severe pain, ectopic pregnancy, and sterility.

There's no reason to use douches. Unless specifically suggested by a doctor, douching doesn't relieve symptoms of reproductive-tract infections. In fact, it can lead to infections and allergic reactions. Douching may also push infections in the vagina into other parts of the reproductive system, which can lead to PID. Douches do not work as birth control and should never be relied on to prevent pregnancy. And we don't need douches to clean our vaginas. The vagina has its own natural cleansing process.

Avoid scented tampons, bubble bath, vaginal sprays, and douches. All of these can irritate the vagina.

Have your male partner wear a condom. Even though vaginitis is not generally thought of as an STI, some types can be transmitted sexually.

Make sure that your partner's genitals are clean. A man should wash his penis before lovemaking. Abstain from intercourse if your vaginal area is irritated. Having sex can make it worse.

If you have repeated bouts of vaginitis, don't use tampons; choose napkins instead.

Keep yourself healthy. That means eat right, drink lots of water, control stress, and get plenty of rest so that your immune system can ward off infections.

Some kinds of vaginitis generally require medication. Untreated they can lead to more serious kinds of reproductive-health problems. It's very important to know their specific symptoms and treatment.

Bacterial Vaginosis

Bacterial vaginosis or BV may be the most common RTI. It can have many symptoms or no symptoms at all and is often mistaken for other types of RTI's. In the past doctors called it "nonspecific vaginitis" or referred to it by the names of the bacteria—generally *Gardnerella* or *Haemophilus.* Untreated it can lead to problems during pregnancy and other more serious reproductive-health ailments such as PID.

BV has been called "an ecological disaster of the vagina" because it occurs when normal bacteria found in the vagina grow out of control. In fact, women with the infection may have one hundred to one thousand times more bacteria than normal. No one understands exactly what causes it, but it is generally not a result of sexual intercourse or sexual contact.

Detecting BV.

Although some women show no signs of BV, the most common symptom is a whitish, grayish white, or yellowish discharge that has an odor sometimes described as foul or fishy. The smell is generally stronger after washing with soap or after sexual activity. It's very important that you describe the consistency and odor of your discharge to your doctor, who can then properly diagnose BV by examining your vaginal secretions under a microscope. BV cannot be reliably detected by a Pap smear.

Treatment.

Unlike yeast infections, BV cannot be gotten rid of with over-the-counter products. Don't use douches or sprays to try and hide the odor; that can only make the problem worse and harder to diagnose. The standard treatment is an antibiotic used as a cream, gel, or suppository, which must be prescribed by a physician. The most common is metronidazole.

Yeast Infections

Yeast infections are extremely common; just about every woman has had one. They aren't life threatening, but they are confusing. In fact, many women may be confusing yeast infections with more serious gynecological problems and receiving improper treatment. That's why it's imperative to understand yeast infections and learn how to recognize them in your own body.

Yeast infections occur when *candida albicans,* a type of yeast that occurs naturally in the vagina (and in the mouth and intestines) grows out of control, resulting in infection. Though we all have yeast infections from time to time, some women get them chronically; as soon as one has cleared up, another is on its way. Depressed immunity is often the cause. In some women, stress, poor eating habits, not getting enough sleep, and other illnesses cause the pH balance of the vagina to change, and yeast begins to thrive. Taking antibiotics such as penicillin or ampicillin to combat infections such as step throat can also cause yeast infections. These antibiotics are meant to kill disease-causing bacteria, but they also kill protective bacteria, thus allowing yeast to grow.

Untreated yeast infections can be more than just annoying for pregnant women. During birth, a woman can pass the infection to her child; this is called thrush when it infects the mouth and tongue.

Detecting Yeast Infections.

Telling the difference between yeast infections and other gynecological problems often comes down to subtle distinctions in vaginal discharge. The discharge associated with yeast infections is lumpy and white. Some women describe it as the consistency of cottage cheese, sometimes with a breadlike smell. Women with yeast also generally have itching or irritation of the vulva and sometimes pain during intercourse and burning during urination. To tell for sure whether the infection is yeast, a doctor must examine vaginal secretions under a microscope.

Treatment.
Over-the-counter treatments such as Monistat 7 and Gyne-Lotrimin are generally used to treat yeast infections. The medication is inserted directly into the vagina once a day (preferably at night), and the infection takes about a week to clear up.

However, you must not use these medications unless you know *for sure* that you have a yeast infection. You must either have been tested by a doctor or have had a previous test and been paying close attention to your body so that you know exactly how to recognize the signs. Using yeast medication for other problems isn't just a waste of time and money, it's also dangerous. If you have something other than yeast, such as an STI, taking over-the-counter yeast medication may cause the symptoms to subside, but at the same time you may be passing the infection to a sexual partner or it may be spreading dangerously to other parts of the reproductive system.

Sometimes yeast infections go away on their own. Other times, women use self-help methods to get rid of yeast and keep it away. The following methods are two of the most common.

Boost the immune system. Learn to control stress; eat a balanced diet that includes plenty of fruits, vegetables, and whole grains and is low in salt, sugar, and fat; and get as much sleep as your body needs. Also take 500 milligrams of vitamin C twice a day.

Try eating low-fat yogurt that contains "friendly" bacteria. (Some women also benefit by putting yogurt into the vagina.) Only yogurt with live bacteria is effective, so check the label for the phrase "contains active lactobacillus acidophilus." You can eat one cup a day or take acidophilus in tablet form. Women who are particularly susceptible to yeast infections caused by antibiotics should eat yogurt or take acidophilus with the medication.

A Special Note of Caution.
Women who have been infected with HIV are often plagued by chronic yeast infections both in the vagina and in the mouth. The suppressed immune system allows the yeast to thrive, and a yeast infection is sometimes the first symptom that shows up in women who have the AIDS virus.

This does *not* mean that if you have chronic yeast infections, you have AIDS. In most cases, these infections are triggered by less serious problems of immunity or by antibiotics. However, if you can't explain stubborn yeast infections that come back again and again *and* you suspect

I had never liked the way I smelled "down there." Since I was a teenager, I thought that the odor could creep through my panties out into the world. Because of that, I was always careful to wash my genitals every day, and I used a douche maybe once a month.

But about six months ago, I noticed that the odor was stronger than usual and the discharge heavier. I assumed it was normal, perhaps a reaction to stress. So I took extra special care to wash myself frequently and thoroughly. I also tried a medicated douche. The product was messy and left a brown stain in my shower, and it didn't work either. A day after I would douche, the smell would be back.

In the back of my mind I knew I should go to the health clinic on campus and get this checked out. But I really didn't have time, and I hated the long wait. Besides, I didn't feel as though many of the doctors—especially the men—really knew that much about women's bodies. Instead of going, I convinced myself that this was a yeast infection, and that some medicine I could get at the drugstore would make it go away. I was taken aback by how much Monistat costs—about $15—but I figured I'd better use it and get rid of whatever I had and be done with the unpleasant smell.

I used the medication for about a week, and when I was using it, I didn't notice the smell. About a week after I completed the dose, however, the smell was back. I knew it was time to really look into this.

I went to the library and paged through a copy of a women's medical book. I read the descriptions of the different gynecological problems and the kinds of symptoms that went along with them and jotted down some notes. Once I got home I went into the bathroom—notes in hand—and decided I needed to get a good look and a good whiff of the discharge that was staining my underpants. Instead of getting grossed out, I touched and sniffed the discharge. It didn't seem like cottage cheese, which was what went with yeast infections, and it didn't seem thick and green, thank God, like the discharge that went with gonorrhea. Instead it had a fishy odor and was kind of gray. It seemed like I had bacterial vaginosis, a term I had never heard of.

With information in hand, I got myself into the health clinic. The doctor checked the discharge and suggested that it was normal. I insisted that it wasn't and described the smell. He then said he would give me a Pap smear. I told him about the bacterial vaginosis, remembering that the book had said that it wouldn't show up on a Pap. I know he felt annoyed with me, but eventually he did test me for what he called "nonspecific vaginitis." Sure enough, I had it, and was given the proper treatment.

"I now understand that discharge is natural, not nasty."

—NAME WITHHELD, STUDENT, QUEENS, NEW YORK

I really learned a good lesson. I'm no longer so worried about my normal smell, and I've gotten to know when the odor is telling me that something is wrong. Also, I now understand that discharge is natural, not nasty.

that you may have contracted HIV, get tested. For more on AIDS, see chapter 31, "HIV and AIDS."

For more information on yeast infections contact the Human Ecology Action League (HEAL), P.O. Box 49126, Atlanta, GA 30359; (404) 248-1898. HEAL is an international support group for sufferers of illness caused by environmental factors and chemical sensitivity, including yeast infections. The organization has chapters in many cities and publishes a newsletter, *The Human Ecologist,* which includes recent trends in research and medical news.

You can also read *The Yeast Connection: A Medical Breakthrough* by William G. Crook, M.D.

Urinary-Tract Infections

Anyone can get a urinary-tract infection (UTI). The best-known type is called cystitis; this is what we think of as a bladder infection. Women get UTI's more than men because the female urethra connecting the bladder to the urinary opening is shorter than it is in males. That means that bacteria don't have to travel far to get to the bladder.

UTI's are caused by bacteria traveling from the large intestine to the urethra and bladder, and they often occur when a woman wipes herself from the back to the front when using the toilet. Although they are not considered to be sexually transmitted infections, UTI's are often caused by sexual intercourse. Sexual thrusting can push bacteria into the bladder. They can also be triggered when the bladder is not emptied completely. For instance, some women who use the diaphragm contract bladder infections because the contraceptive exerts pressure on the urethra and can obstruct the bladder from emptying completely. Pregnant women are also susceptible because the fetus puts pressure on the bladder.

Detecting UTI's.
Pain and burning during urination is a common sign of a bladder infection. People who have them also feel as though they have to urinate fre-

quently, but when they do, only small amounts of urine come out. The urine may also look cloudy or have an unusual odor. Sometimes blood is present in the urine.

It's very important to see a doctor if symptoms persist for more than forty-eight hours. To diagnose a bladder infection, a physician will request a urine sample and examine it under a microscope.

Treatment.

Sometimes UTI's go away by themselves, or they may disappear if you follow the self-help suggestions below. In other cases, you'll need to take antibiotics.

To prevent and treat mild UTI's, try these suggestions:

After urinating or moving your bowels, wipe yourself from front to back to keep fecal materials out of your urinary tract. Be sure to teach your daughters the correct way to wipe as well. Keep the genitals clean by washing (again from front to back) with a mild cleanser or soap.

Drink at least six to eight glasses of water every day. Cranberry juice also helps, or cranberry tablets (sold in health-food stores) can be taken. Avoid alcohol and caffeine.

Urinate frequently rather than holding it in. And make sure to empty your bladder completely each time.

Keep your immune system strong by controlling stress, eating healthfully, and getting plenty of rest.

Make sure you're well lubricated during sexual activity. If you have a problem with lubrication, use a water-based lubricant such as K-Y jelly. Also try to urinate after intercourse to flush bacteria out of the bladder.

For more information, contact the National Kidney and Urologic Diseases Information Clearinghouse, Box NKUDIC, 9000 Rockville Pike, Bethesda, MD 20892; (301) 654-4415. Ask for the brochure "Urinary Tract Infections in Adults." Or contact the National Kidney Foundation/UTI, 30 E. 33rd St., Dept. UTI, New York, NY 10016; (212) 889-2210. Ask for the booklet "Urinary Tract Infections."

Sexually Transmitted Infections

STI's are viral and bacterial infections that are passed through sexual activity—intercourse as well as oral and anal sex. Untreated, STI's can be very serious and are the chief cause of pelvic inflammatory disease, which infects one in four Black women. PID can lead to tubal or ectopic pregnancy and infertility.

To prevent the spread of STI's, including AIDS, all of us must have sex safely. Though women are often blamed for spreading STI's, in reality, we are more likely to be on the receiving end. So protect yourself. The best way to avoid contracting an STI is by using condoms, and barrier contraceptives (such as the diaphragm) can also prevent the spread when used with a spermicide. (But to prevent the spread of AIDS, you must use a diaphragm or other barrier contraceptive *with* a condom.) Heterosexual women are not the only ones who contract STI's: Women can also pass them to each other. For information on safer sex, see chapter 27, "Sexuality and Having Sex Safely."

Remember that most STI's cannot be detected by a Pap smear, so you must report any unusual symptoms to your health-care provider. Never let any doctor make you feel guilty for having an STI; sexually transmitted infections are health not morality problems.

There are some thirty STI's; following is a discussion of the most common (AIDS is not discussed here; see chapter 31, "HIV and AIDS").

Chlamydia

Chlamydia is the most common STI, affecting 4 million men and women each year. It is also the most mysterious. Because it sometimes has no symptoms at all, it has been referred to as "the silent venereal disease."

Chlamydia is a bacterial infection that is spread through vaginal and anal intercourse. The Alan Guttmacher Institute reports that in a single act of unprotected sex with an infected partner, women have a 40 percent chance of contracting chlamydia. Pregnant women can also pass it to newborns through the birth canal. More than 100,000 babies are born each year infected with the disease, and these babies may develop eye infections or pneumonia.

Detecting Chlamydia.

Early symptoms of chlamydia are often absent or very mild. The American Social Health Association reports that up to 75 percent of women and 50 percent of men experience no symptoms, which means that the disease often goes undetected and untreated. Many women discover they have chlamydia only after their partners find out they have it. When symptoms do arise, they include abdominal pain, pain or burning during urination (especially in men), abnormal discharge, and painful intercourse.

A new test offers quick detection of chlamydia during a routine office visit. Ask for a test, especially if you are sexually active or have any suspicion that you've been exposed to the disease. The Centers for Disease Control recommends that pregnant women get tested for chlamydia during the first trimester.

Treating Chlamydia.
Chlamydia is easily treated with oral antibiotics, generally doxycycline. The newest treatment for chlamydia is zithromax, which is taken in one dose. Sexual partners should be tested and treated together to prevent spreading it back and forth.

Crab Lice
Crab lice, which are also called pubic lice or simply "crabs," are more annoying and embarrassing than dangerous. Every year 3 million people get them. Tiny creatures that look like crabs, they live in the pubic hair and sometimes in the hair on the chest, armpits, and face. Their eggs are white and are deposited in small clumps near the roots of pubic hair. They are passed from person to person through intimate and sexual contact and through infected towels, sheets, clothing, and even toilet seats.

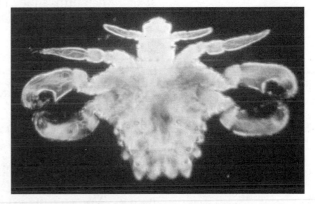

Detecting Crabs.
The most common symptom of crabs is intense itching caused by their bites. Using a magnifying glass, you can see the tiny creatures move or find eggs fastened to the pubic hair. A doctor can diagnose them easily using a microscope.

A greatly enlarged photo of a crab louse. *(Photo: Terri L. Meinking)*

Treating Crabs.
Despite the discomfort, try not to scratch the area; that may encourage their spread. According to new research, the most effective treatment for crabs is an over-the-counter product called NIX. If you use other kinds of over-the-counter medications such as RID, you must use the treatment twice in order to get rid of all crabs and eggs. Whichever you use, remember that these products contain strong ingredients, so use them carefully and correctly. Partners must be treated at the same time, and all clothing, towels, and bedding should be washed in hot water.

Genital Warts

Genital warts are caused by the human papilloma virus (HPV), which some 24 to 40 million Americans carry in their bodies. HPV can be very serious and can cause cervical cancer. The virus that causes warts is spread through vaginal, anal, and oral intercourse. Some forms of the virus can be transmitted sexually even when no lesions are visible.

Detecting Genital Warts.

The warts thrive in warm, moist areas, and they grow on the genitals, in the urethra, and around the anus. They are usually raised, soft to the touch, and sometimes itchy. Genital warts look like warts that grow on other places on the body, and as they grow larger they begin to resemble miniature cauliflower florets. In men they grow on the head of the penis, under the foreskin, and on the shaft.

A doctor can detect warts by looking at them, even though they are sometimes confused as herpes lesions. Some practitioners use a vinegar soak, which turns hidden warts white, to detect them. Magnifying equipment can also help spot warts. A Pap test can identify HPV for sure.

Treating Genital Warts.

There is no cure for HPV, but there are ways to get rid of warts. However, they can recur, especially during times of stress and illness. Doctors treat warts with a chemical called podophyllin. Though effective, it can be very irritating to the skin surrounding the warts. It is applied to the warts and then washed off thoroughly several hours later. It sometimes takes several applications—and trips to the doctor's office—to get rid of warts. (This option should not be used during pregnancy.) Women can also treat warts themselves with a prescription medication called podofilox, but it must be used with care. Medical providers also can also freeze them off using dry ice, burn them using acid, or remove them with laser surgery.

Gonorrhea

Every year about 1 million cases of gonorrhea are reported. Left untreated, the disease has serious consequences, including sterility, arthritis, heart problems, disorders of the central nervous system, pelvic inflammatory disease, complications during pregnancy, and eye infections in newborns.

A bacterial infection, gonorrhea is spread through vaginal, anal, and oral intercourse. It can invade not only the genitals, but also other warm, moist areas of the body such as the eyes and throat.

Detecting Gonorrhea.

As with chlamydia, the majority of women who have been infected with gonorrhea show no symptoms; they often find out they have it when their male partners are diagnosed. Women who do have symptoms notice a greenish yellow discharge and burning or pain when urinating. Men, who are more likely to experience symptoms, also have discharge (from the penis) and pain or burning during urination. If the disease has spread, severe symptoms such as abdominal and pelvic pain and swelling, low back pain, and vaginal bleeding can occur.

Your doctor can test for gonorrhea immediately by examining discharge under a microscope. This test is less accurate, however, than a culture test. Cultures usually have to be sent out to a lab, so results aren't available for a day or two.

Treating Gonorrhea.

Gonorrhea can be treated effectively with antibiotics, generally penicillin or rocephin, which are both given as shots. Because many people who have gonorrhea also have chlamydia, the CDC recommends treating both diseases at once. Sexual partners should be tested and treated at the same time.

Hepatitis B

Every year 300,000 Americans are infected with hepatitis B, a dangerous STD that in rare cases can lead to liver disease and death. Though most people don't know it, hepatitis B is the only STI that can be prevented through a vaccination.

Hepatitis B is highly contagious, much more so than most other STI's; in fact, it is one hundred times more contagious than HIV. It is spread through intimate sexual contact including oral, vaginal, and anal intercourse as well as kissing. It can also be transmitted through shellfish and unclean needles used to shoot drugs or in the health-care setting. In the majority of cases, pregnant women infected with the disease will pass it on to their unborn children.

Detecting Hepatitis B.

In some people there are no symptoms, even when the disease is in its most contagious stage. When symptoms do occur, they include extreme fatigue, headache, fever, nausea, vomiting, lack of appetite, dark urine, light-colored stools, skin rashes, tenderness in the lower abdomen, and yellowing of the skin (in light-skinned women) and whites of the eyes.

Doctors diagnose the disease by looking for the most obvious symptoms and use a blood test to confirm the diagnosis.

Treating Hepatitis B.
No treatment exists for this disease. In most people the body fights it, and eventually it goes away. In about 10 percent of cases, however, those infected become chronic carriers of the disease.

With no medical treatment available, prevention becomes extremely important. Because it is so highly contagious, hepatitis B cannot be prevented as easily as other STI's. The vaccination, then, is the best way to avoid the disease. The CDC recommends that all infants get vaccinated against hepatitis B and suggests it as well for adolescents and adults who are sexually active. The vaccine, which is administered in a three-shot series, can be costly—several hundreds of dollars—but the shots are cheaper and safer than treating the disease.

For more information, call the National Foundation for Infectious Disease's Hepatitis B Hotline, (800) HEP-B-873.

Herpes
Over 30 million Americans carry the herpes virus, and approximately 200,000 to 500,000 cases are reported each year. Herpes comes in two types: herpes simplex virus type I, which causes cold sores around the mouth or on the lips and is little more than a nuisance, and herpes simplex virus type II, which causes sores on the genitals, thighs, and buttocks. Type I can be transmitted from the mouth to the genitals during oral sex; type II is passed during anal and vaginal sex and is the most distressing. Herpes can also be passed from mother to baby during childbirth. In newborns it can cause severe problems and in some cases lead to death.

Both types of herpes are incurable. Once contracted, the virus lies dormant in a nerve root in the base of the spine and kicks into action during menstruation, pregnancy, illness, and times of stress.

Detecting Herpes.
The first outbreak after the virus enters the body is generally the most severe. An outbreak begins with tingling, soreness, itching, burning, or pressure in the genital area or on the mouth for type I. Because herpes is

During the late 1970s, when I was seventeen and everything was free and easy, I had two one-night stands. Shortly afterward, I went on vacation out of town. And all of a sudden, I had this incredible discharge and pain. When I got back from my vacation, it hadn't gotten any better. It hurt and it itched. Whenever I went to the bathroom, and my urine touched my genitals, I wanted to scream. It burned so much. And I couldn't scratch, because it was in this incredibly personal place.

I was only a kid, and back then the only problems we had to worry about were syphilis and gonorrhea. I figured I would get a shot and that was it. Out of body, out of mind. When I went to the doctor, she took one look and said it was herpes. She said it very, very calmly. I didn't know what that meant. I said, "Give me something and make it go away." She said, "I can't." I said, "I don't get it." She said, "You've got it and it's a virus that will always be in your body. It's yours forever." I felt like I was being punished for my one-nighters. No one had ever told me that they had herpes. No one had ever told me this could happen. I was furious. I was scared. But I didn't have anyone to talk to about it. My mother was dead. Telling my father was out of the question.

I asked my doctor what I could do. She said, "Well, what I do, I mean, what other people tell me they do . . . " I interrupted her, "Wait a minute, you said what you do." She admitted that she had it too. Having herpes made me feel less like a person. I really felt like a slut. To find out that my doctor had it made me less like a scarlet woman.

When the famous Newsweek *article came out in the 1980s with the scarlet* H *on the cover for* herpes, *I really felt like a pariah. Now everybody knew what it was, and there was such a stigma. About that time, I was honest with a man I was dating. I told him I had herpes, and he split.*

The last thing I want is to give it to someone else. If the blisters are inside, they hurt like hell. It's like you run a fever and you're all over uncomfortable. When you have it, there's that feeling that whoever gave it to you didn't care at all about whatever happened to you and has gone on with their life leaving you with a permanent reminder. It's with me for life. If I ever have children, I will most likely have to have a cesarean section during labor so that I won't pass it on to the baby. Now I always use condoms. And I make sure that I get Pap smears every year to screen for cancer.

Still, it is easier to deal with now. The virus is older and it's more dormant. My outbreaks aren't as bad, and I don't get them as often. I tell anyone it looks like I'm going to have an intimate relationship with up front. Nowadays, people are pretty accepting about it. Now there's AIDS. Herpes

"This is the one body I have. Herpes is a part of me now."

—NAME WITHHELD, WRITER, CINCINNATI

doesn't look so bad in comparison. Either the stigma surrounding herpes isn't as bad or I'm more comfortable with my life. A lot of times I used to sit back and say, "Why did I get herpes? I'm horrible and dirty." But now I say, "This is the one body I have. Herpes is a part of me now." And whenever I enter into a new relationship, worrying if my herpes will be accepted isn't the first thing I'm concerned with. I'm concerned about whether the person is mentally healthy, someone who is good. If someone really cares about you as a person, herpes just isn't going to be a big stumbling block.

a virus, it often brings flulike symptoms such as headaches, mild fever, and fatigue, as well as painful urination.

The next stage is signaled by red bumps that develop into water blisters. Eventually they evolve into open sores that crust over and heal. A typical outbreak lasts about ten days to two weeks.

Doctors can sometimes diagnose herpes by examining the lesions. However, this method is not foolproof, because other STIs—such as genital warts—can look like herpes. Laboratory tests provide certain diagnosis.

Treating Herpes.

Herpes has no cure, but there are ways to shorten outbreaks and ease discomfort. (Pregnant women must take special care to avoid outbreaks because herpes is so dangerous to babies being born.) An antiviral medication called acyclovir—brand name Zovirax—can help reduce the length and severity of outbreaks. Some people take the medication between outbreaks to prevent them. The drug is expensive and can be very costly for those who are taking it to prevent outbreaks.

A cheaper option is lysine, an amino acid that can be purchased over-the-counter where vitamins are sold. Recent studies show that lysine can shorten and reduce the severity of outbreaks and can be used as a preventive method. During an outbreak, take 3 grams per day, and between outbreaks—especially during times of stress—take about half that amount.

Vitamin C and zinc, which help boost the immune system, can also ease and prevent outbreaks. Keeping stress to a minimum helps, as does avoiding foods that can trigger outbreaks such as chocolate, nuts, and cola.

When herpes sores are active, keep the genital area clean and dry.

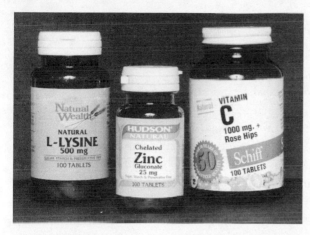

Lysine, zinc, and vitamin C cannot cure herpes but can help ease, shorten, and even prevent outbreaks. *(Photo: T. L. Litt/Impact Visuals)*

Wear loose-fitting cotton underwear and clothes that can "breathe." Pregnant women who have active sores at the time of delivery generally must deliver by cesarean section.

With no treatment, it's best to avoid contracting the herpes virus. Do so by practicing safer sex when a partner is having an outbreak. Even between outbreaks, have sex with a condom, because the lesions can be hard to spot or feel for some people. Don't touch an open lesion with any part of your body. That means don't kiss, have oral sex, or even use your hands without using a latex barrier for protection. If you do, wash the area immediately.

Avoid sharing towels or linen with someone who has active lesions. Soap and hot water kill the virus.

For more information, contact the National Herpes Hotline at (919) 361-8488, or write to the Herpes Resource Center in care of the American Social Health Association, P.O. Box 13827, Research Triangle Park, NC 27709. Or write or call the Herpes Advice Center, The Stanford, 51 E. 25th St., New York, NY 10010; (212)-213-6150.

Syphilis
Syphilis is a serious STI that affects about 120,000 Americans each year. It is caused by a bacteria that dies very quickly outside of the human body and can be easily treated with penicillin. It is passed through open sores and can be spread through vaginal, anal, and oral intercourse and even kissing. Untreated, it can damage the heart, brain, eyes, nervous system, bones, and joints. Pregnant women can also pass it to their unborn babies, causing blindness, facial abnormalities, bone disease, and deafness.

Detecting Syphilis.

The first sign of syphilis is usually a painless sore called a chancre, which appears from three weeks to ninety days after infection. The sores can appear on the genitals, anus, the mouth, or wherever the bacteria entered the body. They ooze clear liquid and last anywhere from three to five weeks. At this stage, the bacteria is very contagious.

The next stage occurs about a week to several months later. Even though the sores have healed, the bacteria is still in the body. This stage is marked by flulike symptoms and also a rash on the body, especially on the palms of the hands and soles of the feet. Lesions may also appear.

The latent stage follows, and it may last for years as the bacteria invades the organs. It has no symptoms and is generally not contagious. The last stage of the disease produces serious illness and can lead to death.

Several tests can diagnose syphilis, depending on the stage of the disease. A doctor can examine fluid from the sores to identify the bacteria, or a blood test can be used to detect its presence or the presence of disease-fighting antibodies. In the later stages, spinal fluid may be examined.

Treating Syphilis.

Syphilis is treated with penicillin, injectable or intravenously, depending on the stage. Other kinds of antibiotics are given to people who are allergic to penicillin. Both partners should be diagnosed and treated at the same time. Treatment should be followed up with a blood test to make sure that the disease has been cured.

Trichomoniasis

Trichomoniasis or "trich" is a parasitic infection that affects 3 million Americans each year. It is spread by vaginal intercourse and also by sharing towels or washcloths. It is sometimes difficult to recognize, often mistaken as a yeast infection, bacterial vaginosis, or another problem.

Knowing Your Discharge

Bacterial vaginosis (BV), yeast infections, and trich produce discharges that are often confused. However, the treatments for each problem are different: BV and trich are treated with prescription medication, while self-help remedies and over-the-counter products cure yeast. Too often women take yeast remedies to cure BV or trich because they are easy to find and don't require a doctor's visit. But they don't work.

Here's a quick look at the different kinds of discharge:

Infection	Discharge
Trich	foamy, yellowish or gray, musty-smelling that can cause itching around the vagina
BV	whitish or grayish white, with an odor sometimes described as foul or fishy that is increased after intercourse
Yeast	consistency of cottage cheese, sometimes with a breadlike smell, that can cause itching and irritation

Detecting Trich.

In men and in some women trich has no symptoms. For women the most common symptom is a foamy, yellowish or gray, musty-smelling discharge that can cause itching around the vagina. Spotting, swelling in the groin, and frequent urination can also occur.

To diagnose trich, vaginal discharge is examined under a microscope.

Treating Trich.

The standard treatment is metronidazole (brand name Flagyl) taken orally. Many women taking the drug notice side effects such as headache, nausea, and diarrhea. Alcohol cannot be used while on the medication because it will cause serious illness. Ask your doctor about the single oral dose, which is more effective than taking pills over a longer period of time. Sexual partners should be diagnosed and treated simultaneously.

For More Information

ORGANIZATIONS

AMERICAN SOCIAL HEALTH ASSOCIATION, P.O. Box 13827, Research Triangle Park, NC 27709; (919) 361-8400. For information on all kinds of STI's.

NATIONAL FOUNDATION FOR INFECTIOUS DISEASES, 4733 Bethesda Ave., suite 750, Bethesda, MD 20814; (301)-656-0003. For information on all kinds of STI's.

NATIONAL STD HOTLINE, (800) 227-8922. For answers to general questions about STI's.

PLANNED PARENTHOOD FEDERATION OF AMERICA, 810 Seventh Ave., New York, NY 10019; (212) 541-7800. Ask for the pamphlets "Sexually Transmitted Diseases—The Facts," "HPV and Genital Warts: Questions and Answers," "Vaginitis: Questions and Answers," "Herpes: Questions and Answers," and "Chlamydia: Questions and Answers."

WOMEN'S HEALTH RESOURCE CENTER, 2440 M St. NW, Washington, DC 20037; (202) 293-6045. Ask for a free copy of "Sexually Transmitted Diseases: What Women Should Know for the 90s."

BOOKS

What Women Should Know About Chronic Infections and Sexually Transmitted Disease, Pamela P. Novotny, Dell Publishing, 1991.

13

Fighting Fibroids

In contrast to our glorious diversity of skin color, size, and other physical traits, there is one characteristic that far too many Black women share—uterine fibroid tumors. When groups of sisters gather, it seems like just about everyone has one, has had one, or knows several other women who have. Given their prevalence among us, it's surprising how little is known about how they are caused.

What Are Fibroids?

Fibroids are benign, generally nonmalignant tumors that grow in the uterus. About 40 percent of women in their late twenties to midforties have them. Bundles of smooth muscle and connective tissue with their own blood supply, fibroids are usually found in one of three locations: within the muscle layer of the uterus; outside the uterine wall; and inside the uterus. Often changing their size and shape, the single or multiple growths can range in size from that of a pea to larger than a grapefruit. Though they generally are not cancerous, they can be frightening to women who have them and can cause numerous health problems. In fact, 50 percent of women with fibroids have symptoms severe enough to affect their quality of life.

No one knows what causes fibroids, though researchers believe the tumors thrive on the hormone estrogen, because they seem to enlarge

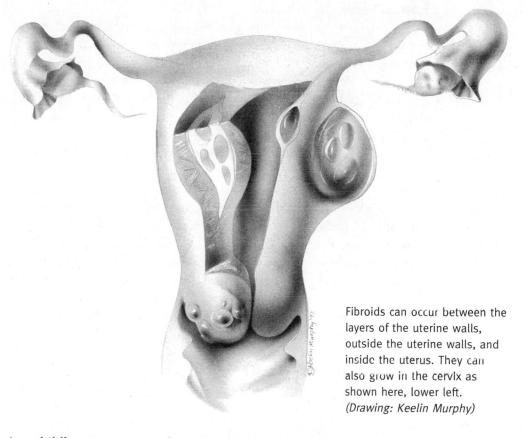

Fibroids can occur between the layers of the uterine walls, outside the uterine walls, and inside the uterus. They can also grow in the cervix as shown here, lower left.
(Drawing: Keelin Murphy)

during childbearing years and usually shrink after menopause when the production of estrogen decreases. Fibroids are also more common in women who have not had children and women who have taken birth control pills that contain high doses of estrogen. Medical experts also know that Black women have a 50 to 75 percent chance of developing the tumors, compared with a 33 percent chance for white women. It is not uncommon for several generations of women in the same family to suffer from the problem.

While there may appear to be a hereditary factor in the prevalence of fibroids among women of African descent, no definitive medical evidence exists to support the theory that Black women are genetically predisposed to the growths. Rather, experts hypothesize that Black women suffer a higher rate of fibroids and more complications from the tumors because we do not get routine checkups early or often enough. Far too many Black women delay getting basic gynecological exams, so that by the time we get into a physician's office, the fibroids are numerous and large.

How to Recognize Fibroids

Often detected during routine gynecological examinations or by a pelvic ultrasonic scan (which produces a sound-wave picture), most fibroids are small, harmless growths that can cause no symptoms and require no treatment at all. However, if left unchecked, the tumors can create a dominolike effect of reproductive-health problems ranging from excessive bleeding to infertility and may call for hysterectomy, the surgical removal of the entire uterus.

Heavy or prolonged menstrual bleeding is one of the early warning signs of fibroids. Some women complain of bleeding so heavily that they go through pads and tampons by the boxful. The bleeding can become so severe that the women become anemic and have to be transfused to get their low blood counts back to normal.

In addition to heavy bleeding, large fibroids can cause abdominal swelling (many women mistake large fibroids for unexplained weight gain), lower-back pain, painful sexual intercourse, fatigue due to iron deficiency, and a sensation of pressure on the back, legs, or lower abdomen. A large tumor can also exert pressure on the bladder and/or bowel, causing frequent urination or constipation.

For women trying to conceive, fibroids occasionally interfere with the implantation of the egg in the womb. For pregnant women, the growths can distort the uterine cavity, leading to recurrent miscarriage or complicated delivery.

Preventing and Managing Fibroids

The best protection against fibroids is to pay close attention to your body and get regular gynecological exams. Many experts also say that changes in diet can help women avoid or shrink fibroids. Studies show that eliminating (or at least reducing) caffeinated drinks (coffee, tea, chocolate, cola drinks), whole-milk dairy products, salt, alcoholic beverages, and fried and sugary foods can boost overall health and may fight fibroids. Many women have found success by eliminating all meat, including chicken, from their diets. Some holistic practitioners speculate that the hormones injected into animals cause or worsen fibroid tumors. Pesticides and chemical additives have also been implicated. Soy products are a good alternative to dairy, and fish can be substituted for poultry and red meat. A healthy diet should also include plenty of fresh vegetables, fruit, potatoes, pasta, nuts, beans, whole-grain rice and cereals, and water to help keep fibroids at bay.

Since I first started my period during adolescence, I've suffered from constant pain at the time of my menstrual cycle. But beginning my sophomore year in college, the pain and other symptoms became extreme. I was hospitalized almost monthly with pelvic discomfort so severe that I couldn't sleep for days because the pain would wake me up in the middle of the night. On several occasions I became dehydrated, couldn't eat, and had to be fed intravenously. My weight decreased drastically to 100 pounds, down from my normal weight of 120.

My periods were so heavy and the pain so debilitating that my menstrual cycle controlled my life. I took a job in sales so that I could tailor my work schedule around my menstrual cycle in order to cope with the problem. I worked frantically to reach my quota because I knew that when my menses began, I would be incapacitated.

Perhaps as bad as the pain was the mystery: I had no idea what was causing this problem. I sought relief from five different doctors, each with a different—erroneous—diagnosis. I was told that I had endometriosis. I was constipated often and suffered from frequent gas and urination, so I thought the problem was in my colon. I was given Tylenol with codeine, which made me tired and more constipated.

Finally I reached a frightening turning point. I woke up from anesthesia into the cold eyes of the gynecologist telling me that I may never have children. His diagnosis from an exploratory procedure revealed that my entire uterine cavity was deformed. I had at least one fibroid the size of a grapefruit and twenty-six others on the outside, inside, and embedded in the walls of my uterus. They had been pressing down on the nerve endings in my pelvic region, causing my pain. The doctor suggested I get pregnant, which might alleviate the pain, or better yet, have a hysterectomy. I was only twenty-two years old and alone. I knew I had to get more information and find a better, more sympathetic doctor.

Eventually I found a woman doctor, who was much more sensitive, thorough, and supportive. We decided I would undergo a polymyomectomy, which would remove the fibroids but leave my womb intact.

Three years have passed since the surgery, and I have finally been able to live a more normal life. However, recently I've noticed that some of the old symptoms have been sneaking up, and I'm afraid that the fibroids have begun to reform.

I'm not ready to conceive, but I also refuse to let these tumors control me again. I'm talking to my sisters openly about this problem because of the six of them, four have had surgery for fibroids. I'm also looking into making

> "I refuse to let these tumors control me."
>
> —Jean Jones, Jacksonville, Florida, hospital development manager

dietary changes. Right now I eat red meat and also lots of fried foods and tons of dairy. I also drink coffee and soda and eat sweets. Though I've tried unsuccessfully to cut down in the past, this time I'm going to make it happen.

Holistic Alternatives

Daya Oliver, a holistic-health consultant and director of Daya Associates in Harlem, treats fibroids by detoxifying the body through nutrition counseling and colonic irrigation, which clears the bowel tract of impurities. She bluntly states the importance of a healthy diet: "About 70 percent of my female clients have fibroids, which I believe are an accumulation from high-fat, high-cholesterol diets. Black women need to spend their money on juicers and organic vegetables. You either pay now to prevent fibroids or pay later for surgery that might prevent you from having a child."

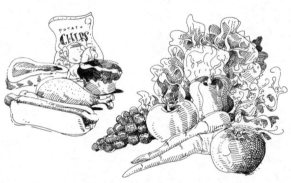

To prevent fibroids, cut down on meat and junk food, and eat more fruit and vegetables.
(Drawing: Yvonne Buchanan)

In a moving article in *Essence* magazine, poet and writer Alexis De Veaux told of using nontraditional alternatives to heal her fibroid tumors. "I discovered alternative systems of natural healing: herbology, meditation, massage, homeopathy, t'ai chi. Initiated into natural living, I fasted and detoxed with enemas and colonics. I ate 80 percent of my food raw. Cut out all dairy and flesh food products. Got myself a juicer and drank delicious, fresh juice daily. I believed that I could heal myself. That 'you are what you eat.' That food is medicine." De Veaux also added exercise to her daily schedule and worked hard to put her emotional and spiritual lives in balance by dissolving old hurt and pain. Thanks to these changes in her lifestyle she was able to manage her fibroids for six years; eventually, however, she opted to have the tumors removed surgically.

De Veaux and others understand that the relationship between mind and body can be critical in the prevention and management of fibroids. Studies suggest that like fatty, cholesterol-packed foods, stress and negative mental attitudes contribute to illness. For Black women, learning how to deal positively with racism and sexism can help reduce the stress many of us live with. Meditation, yoga, and regular exercise such as walking, aerobic dancing, and running are some of the holistic techniques African-American women can use to "cool out."

In addition to vitamins A, B, and E, which help balance estrogen levels, many women include herbal-medicine treatments in their battle plan against fibroids. Wild yam, chaste berry, raspberry leaf, and damiana are all herbs that have proven effective in the reduction of fibroids, according to experts. (While a variety of vitamins and herbs are widely available, be sure to get expert advice before taking them. It can be dangerous to self-medicate without the supervision of a health-care professional.)

How to Treat Fibroids

In some cases fibroids shrink on their own and require no treatment at all, especially if you are following a healthy diet and exercise regimen. Also, fibroids tend to shrink during and after menopause when estrogen levels (which fibroids thrive on) drop. But even if you are approaching menopause, or have small fibroids that are not growing or not growing rapidly, you must visit a gynecologist who will monitor them. Though you may notice some positive signs (such as lighter menstrual periods), only a health-care professional can tell you for sure the exact state of your fibroid tumors.

Studies show that a type of medication called GnRH analogs (most commonly prescribed as Lupron) can reduce fibroids by temporarily shutting down the body's production of estrogen, the hormone that feeds fibroid growth. The medication, generally given as an injection, shrinks the fibroids, allowing physicians to better monitor them or to remove them using less invasive procedures.

This type of drug treatment, however, is not without its drawbacks. It is only a temporary stopgap measure; when the medication is discontinued, the fibroids grow back. Plus, it can be much too expensive for some women. Also, because it inhibits the release of estrogen, it can induce a temporary menopausal state with such side effects as hot flashes, vaginal dryness, and mood swings.

If your fibroids are large and causing major health problems, chances are you will have to consider undergoing some form of surgery to remove them. For example, you may need surgery if the fibroids are:

- Causing bleeding heavy enough to lead to anemia
- Growing rapidly, which may suggest malignancy (this is extremely rare)
- As large as the size of a fourteen-week-old fetus, which may obscure more serious problems such as ovarian cancer

- Causing severe pain or pressing on the bladder or urethra, which could result in kidney failure

If the fibroids are inside the uterus and small—less than 1.5 centimeters in size—a doctor may use an instrument called a hysteroscope to remove them. In this procedure, the fibroids are either burned away with a laser or scraped off. This procedure is generally done on an outpatient basis, and there is no scar or severe pain. Small fibroids on the outside of the uterus can be removed with a laparoscope, a telescopic instrument inserted through an incision in the abdomen.

If the fibroids have caused the uterus to swell to the size it would be in a twelve-week pregnancy or larger, *myomectomy* might be recommended. In this procedure, the physician surgically removes the fibroids while leaving the uterus intact—which means that a myomectomy shouldn't affect your ability to conceive. The surgery can be done with a scalpel, but the newest option is laser myomectomy. In this procedure, the surgeon removes the fibroids, generally with a laser beam via a small incision in the belly. Some surgeons will not perform myomectomies because the fibroid or fibroids are too large or there are too many. A complicated operation may be beyond the skill level of the surgeon. It's important to remember that a surgeon's skill makes a big difference when it comes to myomectomy, so don't be afraid to ask how many of these procedures your doctor has performed.

Between 15 and 45 percent of women who undergo myomectomies also report subsequent regrowth of the tumors. The best way to find out whether myomectomy is for you is to openly discuss all of the advantages and disadvantages with your physician. Myomectomy is a more complicated procedure than hysterectomy, and many physicians don't know how to perform it; this prompts some to disregard it as a treatment option.

Hysterectomy, the surgical removal of the uterus, is still the most common treatment for fibroids. But it shouldn't be: With the alternatives to hysterectomy, it should only be considered after you've discussed other treatments with your doctor. Hysterectomy will forever rid your body of fibroids, but it also ends the possibility of giving birth.

Every year physicians perform over half a million hysterectomies, making it the second most frequent major surgery performed in this country; only cesarean sections are performed more often. Doctors in the United States perform hysterectomies more than doctors in European countries, and they remove ovaries in greater numbers than

I knew something was wrong. My periods weren't supposed to be five or six days of heavy flow coupled with clotting and pain. But I told myself that the problem was due to lack of exercise, not something more serious. I didn't have time to be sick. A single mother with four small children, I was also in the process of starting my own business. I put my children's needs and the business ahead of my own. As long as I felt fine and could get out of bed every day, there was no need to worry.

But the thought of my health failing crept into my consciousness from time to time. If I were bedridden, who would care for my children? So I went to the doctor.

"Don't worry about them; if you don't bother them, they won't bother you," he said of the fibroids he found in my uterus. Because I had sought help early, they were small, less than the size of a four-week-old embryo. But the fact that something foreign was growing in my body, capable of multiplying, unnerved me.

For a while I had been reading books and articles on nutrition in an attempt to lead a more healthy lifestyle, and I had cut red meat out of my diet after encountering facts about the negative effects meat has on the body. The more I read, the more I leaned toward making a drastic dietary change. If fibroids are linked to poor eating habits, I could certainly benefit—and save thousands of dollars on medical care—by eating properly.

I gave up chicken, white flour, sugar, salt, and all dairy. I also fasted twice during a three-week period and practiced yoga and meditation every day to relieve stress. I also attended a seminar on fibroid tumors sponsored by Daya Associates in Harlem, a progressive gynecologist from Brooklyn, who is interested in holistic methods of healing.

After a few months, I noticed a dramatic change. I no longer felt moody and depressed, and my cramps disappeared. My period became much more regular, with no clotting. The flow has decreased and is bright red in color.

I had been healing my own body without professional help and decided it was time to have a doctor monitor my fibroids and my diet. To my surprise, when she examined me, my fibroids were gone. At that point, I became a true believer in healthy living.

> *"I had been healing my own body without professional help and decided it was time to have a doctor monitor my fibroids and my diet. To my surprise, when she examined me, my fibroids were gone."*
>
> —Bette Vargas, entrepreneur, Brooklyn

they did twenty years ago. Hysterectomies are most often performed for fibroid tumors.

Yet a number of experts believe that many, if not the majority, of hysterectomies may be unnecessary. Black women receive a disproportionate number of hysterectomies, and the mortality rate for the operation is twice as high for Black as for white women. What's more, in the state of Maryland, one study showed that 67 percent of hysterectomies performed on Black women were for fibroids, compared to 30 percent for white women.

If a doctor tells you that you must have a hysterectomy to rid your body of fibroids, consult another physician. Some doctors will automatically recommend hysterectomy because they are unaware of or not proficient in some of the newer techniques to rid the body of fibroids. At about $3,000 to $6,000, hysterectomy is much more expensive than other procedures. That, suggests many health activists, is why doctors are sometimes eager to perform them. On the other hand, if your fibroids are severe, you've had a myomectomy and they've grown back, *and* you've had all the children you want or you don't want any, then having a hysterectomy may be a viable choice for you. But before you decide, be sure you know what the operation entails, its risks and its side effects. (For more information on hysterectomy, see chapter 16, "The Hysterectomy Decision.")

You Can Be Healed

One of the most important things for Black women to remember about uterine fibroid tumors is that we can manage or perhaps avoid them, and we don't have to do it alone. Though there hasn't been enough research conducted on the cause, growth, treatment, and prevention of fibroids (given how widespread the problem is), you can find information about natural healing, surgery, and other treatment options that are available to you. If you have been diagnosed with fibroids, talk to other Black women friends and family members about the problem. And most important, choose health-care providers who treat you as a partner and allow you to determine your medical destiny. If you have fibroids, here are some questions to ask your doctor:

Do you think my fibroids should be removed? Why?

What diagnostic tests have you done to rule out other causes for my symptoms?

If the fibroids aren't causing any problems, what are the risks if I don't have surgery?

Is there any way to treat them without surgery?

Can I shrink the fibroid with medication? Would the resulting smaller fibroid lessen the complications of surgery?

If minor surgery is required, are you comfortable doing the procedure? How many times have you done it before? Can you recommend someone else?

What are the risks if I decide to postpone or rule out surgery? How often should I monitor the fibroid with checkups?

If I decide to have surgery, what is the estimated cost and recovery period?

In the October 1991 issue of *Vital Signs* (No. 3, "The Politics of Black Women's Health"), the newsletter of the National Black Women's Health Project, Marsha Carruthers wrote about her struggle with fibroids and her decision to change her eating habits as a step toward healing. She offers the following advice as you start your own healing process:

- Find out as much as you can about fibroids. Not a lot has been written, but read whatever information is out there.
- Compare the cost of good, healthy, vital food to that of extra sanitary pads, painkillers, possible surgery, and your own pain and suffering. Healthy food is sometimes more expensive and more time-consuming to prepare than fast food and highly processed choices, but taking other "costs" into consideration, it's worth the time and expense. And don't forget: You're worth it.
- Begin a new regimen at the beginning of a menstrual cycle, so you can monitor your progress.
- Take it easy. Realize that rest is an important component of the healing process.
- Monitor your physical and emotional symptoms so you know as much as possible about your own body and its responses.
- Allow yourself time to heal. Consider this a wellness vacation that you deserve. Otherwise, your regimen could turn into just another stressful problem.
- Keep a journal. This is an empowering experience, which you will want to remember and possibly share with other sisters.

For More Information

ORGANIZATIONS

THE HYSTERECTOMY EDUCATIONAL RESOURCES AND SERVICES (HERS) FOUNDATION, 422 Bryn Mawr Ave., Bala Cynwyd, PA 19004; (215) 667-7757. HERS has a wide range of information on hysterectomy, how to avoid it, and the consequences of and alternatives to surgery.

WOMEN'S REPRODUCTIVE HEALTH NETWORK, P.O. Box 301607,

Portland, OR 97230-9607; (503) 252-9024. The organization provides free information and support for women who are contemplating hysterectomies or have had hysterectomies and are suffering side effects.

TREATMENT AND SUPPORT

CIVILIZED MEDICINE INSTITUTE, J.E.W.E.L. (Justifiably Enchanted with Enlightened Living) Publications, 8469 E. Jefferson Ave., Detroit, MI 48214; (313) 331-8747. The Institute, run by Dr. Jewel Pookrum, offers a Uterine Fibroid Support Group that helps members cope with emotional issues surrounding fibroids and offers holistic treatment and prevention advice. There are currently chapters in Detroit, Atlanta, and New York (mentioned below) and plans to open a Cleveland chapter.

DAYA ASSOCIATES, 76 W. 125th St., New York, NY 10027; (212) 722-2194. Daya Oliver, a holistic-health practitioner, holds weekly support-group meetings for women with fibroids for a nominal fee. She also sponsors a health symposium every spring for women only, which addresses holistic methods for healing fibroids. Says Detroit group member Verda Turner: "The group has given me a better understanding of myself. I still have a lot of growing to do, but I think I'm on the right path spiritually."

BOOKS

Fibroid Tumors and Endometriosis: A Self-Help Program, by Susan M. Lark, M.D., Westchester Publishing Company (Los Altos, Calif.), 1993.

ARTICLES in *Essence*

Essence magazine has covered fibroids frequently. These articles deserve special mention:
"New Body, New Life," Alexis De Veaux, June 1988
"The Fibroid Epidemic," Evelyn C. White, December 1990
"More on Fibroids," Evelyn C. White, December 1991
"Fibroids: A Report," Rachel Jackson Christmas, January 1994

14

How to Get Pregnant: Reproduction and Infertility

Every would-be mother dreams of bearing a healthy, normal child. Wishing alone, however, will not make it so. In recent years, a wealth of medical evidence has established that the physical and emotional health of parents has a major impact on the well-being of an unborn child not only during pregnancy but also prior to conception. For some couples, conception seems impossible. After months or even years of trying, they still can't conceive. And, surprisingly, given the unfair image of Black women as "baby-making machines," infertility may be more common among Black couples as compared with white. Some give up and decide to remain childless, while others happily adopt Black children from among the many that need homes. If you've recently decided to conceive, you'll need to know how to raise your chances of getting pregnant and having a healthy pregnancy. If you've been trying to conceive without success, it's important to understand why you may be having trouble making a baby and learn what you can do about it. You'll also need to know where you can get information and emotional support and what you need to know if you want to adopt a child.

Should You Get Pregnant?

Can you afford a child? This means both financially and emotionally. Many women, especially young ones, think a baby will give them the love they crave and didn't get from parents or partners, but babies are not equipped to give. They take and take. Having a child requires that you not only buy the diapers and the food, but that you nurture them and keep them clean and comfortable and healthy.

If you are partnered, is your relationship ready for a child? You may be pressured by your man to have "his baby" to prove something. Don't. A man who needs for you to "bear his seed" so that he can feel secure isn't the kind of man you want. Take your time in getting to know him. A baby puts a strain on the best of relationships—you were two and now you're three, and that third person needs all of your attention. To raise a child together is tough; it requires maturity and understanding. Think long and hard about this one.

Do you and your partner have similar ideas about educating the child? What about religion? Discipline? Most people figure that if they're in a good relationship, then they'll be good parents, but this ain't necessarily so.

Is your relationship shaky? Many people think a baby will fix things between them. This is so wrong. What ends up happening is the baby further exacerbates whatever problems there were. Fortunately, those relationships that are strong tend to blossom after a baby is born.

Do you like children? This may seem like a silly question, but you should really consider it. You don't have to turn to mush every time you see a child walking down the street, but you should be able to be around children, with their demands and uncivilized behavior, without wanting to scream. You should be able to talk with them, establish a rapport and a relationship. If you can't think of any child you've liked and spent time with, maybe you should think longer about becoming a parent. One way to test your feelings about children is to go out of your way to be around them. Of course, you'll react differently to your own, but you'll get a good sense of what it's like spending a weekend alone with a niece or nephew. If you like the idea of sharing your life with a child, that's a good sign.

Can your life—the way it is now with school or work—sustain the strain of a child? Are you working on a degree or trying to break out of the secretarial pool into management? If so, maybe now isn't the best time to have a baby. If, however, you've accomplished some of the things you've set out to do, then you may be ready to make space in your life.

Are you the right age to have a child? For many young women, having a baby before the end of high school can create a lifetime of burdens. Teenagers tend to have babies with lower birth weights, babies born with defects, and more difficult labor and deliveries.

Pre-Conception Checkup
Approximately three to six months before you start trying to conceive, you'll need to visit your doctor or nurse-midwife for a prepregnancy or pre-conception exam. This will allow you, your doctor, and your mate to identify any potential problems your health, history, or lifestyle may present to your fertility and/or pregnancy and will give you ample time to correct them.

Most gynecologists and family doctors in private practice and HMO's perform prepregnancy exams, as do health care practitioners at a number of health clinics. For specific recommendations, you may want to check with friends who have recently had children, Planned Parenthood, or your local hospital or medical society. Depending on where you live and who you see, the cost of a pre-conception physical could range anywhere from $75 to $200. You may want to check with your insurance company, however, as many of the costs associated with this exam may be covered.

Stopping Birth Control
When you're ready to get pregnant, you must stop using birth control. Some types take longer than others to leave your system.

The Pill. The birth control pill makes your menstrual cycle regular, so when you stop taking it, your next couple of periods may be irregular. But your cycle should normalize within a few months.

Norplant. These implants, which are placed under the skin in the arm, prevent contraception for up to five years. If you decide you'd like to become pregnant before that time, your doctor can take them out. Once they've been removed, you should be able to get pregnant anytime.

Depo-Provera: This injectable contraception generally lasts about three months, but even after the shot is discontinued, some women have trouble getting pregnant. Lingering effects of the shot may inhibit ovulation for three to nine months.

(Please note: The National Black Women's Health Project does not recommend either Norplant or Depo-Provera. For more information see chapter 10, "Birth Control.")

Conception and Women Over Thirty

Not too long ago, conventional wisdom had it that women in their late thirties and early forties should be setting their sights on becoming grandmothers rather than experiencing motherhood. In the last twenty years, however, the number of women waiting to conceive has increased markedly. Careers, late and second marriages, finances, and personal preference have made waiting until after age thirty to have a baby commonplace.

As a woman ages, the risks of her having problems during pregnancy increase, and it may be more difficult for her to have a healthy child. Chromosomal abnormality and Down's syndrome are some of the potential disorders we hear about most often being associated with advanced maternal age. For women over thirty-five, spontaneous abortion (miscarriage) during the first three months of pregnancy is also more prevalent, as are high blood pressure during pregnancy, gestational diabetes, and premature delivery. A decrease in muscle tone and flexibility can also make delivery more difficult.

It may also take a woman over thirty-five longer to get pregnant. Fertility declines as we reach our midthirties because there are fewer eggs available for fertilization. Still, even if it takes longer to conceive and despite the risks, the overwhelming majority of women in their thirties can and do get pregnant and have healthy babies and few complications.

How Reproduction Works

Every month a woman ovulates and an egg is released from her ovaries into one of her fallopian tubes. During that period of about twelve to twenty-four hours the egg travels through the tube toward her uterus. If that egg comes into contact with fresh sperm during that period, it may be fertilized, implant on the lining of the uterus, and grow into a fetus. If it isn't fertilized, the egg is absorbed into the woman's body.

Fertilization can occur during sexual intercourse. At the peak of sexual excitement, a man ejaculates, sending semen (a mixture of fluid and millions of sperm cells) into the woman's vagina. (Though a man has to have an orgasm in order to ejaculate, a woman doesn't have to be aroused to conceive, which is why women who are raped can get pregnant.) Once the sperm enters the vagina, they travel up through the

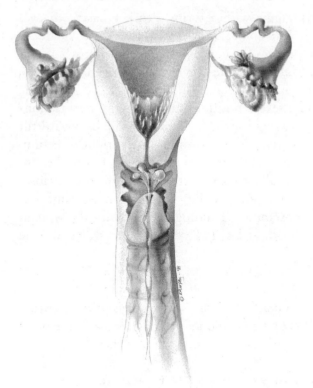

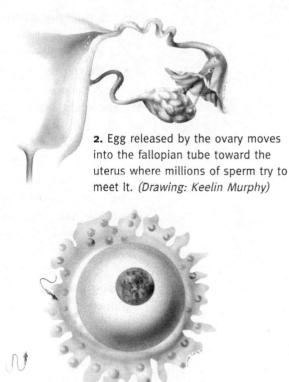

2. Egg released by the ovary moves into the fallopian tube toward the uterus where millions of sperm try to meet It. *(Drawing: Keelin Murphy)*

1. Ejaculation inside the vagina. *(Drawing: Keelin Murphy)*

3. Fertilization occurs when a sperm (enlarged) succeeds in penetrating the egg. *(Drawing: Keelin Murphy)*

cervix, into the uterus, and out into the fallopian tubes. It only takes one sperm cell to meet up with the egg in order for fertilization to occur.

If a man and woman have sex when she's not ovulating, she won't become pregnant, because there won't be an egg available for fertilization. However, sperm can live in a woman's body two to three days or longer. So, if she has intercourse a few days before ovulation, sperm may still be present by the time she ovulates and she can become pregnant.

A woman can get pregnant without sexual intercourse. For example, when a man's penis is erect, it can leak preejaculatory, fluid which contains semen. If that semen finds its way into the vagina, it can impregnate the egg. Pregnancy can occur when the penis is not inside of the vagina, but the man ejaculates near it. That's why withdrawal—pulling the penis rapidly out of the vagina before ejaculation—sometimes results in pregnancy. Heterosexual women whose mates have fertility problems use alternative insemination, which is also called donor or artificial insemination; lesbians also use this method. In this procedure sperm is injected into the woman's vagina with a syringe, turkey baster, or eye-dropper as an alternative to intercourse.

You can improve your chances for conceiving by knowing when and how to have intercourse. Male hormones are at their peak in the morning. Sperm counts are also highest then, assuming you have not made love the night before. Some sexual positions are also more fertilization-friendly than others. When having sex, try to increase the backward tilt of your vagina to get the sperm off and running in the right direction. The woman-on-bottom, man-on-top missionary style is a good bet; so are the rear-entry style (which allows your partner to get his sperm closer to the cervix) and lying on your side. While you are trying to conceive, try not to make love sitting, standing, bending over, or with the woman on top, as these positions make it less likely that sperm will enter the cervix.

Charting Ovulation

The ideal time to attempt to conceive is one or two days prior to ovulation, so that sperm will already be positioned in the fallopian tube waiting for the egg to arrive. That means you must know when your ovulation is about to occur.

Doctors estimate that most women ovulate thirteen to fifteen days after the start of the menstrual cycle (the first day that bleeding occurs). This is not an exact science, however, and many women who want to pinpoint ovulation do so by keeping a basal body-temperature guide, a chart that records the fluctuations of reproductive hormones. Just before and during ovulation, the body temperature dips to slightly below normal (98.6 degrees F.) and then rises to slightly above normal just after ovulation. So by taking your temperature every day for two to three months, beginning with the first day of a new menstrual cycle, you can determine specific drops in body temperature that generally indicate that ovulation is taking place.

You can also learn to recognize changes in your cervical mucus to help determine when ovulation is about to occur. All women have discharge, which changes during different times in the menstrual cycle. During ovulation, cervical fluid increases and becomes thinner, wetter, and more slippery. Just after ovulation it is more sticky and rubbery.

You can also determine when you are at your most fertile with one of the commercial ovulation-predictor kits for sale in most drugstores. To predict ovulation, you mix an early-morning urine sample with a chemical solution; if you are about to ovulate, the solution will change colors

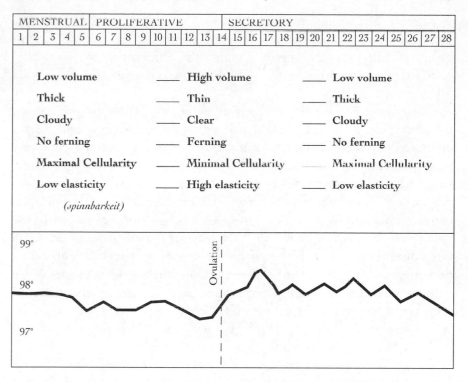

MENSTRUAL	PROLIFERATIVE				SECRETORY											
1	2	3	4	5	6	7	8	9	10	11	12	13	14	15	16	17	18	19	20	21	22	23	24	25	26	27	28

Low volume	___	High volume	___	Low volume
Thick	___	Thin	___	Thick
Cloudy	___	Clear	___	Cloudy
No ferning	___	Ferning	___	No ferning
Maximal Cellularity	___	Minimal Cellularity	___	Maximal Cellularity
Low elasticity	___	High elasticity	___	Low elasticity
(spinnbarkeit)				

This chart describes the changes the body goes through during the various phases of the menstrual cycle. For example, about fourteen days into the cycle, ovulation occurs; this is the best time to try to get pregnant. During this phase, hormonal levels change; body temperature drops, then rises; cervical mucus increases and grows thinner and more elastic; and symptoms such as spotting and mild pain may appear.

because of hormones that are released into the urine prior to ovulation. (Women over forty should note that the early stages of menopause can affect test results, as can fertility drugs.)

Practical Tips to Encourage Conception

It's extremely wise to make sure your body is at its best when you're ready to try to get pregnant. It takes two to make a baby, so your mate has to keep healthy, too. Both of you should follow this practical advice:

Eat right. Good nutrition may be the most essential prerequisite for conceiving and delivering a healthy child. Studies show that women who are well nourished when they conceive are more likely to have stronger bodies that are better able to cope with the demands of pregnancy and more nutrient resources for the growing child. That means sticking to a diet low in fat, sugar, salt, and processed foods. Eat plenty of fish, lean meat, vegetables, fruit, grains, and cereals. Drink at least six glasses of water per day.

Manage any medical problems. If you have an illness that could complicate pregnancy—such as diabetes or high blood pressure—talk to your doctor about how you can get it under control.

Keep fit. The stronger your body is, the better you'll be able to handle pregnancy and childbirth. But be careful not to exercise too strenuously—as in serious training for a marathon. Sometimes strenuous exercise leads to amenorrhea or the absence of menstruation, and temporary infertility results.

Watch your weight. Try to keep as close as possible to the recommended weight for your height and age. (Because height and weight charts have recently been under scrutiny, it's best to discuss your case with your health care provider.) Women who are underweight sometimes have irregular periods or lose them altogether, which can prevent pregnancy. Those who are 10 percent below their optimum weight also run a greater risk of delivering low-weight babies. Obese women (those more than 20 percent above ideal weight), of which there are many in our community, run a higher risk of developing diabetes, high blood pressure, and toxemia, and delivering low-birth-weight babies. Even women who are just slightly overweight may experience discomfort as they begin to put on the added weight that comes with pregnancy. It's best to either gain or lose weight before conceiving and to give your body some time to adjust to the new size.

Control stress. It's not that your worries and concerns should not be important to you, they simply should not be allowed to overwhelm you to the point that they affect your emotional and physical health. In women of childbearing age, stress, left unchecked, can affect your fertility. If you do get pregnant, it may cause problems for your unborn child. Keep stress in check with long walks, yoga, meditation, therapy, support groups—or any way that works for you.

Don't smoke. According to *Alcohol, Tobacco and Other Drugs May Harm the Unborn,* a report published by the U.S. Department of Health and Human Services, women who smoke regularly are "more likely than nonsmokers to take a year or more to conceive. Male smokers run a greater risk of lowering sperm production and motility and increasing the amount of sperm that are abnormally formed." Plus, if you do smoke, it's best to quit before you get pregnant, because you absolutely *must* stop once you've conceived: Smoking can lead to miscarriage and low birth weight in babies.

Stop drinking and don't use drugs. Women who have more than three drinks a day are more likely to experience menstrual irregularities, hormonal dysfunction, the stoppage of ovulation, and early menopause. Among men who drink heavily, testosterone levels and sperm counts are lowered, sexual drive is diminished, and impotence may occur. Drugs

I'd been married about seven years and was raising two of my husband's children. They called me Momma, and I knew they loved me, but it wasn't enough. To me there is no greater love than having your own.

So even while I was playing mommy to his kids, my husband and I had been trying to have a child since a year after we were married. After trying for three years to conceive, I decided to swallow my feminine pride and sought the services of an infertility specialist. The verdict: a hormonal imbalance—my prolactin level was too high. My doctor prescribed a treatment, and afterward my menstrual cycle regulated itself. I thought to myself, all right, now I could have a child! Wrong. Dead wrong.

We tried again to conceive, to no avail. I was desperate. I felt like a failure as a woman. I went again to see my OB-GYN, and she assured me that I was just fine and to just keep trying. We did. Nothing happened for several years. Well, one day I had a good cry—emptied myself out, as a matter of fact—and convinced myself that I would get over it. By this time, I had grown used to the constant questioning from family and friends about when I was going to have a baby of my own. I became expert at dodging their questions at family gatherings and stayed out of the range of maternal group conversations at work. I also learned to deal with the depression that comes with feeling inadequate because I was unable to give my husband and, most importantly, myself, a child.

During this time, I went on a diet and lost a considerable amount of weight. I did so by getting rid of my wayward eating habits and switching to a healthy diet. Well, in June of 1992, I began to feel very strange. I attributed my abdominal pains, light-headedness, sleepiness, and nausea to the fact that I was getting my period. Then days passed—fourteen, to be exact—and I still wasn't "seeing red." I thought that I was experiencing an irregular cycle again. No big deal. I mentioned my symptoms to my best friend, who's a major hypochondriac, and she insisted that I get one of those home pregnancy tests.

I did so just to humor her. To my surprise, I was pregnant. In March of 1993, at age thirty-five, I gave birth to a little boy, 7 pounds, 13 ounces, 21 inches long. After trying so hard, for so long, I still can't quite believe he's mine. I am so proud.

"After trying so hard, for so long, I still can't quite believe he's mine."

—NAME WITHHELD, RENT EXAMINER, BROOKLYN

such as marijuana, heroin, and cocaine can reduce sperm counts and cause menstrual and ovulation irregularities, a decrease in sexual desire, and, in some cases where the couples are marginally fertile, temporary sterility. Again, it's best to stop now, because you cannot drink or use drugs during pregnancy without risking serious harm to your baby.

Look out for other health risks. Prescription medications, caffeine, over-the-counter remedies, vitamins, industrial chemicals, and other environmental pollutants can keep you from getting pregnant. It's best to be a natural woman: Try to stay as chemical-free as possible, before and during pregnancy.

Warn your mate about becoming overheated. He should steer clear of very strenuous workouts in warm areas because high temperatures can lower his sperm count and the sperm's ability to travel. Tight clothing or clothes that hold the heat, especially during exercise, are also potentially harmful, and the same goes for saunas, steam baths, Jacuzzis, and hot showers.

Infertility

For couples who look forward to having children, few disappointments are as crushing as not being able to conceive. A clinical condition, infertility strikes at the heart of our dreams, values, and visions of ourselves. And while it is increasingly treatable, overcoming infertility can also be a trial requiring vast physical, emotional, and financial reserves.

Experts diagnose infertility when a couple has had unprotected intercourse for one year without the woman becoming pregnant or the woman is unable to carry the pregnancy to live birth. (Look for a discussion of miscarriage in chapter 15, "Having a Healthy Baby.") Often couples think they're infertile after attempting to conceive without success for a few months, but actually they may just need to keep trying. In fact, only one-fourth of all women get pregnant in the first month after they've stopped using birth control. According to specialists in the field, more than 15 percent of American couples—four and a half million—are plagued by infertility, with Blacks affected nearly one and a half times more often than whites. These statistics may seem frightening, but there is good news. After a year of treatment, more than half of all couples who experience problems conceiving are able to become fertile.

Causes of Infertility

Infertility is generally blamed on the woman, although, in reality, 40 percent of the time it's caused by factors affecting the female, 40 percent by factors attributed to the male, and 20 percent by a combination of male and female factors. In the remaining cases, experts can't find a cause, although only 3.5 percent of the time does infertility continue to

The Horror of DES

In 1981 one day before her twenty-fifth birthday, Sonya Wisdom went to a nurse practitioner for a routine pelvic exam and Pap smear. "During the course of the exam I was asked, to my complete surprise, if I had been exposed to a drug called diethylstilbestrol or DES. I had read about the drug briefly, never dreaming a connection to me was even remotely possible."

But after she thought about it, Sonya realized that her mother was a perfect candidate for DES, a synthetic hormone that was given to millions of women all over the world from 1941 to 1971 in the mistaken belief that it would help prevent miscarriage. Desperate for a child after four miscarriages, she had probably been given the drug knowingly or unknowingly. With that revelation came the beginning of Sonya's nightmare.

DES didn't prevent miscarriage. Instead it has caused unforeseen damage to the bodies of many of the children who were exposed to it before birth. These DES daughters (and some DES sons) can suffer from cancer and reproductive problems, *including infertility, miscarriage, ectopic pregnancy, and premature birth. And as more and more of these DES babies are reaching midlife, experts are beginning to link the drug with diseases that cause permanent impairment of the immune system.*

Sonya blames exposure to DES for her difficult pregnancy. "It was through a combination of a very real miracle and sheer determination that my son was born," she says. "I believed during my pregnancy and I believe now that DES was a participating factor in my pregnancy."

DES Action, a group that provides medical information, referrals, and publications, urges men and women to ask their mothers whether they took DES. It's better to know so that health-care practitioners can recommend special care. Many physicians believe that DES daughters should avoid the Pill, and DES mothers should use it cautiously if at all.

For more information • contact DES Action, 1615 Broadway, suite 510, Oakland, CA 94612; (510) 465-4011.

be unexplained once a thorough examination of both partners has been conducted. (In some cases, exposure in the womb to DES, a drug that was given to women in the 1940s, 1950s, and 1960s to prevent miscarriage, has caused infertility in their male and female children.)

Infertility is a medical problem (only a very small percentage of cases involve a psychological factor), with a medical or practical remedy. So it's very important for you and your mate to get checked out by a medical professional if you're having trouble conceiving. If after a year of trying your doctor is saying, "Just relax, you're too tense" or "Stop trying so hard," get a second opinion. Here are some of the causes and solutions.

Factors Affecting Women

Hormonal imbalance, menstrual irregularity, and structural problems of the reproductive organs can all cause infertility and must be checked out by a physician. Other common factors affecting women:

Pelvic Inflammatory Disease (PID).
This severe infection, which may involve the uterus, fallopian tubes, and ovaries, is a leading cause of female infertility. Black women face a particular risk of PID, because too often we contract sexually transmitted infections (STI's) that have no symptoms and allow them to progress unchecked. Untreated STI's can develop into PID. Use of the intrauterine device (IUD) also raises the risk of developing PID.

What to do: All women should have a yearly gynecological examination, which can help detect STI's. Though many STI's have no symptoms (some women find out they're infected after being tested when their partners show signs), you should still pay close attention to your body and notice any changes in discharge or any kinds of sores or irritation in your genital area. Get these checked right away. (For more information on STI's, see chapter 12, "Reproductive-Tract Infections.") If you have PID, you'll notice tenderness or pain in your pelvic region, abnormal or foul-smelling discharge, abnormal bleeding, and perhaps fever and chills. If you suspect you have PID, see a doctor immediately.

Abortion.
The vast majority of abortions don't result in complications. However, in some cases, an infection can occur after an abortion, a common problem in the days before safe, legal abortion and in countries where legal abortion is not available. This infection can lead to damage of the reproductive organs and infertility.

What to do: The National Abortion Federation strongly urges that if you have any of the following symptoms after an abortion, you see a doctor immediately or contact the facility that provided the abortion:

- Severe pain
- Chills or fever with a temperature of 104 degrees F. or more

- Bleeding that is heavier than the heaviest day of your normal period or that saturates one sanitary pad an hour
- Foul-smelling discharge
- Continuing symptoms of pregnancy such as delay (six weeks or more) in resuming menstrual periods.

Gynecological Illnesses.
Endometriosis causes tissue growths to latch on to the outside of the uterus, often blocking the reproductive tract; fibroid tumors and ovarian cysts may prevent conception.

What to do: Yearly gynecological checkups can help prevent and detect problems of the reproductive system. If you suspect you have any of these disorders, see a doctor immediately.

Medication.
A number of drugs can affect fertility, including anticancer drugs and chemotherapy. Illegal drugs of all kinds can prevent conception. Many drugs, both prescription (such as tranquilizers, accutane, which is used for acne, and antiseizure medication) and illegal (especially cocaine and its derivatives), can cause fetal damage. Alcohol can also affect fertility.

What to do: Never adjust or discontinue prescription medication without consulting your physician, but talk to your doctor about any medications you're taking and your plans to get pregnant. Don't drink alcohol if you're trying to get pregnant, and never use illegal drugs.

Factors Affecting Men

STI's.
Untreated STI's, such as gonorrhea or chlamydia, can cause scar tissue in the passageways through which the sperm must travel. In men, STI's are generally signaled by sores on the genitals and/or discharge from the penis.

What to do: If you or he suspect that he may have an STI, he must see a doctor immediately.

Medication.
A number of prescription medications, including drugs to combat high blood pressure, can cause impotence. Antihypertensives and other medications can also affect sperm count and sperm movement. Illegal drugs and alcohol can also affect male fertility.

What to do: He should never adjust or discontinue prescription medication without consulting his physician. Advise him to talk to his doctor about any medications he's taking and mention that the two of you would like to have a child. He shouldn't drink alcohol if you're trying to get pregnant, and no one should use illegal drugs.

Other Sperm-Related Difficulties.
Previous infection or illness (such as the mumps during puberty), extreme stress, and exposure to environmental or workplace toxins all can cause low sperm count and/or problems with sperm motility.

What to do: He must see a doctor if either of you suspects any of these problems.

Sexual Dysfunction. He may have a problem with the structure of his penis, or he may be ejaculating prematurely. Sexual dysfunction is caused by a variety of factors, including problems in relationships, stress, and illness such as diabetes, high blood pressure, and sometimes sickle-cell disease.

What to do: Even though it may be difficult, the two of you must talk about any problems that you're having in your emotional or sexual relationship or that he's having in his life. Simply communicating may help clear them up. And again, he may also need to see his doctor.

Problems You May Be Having Together

Lack of Knowledge.
This is an extremely common reason for infertility. A couple may be having intercourse during a period when the woman isn't likely to get pregnant. Or they may be indulging in poor health habits that prevent conception.

What to do: See the earlier sections in this chapter on charting ovulation and practical tips to encourage conception.

Immunological Problems.
In some cases, a woman develops an antibody resistance to her mate's sperm.

What to do: The two of you must see a doctor. A blood test can generally detect the problem. Some couples solve this dilemma by using a condom during sexual intercourse for several months. When contact between the sperm and cervical mucus is cut off, the level of antibodies that are causing the problem may drop. Then the couple resumes unprotected intercourse. Or she may use his sperm in artificial insemination.

Where to Seek Help

Your physician can recommend a fertility specialist, preferably a doctor who has advanced training and *board certification* in reproductive endocrinology and/or reproductive surgery. Be sure to check into the doctor's credentials before you make an appointment. Most importantly, you should feel comfortable with your physician, and it should be someone with whom the two of you can talk openly and who answers your questions. For more information on choosing a doctor, contact the American Fertility Society, which can send you a list of member doctors in your state and details about their advanced training and certification, or RESOLVE, a national infertility education, advocacy, and support organization. Addresses and phone numbers are given at the end of the chapter.

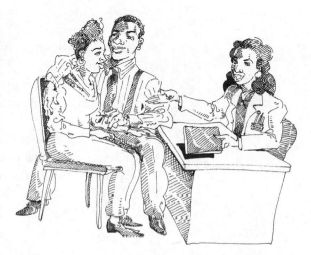

Once you have settled upon a doctor and arranged for a visit, you can expect to undergo a battery of tests. A word of caution: Don't be surprised if your mate refuses to submit to testing. The frankest and most forthright of men have been known to balk at what they consider an invasion of privacy. Many men,

Medical professionals can help couples overcome infertility problems. *(Drawing: Yvonne Buchanan)*

and particularly a number of Black men, equate fertility with masculinity, which can make even a discussion of the subject extremely difficult. You should try to be understanding, but let him know that your goal is not to assign blame but rather to enlist the aid of a professional in identifying and overcoming the problem.

Treatment

Every year, more than a million couples seek treatment for infertility, and most receive medication. In most cases these drugs help to stimulate and supplement the production of the hormones necessary for the development and release of healthy eggs.

You should ask detailed questions (especially regarding cost and side effects) about any drugs that a doctor recommends. Get a second opinion if a doctor recommends any kind of complicated, costly treatment or surgery. For detailed information and advice on drug treatments, contact the American Fertility Society or RESOLVE.

Many new kinds of assisted reproductive technology (ART) are available for infertile couples, but most of these are complicated and expensive. However, it's best that you at least know about them. (For more detailed information, contact the organizations mentioned above.)

Alternative Insemination.

Lesbians, women without mates, and couples with fertility problems may opt to use alternative insemination, which is also called donor or artificial insemination. In this procedure fresh sperm is injected into the woman's vagina with a syringe, turkey baster, or eyedropper as an alternative to intercourse. The sperm may be her mate's or another man's sperm. When using donor sperm from a sperm bank, you *must* insist on knowing whether it was tested for diseases, including HIV.

Intrauterine Insemination (IUI).

A variation of artificial insemination, IUI gives sperm a boost by placing it directly into the uterus, very close to the opening of the fallopian tube. This procedure can be helpful in cases in which infertility is due to,

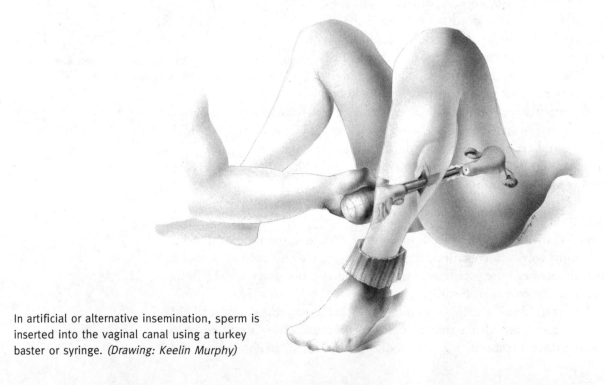

In artificial or alternative insemination, sperm is inserted into the vaginal canal using a turkey baster or syringe. *(Drawing: Keelin Murphy)*

among other things, endometriosis, irregular ovulation, low sperm count, and/or poor sperm movement.

In-Vitro Fertilization (IVF). This is the process that results in what are commonly known as "test-tube babies" and has been in the news frequently in the past several years. In this procedure, an egg is removed from the woman's body, fertilized in a laboratory dish, and then reinserted into the uterus. It can cost thousands of dollars for each attempt.

Gamete Intra-Fallopian Transfer (GIFT). This procedure involves taking mature eggs from a woman's ovaries and placing them together with her partner's sperm in the fallopian tube at the place where fertilization is likely to occur. For this process to have a chance, a woman must have at least one healthy fallopian tube. GIFT can be a viable option in cases of unexplained infertility, endometriosis, cervical-factor infertility, lack of ovulation, and recurring ectopic pregnancy. This procedure can also cost thousands of dollars per attempt.

Zygote Intro-Fallopian Transfer (ZIFT). Similar to GIFT, ZIFT calls for the eggs to be fertilized in the lab, and then the embryo is transferred directly to a woman's fallopian tube, where it is allowed to travel to the uterus on its own and implant naturally. It is also very costly.

There are also other procedures such as surrogate motherhood (in which another woman brings a couple's fetus to term) or using frozen embryos (in which a woman's eggs are fertilized in the lab with her partner's sperm, then frozen and stored away for future use). Such methods are complex and high-priced, and involve sticky legal and ethical issues. You can find out about all types of ART by contacting the American Fertility Society or RESOLVE.

Coping with Emotional Difficulties

Infertility is a crisis that can cause deep conflicts in a relationship and can threaten a man or woman's sense of self and dreams of the future. Infertility treatments can also be stressful. For one, they can be extremely time-consuming and expensive. Unsuccessful treatments can be invasive and exhausting and can make a couple feel victimized by doctors and drugs. Sex may become a battleground, a chore, or clinical, not spontaneous or erotic.

To cope, the two of you must remember that you love each other and that you're trying to create a baby *together*. If you're trying to conceive without a mate, be patient and don't forget that infertility is a medical problem, not a punishment or personal defect. Here are more coping strategies:

Read and learn as much as possible. That way you can avoid needlessly blaming yourself or your partner.

Follow common sense advice together, and then see a doctor together. Getting medical answers will be a big relief.

Share your feelings with your partner, and be sure to listen as well as talk. Try to communicate frequently.

Take the long view. Don't emphasize the short-term ups and downs of the treatments. Set up a timetable, and stick to it.

Get involved in other activities with your partner to take the pressure off baby making. If trying to conceive becomes too stressful, take a break. Or decide to adopt. (Many couples actually conceive shortly after adopting a child, probably because the stress level is less.)

Get help. Contact RESOLVE for referral to a therapist or support group.

Adoption

Many couples and single women decide not to have children but to adopt from the large pool of Black children who need homes. In the United States at any given time there are 75,000 to 100,000 children waiting to be adopted, some 45,000 to 60,000 of them African-American. While the average wait for a healthy white child can be a few years, the wait for Black and mixed-race infants is six months to a year and even less for boys, older kids, and children with special needs.

Your local department of special services, human resources, and/or public welfare can provide you with a list of agencies licensed to oversee adoptions in your state. If you prefer, you can also contact an attorney

---

"Family is in the heart, not in genes or family trees."

—DEBORAH SHELTON PINKNEY, WRITER, CHICAGO

It's a memory etched in the minds of parents everywhere: the moment they saw their children for the first time. For most moms and dads, that unification takes place in a hospital or some other medical setting. My four-month "pregnancy" and two-month "delivery" ended in the living room of my twin sons' foster mother. It was there that the threads of our lives began to weave together.

Because my husband and I chose to adopt, our journey through parenthood hasn't always taken a traditional path. But adoption wasn't a second or third option for us. It was our first choice, something we discussed after meeting in college almost fifteen years ago. We both agreed that it is the responsibility of Black couples to adopt the many Black children who don't have homes. I had planned to bear children also, but time slipped away as I pursued an education and career. At thirty-three, I wasn't exactly excited with the idea of being pregnant.

I haven't regretted those decisions, because it didn't matter to me whose womb my children sprang from. My sons—they were six years old when we met and are nine now—are my children in every way, except genetically. In fact, I sometimes forget that I didn't give birth to them. And they do too!

When we adopted our sons, we had to accept their emotional histories, which includes physical and emotional neglect. The boys fear losing yet another family. They feel unworthy of our love. They feel guilty about the good things in their lives, afraid they will disappear like their first family did. They have a strong need to control and are starved for love. They are confused and sometimes depressed without knowing why. They'll spend their lives trying to fill the hole in their hearts caused by their abandonment.

It hasn't been easy. It won't be easy.

So, while I've shared the questions and doubts of all mothers—Will I be a good parent? Will my sons be happy when they grow up? Can I keep them safe and instill in them a sense of pride and self-respect?—I've had other concerns. Will the boys truly accept me as their mother and grow to love me as much as their birth mother? Will they want and make an effort to remain a part of our family? Will their emotional problems destroy our family-building?

Indeed, the last three years have been a rocky roller-coaster ride. Great highs, real lows. At times we're giddy with joy and revel in the progress our sons have made. However, we've also sought outside help to assist the boys in working through their abusive past.

Through it all, I learned a thing or two about the true meaning of unconditional love, which is giving of yourself without expecting anything in return, not even love. With each crisis, I've had to dig down deeper. To my surprise, I've managed to find pools of water when I thought the well was dry. And I've learned more about myself than I could have ever imagined.

Family is in the heart, not in genes or family trees. Being a family means giving, receiving, and sharing the most valuable possessions you have: love, time, memories.

Maybe that's why I think of my children whenever I listen to one of my favorite songs, a moody tune by the late Nat King Cole. He sang: "The greatest thing you'll ever learn is to love and be loved in return." When I hear those words, I remember the first time I saw my precious sons. They didn't make eye contact at first, but when they did, we all smiled.

specializing in adoptions about private or identified adoptions, through which a birth mother willingly gives up her child to you.

A number of organizations that offer support and information are listed below.

For More Information

ORGANIZATIONS: Fertility

AMERICAN FERTILITY SOCIETY, 1209 Montgomery Hwy., Birmingham, AL 35216; (205) 978-5000. Call or write for general information, referrals, statistics, and publications on reproductive health. You can also send for a list of member doctors in a given state.

RESOLVE, NATIONAL HEADQUARTERS, 1310 Broadway, Dept. GM, Somerville, MA 02144-1731; (617) 623-0744. Offers resources, literature, support groups (for individuals and couples), and a medical hotline (for help in handling medical care and treatment).

ORGANIZATIONS: Adoption

ADOPTIVE FAMILIES OF AMERICA, 3333 Hwy. 100 N., Minneapolis, MN 55422; (612) 535-4829. The AFA offers support and over 300 support groups for families considering adoption. You can also request an information packet that lists over 225 agencies to which families can refer and a catalog of resource materials.

BLACK ADOPTION CONSORTIUM, 5090 Central Hwy, suite 6, Pennsauken, NJ 08109; (800) 552-0222 or (609) 486-0100. The Consortium recruits African-American families to adopt Black children who are currently in the foster-care system.

THE BLACK ADOPTION PLACEMENT AND RESEARCH CENTER, 1801 Harrison St., 2nd floor, Oakland, CA 94612; (510) 839-3678. The Center is a nonprofit organization that recruits African-American or biracial families to be matched with children of the same background for adoption or foster-care purposes. There are no fees to families seeking their services, and the organization offers support groups and activities.

FAMILIES FIRST, P.O. Box 7948 Station C, Atlanta, GA 30357-0948; (404) 853-2800. Offers support and services for families considering adoption or foster care.

NATIONAL ADOPTION INFORMATION CLEARINGHOUSE, 11426 Rockville Pike, suite 410, Rockville, MD 20852; (301) 231-6512. Provides information on adoption and support for families who wish to adopt, who have already adopted children, adult adoptees, women considering giving their child or children up for adoption.

NATIONAL COUNCIL FOR ADOPTION, 1930 17th St. NW, Washington, DC 20009; (202) 328-1200. The Council is an information and advocacy organization for sound, ethical adoption. People looking to adopt and women who are facing a crisis situation can call their National Adoption Hotline at (202) 328-8072. Area referrals are given, and you can also obtain a packet that contains a listing of national referral sources.

Books

Getting Pregnant: What Couples Need to Know Right Now, Niels H. Lauersen, M.D., and Colette Bouchez, Fawcett Columbine, 1992.

How to Be a Successful Fertility Patient: Your Guide to Getting the Best Possible Medical Help to Have a Baby, Peggy Robin, Quill Books, 1993.

In Pursuit of Fertility: A Consultation with a Specialist, Robert R. Franklin and Dorothy Kay Brockman, Henry Holt & Co., 1991.

Love & Fertility: How to Easily Avoid or Achieve Pregnancy . . . Naturally, Mercedes Arzu Wilson, Family of the Americas Foundation (Dunkirk, Md.), 1992.

Planning for Pregnancy, Birth and Beyond, the American College of Obstetricians and Gynecologists Staff, Dutton, 1992.

Pre-Conceptions: What You Can Do Before Pregnancy to Help You Have a Healthy Baby, Nora Tannenhaus, Contemporary Books, 1988.

Preconception: A Woman's Guide to Preparing for Pregnancy and Parenthood, Brenda E. Aikey-Keller, John Muir Publications (Santa Fe, N.M.), 1990.

Pregnancy & Childbirth: The Complete Guide for a New Life, T. Hotchner, Avon Books, 1992.

Pregnancy Over Thirty-Five, Kathryn Schrotenboer-Cox and Joan S. Weiss, Ballantine, 1989.

Surviving Infertility, Linda P. Salzer, HarperPerennial, 1991.

The V.I.P. Program: A Personal Approach to the Art and Science of Having a Baby, Gail Sforza Brewer, Rodale Press, 1988.

What Every Woman Needs to Know: Facts & Fears About Pregnancy, Childbirth & Womanhood, Penny Junor, Random Century, 1989.

Your Fertility Signals: Using Them to Achieve or Avoid Pregnancy, Naturally, Merryl Winstein, Smooth Stone Press (St. Louis), 1990.

15

Having a Healthy Baby

For many a sister, bringing a child into the world is an extremely moving and memorable—if not the most special—event in her life. But having a baby also requires an enormous amount of responsibility, beginning not at the birth of a child but nine months earlier. Prenatal care—taking care of yourself while pregnant—is the key to having a strong, healthy baby.

Too often, however, Black women do not get adequate prenatal care. As was true a century ago, our babies are still more than twice as likely to die before their first birthdays than those born to white women. This high infant mortality rate can in part be blamed on poverty, which keeps many women from getting adequate care when they are pregnant. But studies show that even Black middle-class women are more likely than white women of equal income and education levels to see their babies die. "We can't explain it by income alone," says Paul H. Wise, M.D., director of the Institute for Reproductive and Child Health at Harvard Medical School. "A simple answer is wrong. Other factors, such as discrimination and stress, may play a role. For instance, Mexican-American women have much worse prenatal care than Black women but have far better birth outcomes. We're looking at the very complicated issue of racism and trying to understand its actual clinical expressions."

We can't control discrimination and racism, so it's extremely impor-

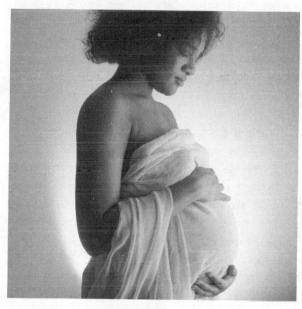

A pregnant woman late in her term. *(Photo: Debbie Egan-Chin/Allford Trotman Associates)*

tant that we Black women take care of our bodies and get proper medical attention during the nine months of pregnancy. Some clinics offer free prenatal care, and prenatal visits are often short—no more than fifteen minutes. Many communities have Healthy Start, a government program that provides medical, social, and educational assistance for infants and pregnant women.

For more information, contact the Maternal and Child Health Bureau, Health Resources and Services Administration, 5600 Fishers Lane, room 18-44, Parklawn Bldg., Rockville, MD 20857; (301) 443-3376.

Are You Pregnant?

If you suspect you're pregnant, you must get that suspicion confirmed. (For information on getting pregnant, see chapter 14, "How to Get Pregnant: Reproduction and Infertility.") Amenorrhea or absence of your period is a classic sign, but it could also be a side effect of stress, intense exercise, hormonal problems, illness, or a change in birth control. In fact, some women still have light periods during the first month or two of pregnancy. Breast tenderness, nausea, and fatigue also signal pregnancy, but again, these symptoms don't confirm it.

To find out for sure, you'll need a pregnancy test. These tests are usually based on the use of monoclonal antibodies to detect HCG (human chorionic gonadotropin), a hormone produced by the placenta early in pregnancy in the urine of a pregnant woman. HCG can be detected in urine or blood as early as seven to ten days after conception. You can get a pregnancy test from your doctor, and free or low-cost tests are offered by family-planning clinics.

Some women choose home pregnancy tests, which are basically the same urine tests you can get from a doctor or at a clinic. When used correctly, these tests are quite reliable and can be used as early as the first day of your missed period (fourteen days after conception). Many come with two tests, so that you can double-check. These tests also come with an 800 number for you to call and speak with a medical person. A single test kit costs about $10; a two-test kit usually costs more. If you get a positive result, you should make an appointment to see your doctor as soon as possible. If you get a negative result but still think you're pregnant, see your doctor to find out for sure.

If you are pregnant, you can calculate your due date or EDD (estimated date of delivery) by taking the date of the first day of your last menstrual period, adding 7 to it, then, from that date, counting back three months. For example, if you started your last menstrual period on April 1, adding 7 to 1 gives you 8; counting back three months from April 8 gives you a due date of January 8.

Considering Your Options
Once you've discovered that you are pregnant, you and your partner need to think very carefully about whether or not you want to have the child. You should ask yourself the questions in Chapter 14 (pp. 234-35).

Having a Baby at Thirty-Five or Older
Twenty years ago, a thirty-five- to forty-year-old woman who was pregnant for the first time or wanted to get pregnant was considered somewhat odd. People in the community used to call the children of older mothers "old babies" and suggested that those children were somehow weird, either mentally slow or just different from other kids. It was also considered high-risk and impractical for the mother and child.

Today, the greatest number of women having babies are in the over-twenty-five group, with the older end growing. Many women are waiting to start their families because of career and other life goals. "Today with modern medical care, maternal risks during pregnancy are manageable and most pregnancies lead to healthy babies and mothers," says

Ronald J. Wapner, M.D., director of the division of Maternal-Fetal Medicine at Thomas Jefferson University in Philadelphia.

Nonetheless, it is important to be aware of the greater risks that come with pregnancy after thirty-five. There is a common risk of developing diabetes, cardiovascular disease, or hypertension (especially if overweight), all of which are more common in older women. There is also an increased chance of delivering a child with a chromosomal abnormality. This problem is often due to an error in cell division during the formation of the egg.

The most common defect is the one that leads to the birth of a child with Down's syndrome. The risk of Down's syndrome is 1 in 900 for the general population; a woman who is thirty-five years old at delivery has a 1 in 270 chance. At forty the chances are 1 in 100, and by age forty-five, 1 in 25.

All women who will be thirty-five at delivery are offered amniocentesis, a test that detects Down's syndrome and some other conditions in the fetus, and some doctors advise all women over thirty to have the test. The test is usually done between the sixteenth and eighteenth weeks of pregnancy (although occasionally performed as early as the fourteenth or as late as the twentieth). The sex of the fetus is also determined by the test. Although complications from the amnio test are rare, there is some incidence of risk including mild cramping, slight vaginal bleeding, a slight elevated chance of miscarriage, and leaking amniotic fluid. Injury to the fetus is rare.

If you are over thirty-five and want to have a child, you should start trying now. It may take a year before you conceive. After a year, if you haven't conceived, you should see a fertility specialist.

Trimester-By-Trimester Guide to Staying Healthy

To have a healthy baby, you *must* follow this advice from the moment you start trying to conceive or find out you're pregnant until well after your baby is born:

- Make and keep your regular doctor's appointments.
- Eat plenty of fruit, vegetables, low-fat dairy or soy-milk products, and protein (beans, fish, nuts), and drink lots of water. Cut caffeine out of the diet or at least reduce consumption to no more than one cup of coffee or tea per day.
- Stay away from all illegal drugs and alcohol and don't take over-the-counter medication without checking with your doctor. But don't

stop taking a prescription drug without consulting your physician.

- Avoid environmental hazards such as lead (for more information see chapter 32, "Our Work, Our World"), X rays, and chemicals such as pesticides.
- Don't smoke.
- Avoid handling cat litter. Cat feces can be infected with toxoplasmosis, a disease that can harm the fetus.

First Trimester: One to Three Months

How You'll Feel.

At this point, you may be the only one who knows you're pregnant. You will probably notice some of these changes in your body:

Weight gain of about 3 to 4 pounds. Normal weight gain during pregnancy is about 25 pounds or more if you're very thin. But don't worry about your weight; eat normally and don't start a weight-loss diet at this time. The weight you gain often includes about 13 pounds of retained water.

- Tiredness and inability to sleep
- Frequent urination
- Excessive salivation
- Heartburn, indigestion, bloating
- Increased appetite, aversions to food and cravings
- Fullness, heaviness, and tenderness of the breasts, tingling and/or darkening of the areola (the darker area around the nipples)
- Constipation
- Mood swings, crying jags
- Dizziness

At this time, many women suffer from morning sickness, the misnamed nausea that can strike any time of the day. For most women, nausea doesn't last past the third month, although a few expectant mothers have it throughout pregnancy. Some women don't experience it at all, others not until the second trimester. No one really knows what causes nausea, but there is no shortage of theories. Morning sickness has been blamed on shifting hormonal patterns, the rapid stretching of the uterine muscle tissue in the digestive tract, and changing dietary needs.

Emotional factors may also contribute to nausea. For example, morning sickness is unheard of in some so-called more primitive societies where a more relaxed lifestyle is more prevalent. There's also some evidence that some women with unplanned or unwanted pregnancies suffer debilitating nausea and vomiting. Mental and physical fatigue also seem to increase the possibility of nausea, as does multiple fetuses.

Your Health Care.

Obstetrician gynecologists, or OB-GYN's, provide most prenatal care and deliver most babies. At present, most are men, and very few are Black. An increasing number of women are opting to become certified nurse-midwives, registered nurses who have additional training in obstetrics. In our community, many families have relied on "granny" midwives to deliver generations of children. Nurse-midwives can provide prenatal care and deliver babies, and their fees are covered by most health-insurance policies. Women who choose this option note that nurse-midwives are generally women, and they provide longer prenatal visits, a greater emphasis on education and birth preparation, and a deeper level of emotional support. Make sure that the midwife you choose is certified and affiliated with an obstetrician in case of emergency. If, however, it has been determined that you have a high-risk pregnancy, you will require the services of an OB GYN, a specialist who is trained to handle every conceivable complication that might arise.

Your first prenatal doctor's visit will be your most comprehensive. While doctors vary in their approaches, there are some basics you should expect in this first visit. First, your doctor will probably confirm your pregnancy. Go to this appointment prepared to answer a battery of family and personal medical history questions. You will have a complete physical exam and blood and urine tests.

After your first appointment, if yours is a low-risk pregnancy, you should visit your practitioner once a month until the end of the thirty-second week. After that you may begin going every two weeks until the last month, when weekly visits are a must. At doctor visits throughout your pregnancy, you may have ultrasounds so that the doctor can observe the fetus. An ultrasound uses sound waves without the dangers of X rays to produce an image

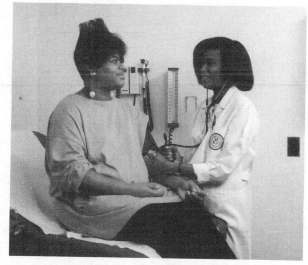

Certified nurse-midwives provide care—from pre-conception counseling to postpartum checkups. (*Photo: American College of Nurse-Midwives, Washington, D.C.*)

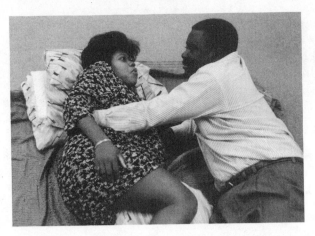

A husband and wife practice breathing and relaxation exercises during a childbirth-education class at Fairfax Hospital in Virginia.
(Photo: Media Center, Fairfax Hospital)

on a screen (sonogram) and to confirm the due date and survey the fetal anatomy. A sonogram can give you a good hint as to the gender of your baby, although it isn't absolutely reliable.

This is also a good time to explore childbirth-education classes. Lamaze classes are the best known.

Named after Dr. Fernand Lamaze, a French OB-GYN, the Lamaze technique combines education about labor and delivery with breathing and relaxation exercises.

Taking Care of Yourself.
During the first few months of pregnancy, you may feel fatigued, so get plenty of rest. To reduce morning sickness, substitute three large meals with several smaller ones throughout the day. These meals should be high in complex carbohydrates—potatoes, pasta, and rice. Fried, fatty foods can make morning sickness worse. To ease nausea, snack on whole-grain crackers or rice cakes and drink lots of water and other fluids, such as fruit and vegetable juices and red raspberry tea.

At this point you should look at your diet and make sure to increase your vitamin and mineral intake and get plenty of rest. You will be given prenatal vitamins, including folic acid, which has been found to lower the risk of birth defects, and B vitamins which can help ease morning sickness.

Upon the advice of your health practitioner, you can continue to exercise during pregnancy. You should do it in moderation, especially if you haven't been exercising. This is not the time to begin a strenuous exercise program. Swimming in shallow water that is neither too hot nor too cold, and walking are probably the best aerobic exercises if you're not in shape. For other exercise options, check with your local community center, hospital, health club, or YWCA for classes designed for expectant mothers.

Second Trimester: Four to Six Months

How You'll Feel.
It's during this period when most women start "showing." These next months are usually considered the easiest because the early discomforts

have disappeared and you've regained your energy. Sometime by the end of the fourth month you may begin to feel the fetus move, although some sources say only very slender women feel anything during the first part of this trimester (the fourth month). By the fifth month the uterus has expanded to reach the height of your navel. You should feel fetal movements now; it's important to let your doctor know when you felt the first movement because this helps determine the delivery date. The sixth month is when you tend to gain the most weight—12 to 14 pounds is the average. If you find your weight has gone way over the average, take sensible action to get back on track, but don't take any extreme measures like dieting. The fetus can't thrive if you diet. You may feel a stitchlike pain at times in the side of your abdomen as the uterine muscle stretches.

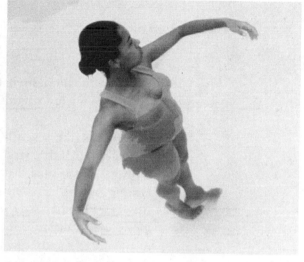

Edema or swelling of the feet and hands and varicose veins on your legs may occur at this time. Because of water retention and extra weight, the legs often swell and cramp during pregnancy. In addition, increases in blood volume can lead to varicose veins. Massage can help reduce this.

Swimming and water exercises are safe during pregnancy.
(Photo: Pascal Secleux/Allford Trotman Associates)

This is also a growth-spurt time for the fetus. A few of the things that are happening to it are:

Fourth month: Fetus is 4 inches long; tooth buds appear; fingers and toes defined.

Fifth month: Fetus is 8 to 10 inches; hair begins to grow on its head; brows and white lashes appear; the fetus is active now, turning from side to side and sometimes moving its head over its heels. By the end of the month it weighs a pound.

Sixth month: By the end of the month the fetus weighs about 1 3/4 pounds and is about 13 inches long. Eyelids begin to part and the eyes open; finger and toe prints are visible.

Your Health Care.
At this point you should be visiting your doctor once a month. Make a list of all your questions and concerns, so you won't forget anything. One symptom you may have during this period is forgetfulness.

Taking Care of Yourself.
Many women complain of constipation at this point, so remember to drink lots of water and fruit and vegetable juices, especially prune juice if you are having difficult bowel movements, and eat plenty of high-fiber fruits and grains.

You may also experience back pain because of the extra weight in the front of your body. Try stretching, yoga, or massage to ease the discomfort.

Third Trimester: Seven to Nine Months

How You'll Feel.
You're in the homestretch! Your fetus is growing bigger and you are getting more uncomfortable, with the biggest increases in your breasts and abdomen.

At about the seventh month you may notice an increasingly heavy whitish vaginal discharge, lower abdominal achiness, heartburn, indigestion, gas, occasional headaches, bleeding gums, shortness of breath, and leaking breasts. The fetus is now exercising by kicking and stretching. It sucks its thumb, opens and closes its eyes, and you may feel it hiccuping. Don't worry about it, hiccups don't cause the same discomfort in babies, in or out of the uterus, as they do in adults. It's now weighing about 3 pounds.

In the final months, your back is probably constantly aching and you feel like moving into the bathroom because you're having to urinate constantly. The fetus is putting pressure on your bladder. The upward pressure on your chest makes it hard to breathe, and sleep may be hard to come by, but it's important that you try to get plenty of rest. Not only will you need to be rested for labor and delivery, but also to sustain yourself physically and emotionally in the early days of motherhood. A few weeks before your delivery date, the fetus settles into position, usually head first in preparation for the trip down the birth canal.

Your Health Care.
You should be seeing your doctor twice a month until the last month, then visits may increase to weekly. Your blood pressure and weight will be checked along with your urine, for sugar and protein, and the fetal heartbeat. The height of your fundus (top of uterus) and the size and position of the fetus, which may give you a rough estimate of the baby's birth weight, will also be examined.

Problems During Pregnancy

Miscarriage

Miscarriage, the most common mishap of pregnancy, affects about one in six women, according to the March of Dimes. It is defined as a pregnancy loss before the fetus is twenty weeks old or before it weighs a pound, and can be extremely devastating. Many women and couples suffer in silence, ashamed and embarrassed, feeling that they've failed in some way.

Most miscarriages occur in the first three months of pregnancy and often before the woman knows she's pregnant. In first pregnancies, about 50 to 60 percent of all these early losses can be blamed on a genetic abnormality of the fetus, and in about 70 to 90 percent of cases, women who have suffered one miscarriage before the twelfth week go on to have a healthy pregnancy the next time.

However, the March of Dimes estimates that every year about 80,000 to 200,000 women experience recurrent miscarriages. After two miscarriages, a woman must get medical treatment, because with each subsequent miscarriage, the likelihood of having a healthy pregnancy drops.

Recurrent miscarriage is caused by a number of factors such as infection stemming from untreated STI's, environmental and industrial exposure to toxins, problems of the immune system, hormonal imbalances, genetic incompatibility of the partners, and structural problems in the reproductive system. Fortunately, many of these difficulties can be treated successfully.

The March of Dimes can refer women and couples to centers or doctors who specialize in diagnosis and treatment of recurrent miscarriage. Call your local office, or contact the National Office of the March of Dimes, 1275 Mamaroneck Ave., White Plains, NY 10605; (914) 428-7100.

Because miscarriage, especially recurrent miscarriage, can be so painful, don't suffer alone. Choose a physician who is compassionate, and find a support group. To find one in your area, send an SASE for information to RESOLVE, 1310 Broadway, Dept. GM, Somerville, MA 02144-1731; (617) 623-0744; or SHARE, St. Joseph Health Center, 300 First Capitol Dr., St. Charles, MO 63301-2893; (314) 947-6164.

You can also read *Preventing Miscarriage: The Good News* by Dr. Jonathan Scher and Carol Dix.

Ectopic Pregnancy

An ectopic pregnancy occurs when the fertilized egg implants itself somewhere outside the uterus. It most commonly occurs in the fallopian

"When the nurse routinely slapped a cuff around my upper arm to take my blood pressure, her eyebrows disappeared into her hairline."

—KAREN GRIGSBY BATES,
JOURNALIST, LOS ANGELES

Until a few days before my son was born, I had had a pretty uneventful pregnancy. I'd read all the basic guidebooks to tell me what to expect as my pregnancy progressed, so it didn't bother me particularly when, around the middle of my seventh month, I had a couple of nosebleeds. When my hands and feet began to swell, I mentioned it to a few friends who had had children, and they shrugged. "Girl, it's August and 90 degrees and you're pregnant—you're going to have some swelling." So I didn't worry about that, either. Nor did I worry when I had a pretty severe headache toward the end of the month. Normal, normal, normal. All that stuff was predicted in the pregnancy books.

I was scheduled for a checkup a few days after the killer headache. It was hot, I was tired and didn't feel like driving, so I asked my husband to take me to the doctor's office. It was a good thing he did, too, because when the nurse routinely slapped a cuff around my upper arm to take my blood pressure, her eyebrows disappeared into her hairline when she read the numbers. "Wait here, I want the doctor to double-check this," she said calmly. "It's probably just this machine." She returned with a new machine and my doctor, Gail Jackson. Dr. Jackson looked up from the new reading and said firmly, "Honey, you aren't leaving here today. Your pressure is sky-high. We're taking you down to admitting, right this minute.

"Hey," I offered brightly, "I'll go home and get a few things and be back in a flash."

"Oh, no you won't!" Dr. Jackson said. "You're getting into a bed and you're getting something to bring that pressure down immediately. I do not intend to have you stroke out on me." Stroke?! That's supposed to happen to people who don't watch their diets, who've gained a bunch of weight, who have problem pregnancies. That wasn't me. But it also happens, randomly, to many women in their first pregnancies. If not treated, it can result in paralysis, blindness, even death. So I found myself being whipped into a hospital gown, gently placed into bed—on my left side, to facilitate better circulation—plastered with monitors (one for me, one for baby) and lying as still as possible for the whole weekend. The doctors huddled, deciding when it would be best for baby to emerge. Thanks to my skyrocketing blood pressure, a nine-month pregnancy had become untenable. (But if pregnancy-induced hypertension is caught early enough, bed rest and medication often allow a woman to go full term.)

Over the weekend, my sight had been getting more and more dim (another warning sign), and on Monday morning, when I couldn't really identify one of my doctors' faces (it was like staring into the sun—you could see an outline, *but not the details), Dr. Jackson decided, "That's it. Tell Bruce to get here by noon if he wants to see his baby being born."*

My husband arrived at noon, changed into scrubs, loaded film into the pockets and cuffs of his scrub suit, and I was wheeled down into O.R. After an epidural was administered, Dr. Jackson and her colleague performed a cesarean section (chattering all the while with Bruce, who was intent on documenting all this), and about a half-hour later, Jordan Alexander Bates Talamon emerged—little (3 pounds, 9 ounces) but healthy, and breathing on his own. Today he's a healthy, rambunctious two-year-old.

The moral of this story? Don't diagnose yourself. Let your doctor do that; it's why she has a medical degree. But if you've been feeling fine and all of a sudden find yourself dragging, if you have fairly dramatic symptoms (a skull-cracking headache is a good example), don't be blasé about it. Call your doctor. Let her decide whether there's cause for concern.

tubes (tubal pregnancy) but can also occur in the ovary, cervix, and in the abdominal cavity. This kind of pregnancy rarely ends in a live birth, and in some cases, having an ectopic pregnancy leads to future infertility.

Ectopic pregnancies are most likely to occur in women over thirty-five and among those with a history of pelvic inflammatory disease or other reproductive-system infection. Black women are particularly prone to ectopic pregnancy because too often we allow untreated sexually transmitted diseases to progress to pelvic inflammatory disease. With that in mind, to avoid ectopic pregnancy always get checked and treated for STI's.

An ectopic pregnancy can be diagnosed with a blood test or ultrasound, and the symptoms are stabbing pains or a dull ache in the abdomen and vaginal bleeding. Left untreated, the tube can rupture, leading to severe loss of blood or shock. If the problem is found early, a doctor can remove the fetus surgically and save the tube. Using laparoscopy, an alternative to major abdominal surgery, a skilled doctor can keep the tube intact, which raises the chance that the next pregnancy will be normal.

Preeclampsia

Preeclampsia is an abnormal elevation of blood pressure, water retention, and protein in the urine that can occur during the latter half of pregnancy (after the twenty-fourth week). Though a rise in blood pressure is normal during pregnancy, preeclampsia is more serious and often requires bed rest and medication. It most commonly crops up in first pregnancies. In its most severe form, it can be life-threatening to both mother and baby, and a doctor may deliver the baby immediately even if it's premature. If you notice a severe continuous headache and/or swelling of your face or fingers, call your physician immediately.

It is crucial to have your blood pressure monitored frequently during pregnancy. Because Black women are particularly prone to high blood pressure, it is very important to keep it in check by avoiding salt and fatty foods, exercising moderately, and keeping stress low.

Having Your Baby

Childbirth Options
Most women still give birth in a hospital operating room, but more and more hospitals are offering birthing rooms, so that low-risk pregnant women can deliver their babies naturally but with the security of technology nearby. These rooms are nicely decorated to make you feel as comfortable as you would in your own bedroom, and your mate and the baby can stay in the same room with you (although usually you will have the option of nursery care for your baby).

There are also birthing centers popping up throughout the country with the same cozy look and feel. These are generally freestanding centers staffed by certified nurse-widwives. They are more intimate and less expensive than hospitals and are a good choice for women who have low-risk pregnancies. To be covered by insurance, the center must be licensed. To find a licensed birthing center in your area or for more information contact the Maternity Center Association, 48 E. 92nd St., New York, NY 10128; (212) 369-7300; or the National Association of Childbearing Centers, 3123 Gottschall Rd., Perkiomenville, PA 18074; (215) 234-8068.

Some women feel most comfortable delivering at home, generally with the assistance of a nurse-midwife. Here are two sources of information on this option: Association for Childbirth at Home International, P.O. Box 430, Glendale, CA 91209; 213 667-0839; and Informed Homebirth/Informed Birth and Parenting, Inc., P.O. Box 3675, Ann Arbor, MI 48106; (313) 662-6857.

I chose to become pregnant at age twenty-five. It was the biggest decision I had made in my life, and I was concerned with my health.

When I called my sisterfriend and asked for her perspective, she gave me the names of a few books to read, Let's Have Healthy Children *by Adelle Davis,* Common Herbs for Natural Health *by Juliette De Bairacli-Levy,* Hygieia: A Woman's Herbal *by Jeannine Parvati, and* Heart and Hands: A Midwife's Guide to Pregnancy and Birth *by Elizabeth Davis. Excellent resources. Reading what other women had experienced during pregnancy also helped tremendously.*

From Let's Have Healthy Children, *the prenatal diet inspired ideas toward a more holistic approach to pregnancy. I became more conscious of my breathing, my physical appearance, and my emotional processes. I gradually changed my eating habits, increasing my protein, B, C, and E vitamins along with combining a macro-vegetarian menu. I gained 44 pounds during my pregnancy, and I was full of energy. I was convinced that it was due to the change in my food intake. I had also stopped drinking coffee and soda a year prior to becoming pregnant. I no longer skipped meals, and I made a strong effort to get a good night's sleep. Dreamtime was essential, so I was always careful about my last meal.*

My perceptions of pregnancy changed also. This society has sent strong messages for women to deny themselves self-love during this time because of the physical changes. It's hard to feel good about yourself when you look so different and when coworkers and family constantly make comments about how "big" or how "fat" you are getting. It's a sensitive issue.

Praying was most important. Alone time. I found comfort in saying simple affirmations and requests to God/Goddess energy. The mystery that lies in your body, you want to protect. It's instinctual. I prayed for the basics: to be alive, healthy, and happy or content.

The next decision I made was to not have my baby in a hospital. I chose The Maternity Center Association located in midtown Manhattan, which was about thirty-five minutes from my home on public transportation. Many people expressed later that they were surprised that I had not chosen a hospital for the fear of complications if a doctor wasn't present. I assured them that I had faith and that the midwives were trained specifically for birthing. If needed, I would be sent to a hospital about ten minutes away.

The Maternity Center Association was efficient and less expensive, since I didn't need extended care. It provided a personal touch. I was not a number in a crowded waiting room. This was important to me. Also, I could invite whomever I wanted into the birthing room at the time of delivery. I chose

"I believe that pregnancy is a rite of passage that is deeply profound."

—JASMINE KETCHAM, POET AND VISUAL ARTIST, BROOKLYN

the orange room, which was designed like a bedroom, and invited a six-year-old friend of mine. I took childbirth classes, meditation, and breathing techniques along with exercise routines. I needed a supportive environment and people to communicate with. The Center provided that. Unfortunately, not many African-American women pass through The Maternity Center Association.

I gave birth to a healthy 7-pound 14-ounce baby boy, with no complications. I needed to experience the whole pregnancy for the perspective it offers; the good, joyful experiences as well as the sad and scary ones. For that I am grateful. I believe that pregnancy is a rite of passage that is deeply profound. There is so much of the inner self that is revealed to you.

Labor and Delivery

Some women choose natural childbirth. That is, they take childbirth-education classes and learn breathing and relaxation exercises. When they are ready to deliver, they receive little or no pain-relief medication. Other women use breathing and relaxation techniques but may also decide to combine this technique with a pain reliever like an epidural or other form of anesthesia. (An epidural is a local anesthetic that is injected into the tissues and spaces surrounding the spine and numbs the body from the waist down to a degree.) You should discuss these options with your health practitioner to decide which is best for you.

There are three stages of labor, and on average, for a first birth, labor usually lasts about twelve to fourteen hours; subsequent births are shorter. When the first stage occurs, you may not even be aware that labor has begun.

First Stage.
Usually the first thing that happens is a plug of mucus that has been in the cervix loosens and passes. This is the dilation stage, and it signifies the cervix is opening. It is also the longest stage, which begins with contractions being about every five to twenty minutes apart. You will probably be walking around, cheerful and talkative, and the pains most likely will be manageable. Contractions gradually become stronger and more frequent, and by the end of this first phase, when you should be headed to the hospital or birth center, contractions should be coming every three to four minutes. This stage ends when your cervix is dilated to 7 centimeters; however, as with everything else about your pregnancy, your

labor will not be the same as anyone else's. You should call your doctor or midwife and speak to her yourself, rather than have your partner do it. It will be easier for her to determine from you how far along in labor you are.

Second Stage.

This is the moment of truth, the one you've been waiting nine long months for. In this phase, also known as transition, your uterus is working to accomplish more in less time, the contractions become stronger, longer, and closer together (two to three minutes apart), and the cervix dilates more until you reach a full 10 centimeters. You may feel the most discomfort during this time, increased lower backache, nausea, rectal pressure, shakiness, and leg fatigue, and you may not be able to talk through your contractions. Pushing starts at this phase. If everything goes well, the fetus will be positioned to come out head first. If the fetus is in a breech position—feet or shoulders heading out first—the doctor may try to turn the fetus so that the head comes first. This procedure is called a ECV (external cephalic version). If this isn't done or it doesn't work, the fetus may have to be delivered through a cesarean, which we'll talk more about later. Your baby is born.

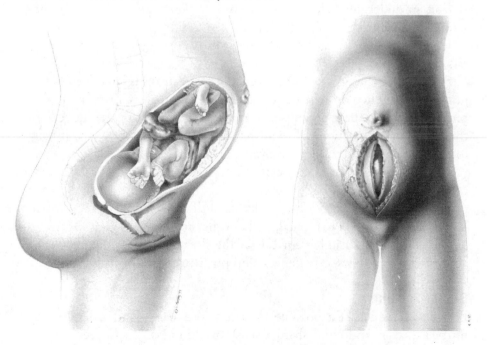

Vaginal childbirth, left; cesarean section, right. *(Drawings: Keelin Murphy)*

Third Stage.

At this time the placenta or afterbirth separates from the uterine wall and is delivered. Many women don't even notice this stage, which generally last anywhere from five minutes to a half hour or longer. You may or may not feel the mild contractions. In most places you will be able to hold and nurse your baby immediately.

After delivery, you'll probably feel excited but exhausted. However, after the initial few days, about half of all women feel sad, a problem known as postpartum depression. The problem may stem from hormonal shifts that occur after childbirth. Some women feel tired and overwhelmed, while others feel that they look awful and miss their old carefree self. This feeling may be confusing to women who have longed to have a baby.

The most important thing to remember is that postpartum depression is normal. To fight it, try to get as much rest as possible, and be sure to eat nutritious foods. Pamper yourself. Don't let the new baby have all the attention; you're important, too.

Cesarean Section

Today one in three births are cesarean, or C-section, as it is called. This is the delivery of a baby through an incision in the abdomen and uterus. A woman undergoing this procedure can either receive general anesthesia or remain awake with an epidural.

Health activists have criticized the overuse of this procedure, which has increased dramatically since 1970.

Studies note that in areas where the rate of cesareans is lower babies fare just as well as they do where the rate is twice as high. Critics say higher physician fees and fear of malpractice lawsuits account for the increase in the procedure. C-section deliveries require a longer hospital stay, usually four to five days, and a longer recovery period, up to eight weeks.

Though in many cases cesareans are not necessary, in other cases they are lifesavers. In instances of severe preeclampsia, serious diabetes, cord prolapse, active herpes lesions, sudden fetal distress, failure of the baby to come down into the birth canal, and at other times, C-sections *are* necessary. But often it's a judgment call of the doctor. Interview your doctor about her or his views, experiences, and practices regarding C-sections.

Breast-Feeding

Breast milk is the best possible food for your baby. And when a baby nurses, mother and child share a sense of closeness. Breast-feeding also provides health benefits—for both of you.

The rewards for the baby are numerous. For instance, breast-fed babies are less likely to get all kinds of infections because when your antibodies pass to the baby through your milk, they help protect the baby. Mother's milk contains the exact balance of nutrients, which adapt to your baby's changing needs. Sudden Infant Death Syndrome (SIDS) is also less common in babies who are breast-fed. Breast-fed babies also tend to cry less because of the skin-to-skin contact, and they develop good jaw alignment and movement.

Many of the benefits of breast-feeding are long-term. Adults who were breast-fed are less likely to develop insulin-dependent diabetes, food allergies, lymphoma, and dermatitis and slower to develop other serious health problems.

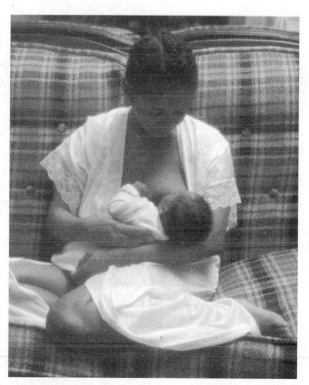

Mothers who breast-feed also reap health benefits. A 1989 study conducted by the *Journal of Clinical Epidemiology* reported that women who breast-fed their babies for twenty-five months or more had a one-third less chance of developing breast cancer than women who didn't. Breast-feeding also protects against ovarian cancer, urinary-tract infections, and even osteoporosis. What's more, women who breast-feed report that they have an easier time losing the extra weight gained during pregnancy. The excess fluids and tissue that have been stored for the baby's benefit are converted into energy for breast-feeding. (It's nature's assumption that the new mother will breast-feed, and the extra fat that was stored while she was pregnant contains nutrients that the baby will need and will receive through the breast milk.) Also,

Breast-feeding fosters a positive bond between mother and baby. *(Photo: Anthony Mills/Allford Trotman Associates)*

breast-feeding is more convenient—no heating bottles in the middle of the night, and you can do it discreetly anywhere—more economical—formula can be quite costly—and better for the baby, who digests breast milk more easily.

Despite the many benefits, many pediatricians are still quick to introduce formula supplement, often for no reason, and some sisters are reluctant to breast-feed. But they needn't be: According to the National

Academy of Sciences Institute of Medicine, it is estimated that the average mother makes about 750 milliliters of breast milk each day. Even very busy women have found ways to fit breast-feeding into their schedules. Breast pumps help. You can use a pump to extract milk from your breasts and feed it to your baby later. Soreness will peak around the third week of breast-feeding and then go away, and leakiness will ease up as the baby settles into a pattern. La Leche League, 9616 Minneapolis Ave., Franklin Park, IL 60131; (800) LA-LECHE and the Lactation Institute and Breastfeeding Clinic, 16430 Ventura Blvd., suite 303, Encino, CA 91436; (818) 995-1913 can answer questions about breast-feeding and offer support and advice. La Leche offers meetings in most areas and will often even send someone to see you if you are having trouble breast-feeding. You can also read *Breastfeeding Your Baby: A Guide for the Contemporary Family* by Carl Jones and Ruth Lawrence and *The Womanly Art of Breastfeeding* by La Leche League International.

For More Information

Nurse-Midwives

THE TRADITIONAL CHILDBEARING GROUP, P.O. Box 638, Boston, MA 02118; (617) 541-0086 (a group of Black midwives); the AMERICAN COLLEGE OF NURSE-MIDWIVES, 1522 K St. NW, suite 1000, Washington, DC 20005; (202) 289-0171; or the Midwives Alliance of North America, P.O. Box 1121, Bristol, VA 24203; (615) 764-5561.

Lamaze and Childbirth Education

THE AMERICAN SOCIETY FOR PSYCHOPROPHYLAXIS IN OBSTETRICS, 1101 Connecticut Ave. NW, suite 700, Washington, DC 20036; (800) 368-4404; or the International Childbirth Education Association, 8060 26th Ave. S., Bloomington, MN 55425; (612) 854-8660.

Cesareans

CESAREANS/SUPPORT, EDUCATION AND CONCERN, 22 Forest Rd., Framingham, MA 01701; (508) 877-8266; or the International Cesarean Awareness Network, P.O. Box 152, Syracuse, NY 13210; (315) 424-1942.

ORGANIZATIONS

AMERICAN FOUNDATION FOR MATERNAL AND CHILD HEALTH, INC., 439 East 51st St., New York, NY 10022; (212) 759-5510. A clearinghouse for up-to-date scientific information on obstetrics and newborn care.

AMERICAN COLLEGE OF OBSTETRICIANS AND GYNECOLOGISTS, 409 12th St. SW, Washington, DC 20024; (800) 762-2264. Distributes educational materials on various women's health issues.

THE BIRTHING PROJECT, 1810 S Street, Sacramento, CA 95814; (916) 442-BABY. A program for pregnant women and young mothers. Pairs a mother-to-be with a volunteer who helps during pregnancy and baby's first year. Has sister projects in Phoenix and Seattle.

HEALTHY MOTHERS, HEALTHY BABIES COALITION, 409 12th St. SW, room 309, Washington, DC 20024; (202) 863-2458. Provides information and education to improve maternal/infant health.

MARCH OF DIMES BIRTH DEFECTS FOUNDATION, 1275 Mamaroneck Ave., White Plains, NY 10605; (914) 428-7100; or contact your local chapter. Provides information on prenatal care, birth defects and their prevention, and healthy pregnancy outcomes guidelines on printed materials available to the public.

NATIONAL CENTER FOR EDUCATION IN MATERNAL AND CHILD HEALTH, 200 N. 15th St., suite 701, Arlington, VA 22201-7802; (703) 524-7802. Provides information and resource materials on pregnancy, childbirth, and maternal and child health services and programs.

NATIONAL COMMISSION TO PREVENT INFANT MORTALITY, Switzer Bldg., 330 C St. SW, room 2014, Washington, DC 20201; (202) 205-8364. A health-care access advocacy organization that provides resources and distributes general-information packets.

NATIONAL MATERNAL AND CHILD HEALTH CLEARINGHOUSE, 8201 Greensboro Dr., suite 600, McLean, VA 22102; (703) 821-8955 ext. 254 or 265. Distributes publications on health issues and provides referrals to various health professionals.

NATIONAL SUDDEN INFANT DEATH SYNDROME RESOURCE CENTER, 8201 Greensboro Dr., suite 600, McLean, VA 22102; (703) 821-8955 ext. 249. Provides grief reading materials for bereaved parents, support-group referrals, fact sheets, and information pamphlets.

BOOKS

Active Birth: The New Approach to Giving Birth Naturally, Revised Edition, Janet Balaskas, Harvard Common Press, 1992.

A Child Is Born, Lennart Nilsson, Delta, 1993.

Childbirth Without Fear: The Original Approach to Natural Childbirth, Grantly Dick-Read, Harper & Row, 1985.

Cradle and All: Women Writers on Pregnancy and Birth, Laura Chester, ed., Faber and Faber, 1989.

Having Your Baby with a Nurse-Midwife, the American College of Nurse-Midwives and Sandra Jacobs, Hyperion, 1993.

The Illustrated Book of Pregnancy and Childbirth, Margaret Martin, Facts on File, 1992.

Planning for Pregnancy, Birth, and Beyond, the American College of Obstetricians and Gynecologists, Dutton, 1992.

Special Delivery: The Complete Guide to Informed Birth, Rahima Baldwin, Celestial Arts (Berkeley, Calif.), 1987.

What to Expect When You're Expecting, Arlene Eisenberg, Heidi E. Murkoff, and Sandee E. Hathaway, Workman Publishing, 1991. (Also, *What to Eat When You're Expecting.*)

16

The Hysterectomy Decision

Each year over half a million American women undergo hysterectomies, the surgical removal of the uterus. And every year, experts say, hundreds of thousands of these women undergo hysterectomies unnecessarily. As Black women, we are particularly vulnerable: A University of Maryland study shows that a disproportionate number of hysterectomies are performed on African-American women, and we tend to have our uteruses removed at a younger age than white women do.

Related to this issue is one of history's worst cases of exploitation of Black women: Even as late as the 1960s in the Deep South, poor African-American women were sterilized against their will or coerced into sterilization in order to keep their public-assistance payments.

Today, for a Black woman undergoing hysterectomy the risks are much greater than they are for white women. Because our access to health care is more limited and we are more likely to suffer from serious illnesses that complicate surgery, Black women are twice as likely to die from the operation as white women, mainly due to our poor health status.

But that doesn't mean that all hysterectomies should be viewed with alarm. Having a hysterectomy can be a blessing or a curse; the choice to have one truly depends on your individual situation. For the woman who's never had a child and wants one desperately, losing her womb may mean losing a vital part of her femininity. But for another woman who already has children or doesn't want any and is living with out-of-control fibroids, doing without a uterus can mean living unencumbered by chronic pain or a gushing menstrual flow. And for yet another woman, faced with the reality of cancer, the choice whether to have a hysterectomy means literally choosing between life and death.

The decision to have a hysterectomy should be taken seriously: It is, after all, major surgery, and any kind of surgery comes with risks and side effects. And like any surgery, it's best to have all the facts before making a decision that will literally change your life—and your body. Black women suffer from fibroid tumors in high numbers, and the majority of hysterectomies are performed to remove fibroids. That makes it especially important for us to be well informed about hysterectomies and alternatives to the operation. For more on fibroids see chapter 13, "Fighting Fibroids."

Cast a skeptical eye on any doctor who automatically prescribes a hysterectomy as the solution to your problems. Insist on getting a second opinion. Read everything you can about your condition, and find out about all available treatments. Ask lots of questions and talk to other sisters who have either had a hysterectomy, considered having one, or found an alternative.

What Is a Hysterectomy?

In the United States, hysterectomy is one of the most frequently performed surgical procedures for women, second only to cesarean sections: More than half of all women over age seventy have had the operation. In the old days, hysterectomies were considered the cure-all for bothersome "female problems." Remove the uterus, the theory went, and chronic gynecological problems such as fibroids, menstrual difficulties, prolapsed uterus, and endometriosis would disappear forever. Some women had their wombs and ovaries removed in an attempt to prevent cancer. Others even used hysterectomy as a form of permanent birth control. One thing is certain: With a hysterectomy, in which the womb is removed either vaginally or through an incision in the belly, the option of bearing children is taken away forever. Doctors sometimes remove both the uterus and the ovaries from women who suffer from or are at risk for ovarian cancer. Women who undergo this operation, called oophorectomy, can count on becoming menopausal no matter how young they are.

No doubt about it, hysterectomy may mean relief from the problems that brought you to the doctor in the first place. Painful periods will be a thing of the past. So will the bladder and bowel problems that result when fibroids begin to press on your internal organs. But understand that in some cases, having a hysterectomy can also mean a long, painful recovery period. The amount of time you spend in the hospital will vary greatly, depending on the type of hysterectomy you have and on your own physical condition, including your fitness level. The side effects of hysterectomy are uncomfortable for some women as well. And the operation is expensive, generally costing between $5,000 and $9,000, depending on the type of surgery. (Health insurance generally covers the operation.)

Vaginal Hysterectomy

For women who have fibroids that are the size of a three-month pregnancy or smaller, the uterus can be removed vaginally, without an abdominal incision. The patient is put under general anesthesia or receives a spinal block, and the doctor separates the uterus from its connecting ligaments, using a clamplike tool. The uterus is then pulled out, using the vagina as a passageway. Because there is no visible incision or visible stitches, recovery time will be quicker and there will be fewer side effects from surgery. Most patients are able to leave the hospital in about two to three days and are feeling better within two weeks' time. Total healing time will take about six weeks. Patients generally can't drive a car for the first two weeks and have to abstain from sexual intercourse for at least six weeks.

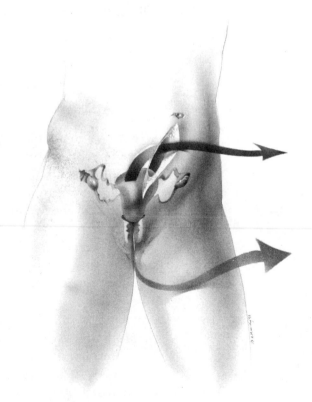

Abdominal Hysterectomy

This option is generally recommended if the ovaries are to be removed, for chronic pelvic disease, and for large fibroids. The doctor will

Hysterectomy: two methods of surgical approach—abdominal and vaginal. *(Drawing: Keelin Murphy)*

make an incision in the abdominal cavity and then remove the uterus. Because the body has been opened, recovering from an abdominal hysterectomy may be more painful than from a vaginal hysterectomy. Patients are generally uncomfortable for about six weeks while the wound heals. During that period, sex (and generally driving) will be out of the question. Some doctors recommend that patients only take showers during that time; baths increase your chances of infection.

Laparoscopic-Assisted Vaginal Hysterectomy

This is a newer option that requires a skilled surgeon. You must ask whether your doctor can perform this kind of surgery, and if so, how many he or she has done.

The doctor makes a tiny incision near the navel, inserting a telescopic instrument called a laparoscope. The laparoscope is attached to a video screen, through which the doctor can see your uterus and work precisely. The uterus is then removed vaginally.

The procedure may take longer than abdominal surgery, but it is considered safer. It is particularly beneficial for women who suffer from endometriosis, because it allows the surgeon to see the area clearly. Recovery time is quicker, too. However, not every woman is a candidate for this surgery.

When Is a Hysterectomy Necessary?

In some cases a woman must have a hysterectomy to save her life. Although each case must be analyzed on its own, these are some conditions that may require hysterectomy:

Cancer of the uterus, vagina, ovaries, fallopian tubes, or cervix, if advanced.

Large fibroid tumors that are extensive or too big to be removed by myomectomy. However, other treatments should be tried first.

Severe bleeding that cannot be controlled and hasn't responded to other treatments. This sometimes occurs after childbirth. If this is your problem, be sure to ask your doctor about a newer procedure called *endometrial ablation.* In this procedure, which is cheaper, less complicated, and has a shorter recovery period than hysterectomy, the surgeon uses an instrument called a hysteroscope to destroy damaged tissue in the uterus.

Advanced pelvic inflammatory disease, which can occur when an infection is left untreated and spreads, infecting the reproductive organs and tissues.

Severe endometriosis, which occurs when fragments of the lining of the uterus are found in other parts of the pelvic cavity, can require hysterectomy, *but only if other methods have failed.* Medication to suppress estrogen or more conservative procedures should be tried first.

A severely dropped uterus, a condition called uterine prolapse. This occurs when the muscles and ligaments that support the womb are stretched. It is considered very serious when the uterus has dropped so far down that the cervix appears outside the vaginal opening. There are alternative treatments for uterine prolapse—such as exercising the muscles or using a diaphragmlike device (called a pessary) to hold the uterus in place. Hysterectomy is called for only in *severe* cases.

Alternatives to Hysterectomy

If you are considering having a hysterectomy, you should know that there are other, less invasive options available. Rapid leaps in technology and research have given us procedures that weren't available to the general public as recently as a year or so ago. Some techniques can preserve fertility for those women who want to have children. Vanessa, a thirty-six-year-old public relations executive, skipped a hysterectomy, opting for another method to remove her fibroids. "I was in my midthirties at the time, and my fibroids were giving me a great deal of trouble. I was bleeding all the time. But I knew I wanted to have children. A hysterectomy was out of the question, so I had a laparoscopic myomectomy. Now my period is back to normal. And thanks to the procedure, when I decide to have kids, I have a better chance of getting pregnant than I did before."

But be aware that each woman's situation is unique; you may not be a good candidate for some kinds of procedures. Check with your doctor. In fact, check with two or three doctors before making up your mind. Here are some alternative treatments for fibroid tumors (for a more in-depth discussion of fibroids, see chapter 13, "Fighting Fibroids"):

Myomectomy
Candidates: Women who have fibroids that are causing problems, but want to keep the uterus intact.

What it is: In this procedure, the fibroid is removed, at times with a laser, through the vagina, or through an incision in the belly. The uterus is left intact.

Drawbacks: Must be performed by a skilled surgeon. Some doctors don't know how to perform the procedure. Many doctors require that

> *"All the*
> *equipment I*
> *needed to have a*
> *child was still*
> *there and in*
> *working order."*
>
> —DIANE WEATHERS,
> WRITER AND EDITOR,
> NEW YORK CITY

Fibroid tumors were sprouting in me like crocuses in springtime. But they weren't the problem. Far more worrisome was the "suspicious uterine mass" detected only on a sonogram. It had to be removed, and there was a possibility that my uterus also might have to go.

I was living in Italy, and my first impulse was to come home. Newspapers were reporting a rash of routine hospital appendectomies and birth deliveries from hell. Furthermore, four years earlier, one of Rome's most prestigious laboratories had misdiagnosed my mysterious mass as an innocent little offshoot of one of my fibroid tumors.

But I was also aware that American doctors had a reputation for being too quick to remove "nonessential" ovaries and uteri in older women. A few months before, a friend had been told by an American doctor that a partial hysterectomy was the best solution for her fibroid-tumor troubles. She declined the offer and returned to Europe where she found a French gynecologist who successfully removed the growths, leaving her reproductive organs in place.

I did my homework. I got second and third medical opinions, perused the medical books, and talked to women who had had similar experiences. I was forty-two years old, single, and was almost ashamed to admit I still had hopes of conceiving a child. Even though I had already decided to adopt, I was willing to fight to keep my options open.

All the advice and research led to the same conclusion: I would have to shop around for the kind of medical treatment I wanted. European gynecologists gave very specific instructions. Since I was determined to have my operation in the States, they cautioned me to seek out a gynecologist who specialized in treating infertility—someone with experience in doing the more complicated surgery often necessary to preserve reproductive organs and who respected a forty-something-year-old woman's wish to become pregnant.

Back in the States, I found such a person. When we talked, it was like talking to a sympathetic girlfriend. He understood perfectly my desire for children. Still, we almost came to blows when he asked me to sign a statement permitting him to remove other organs if necessary. At first I refused. But reluctantly, I conceded that this suspicious mass might be cancerous. I might have to sacrifice an organ or two to save my life.

I will never forget coming out from under the anesthesia and seeing my doctor's pudgy, brown smiling face. The growth he removed was benign, he explained. He also performed a myomectomy and removed the fibroid tumors and did an overall tune-up. All the equipment I needed to have a child was still there and in working order. Then he said something like, "Now stop fooling around—go out and get pregnant!"

you agree to a hysterectomy before you undergo a myomectomy in case the fibroids prove to be too difficult to remove. Before you enter the operating room, find out under what conditions your doctor would perform a hysterectomy.

Lupron

Candidates: Women who are planning to undergo another procedure.

What it is: Lupron is a medication that reduces fibroids by temporarily suppressing the body's production of estrogen, the hormone that feeds fibroid growth. Generally given as an injection, it shrinks the fibroids, leaving physicians to better monitor them or to remove them using less invasive procedures.

Drawbacks: It is only a stopgap measure; when the medication is discontinued, the fibroids grow back. Plus, it can be much too expensive for some women. Also, because it inhibits the release of estrogen, it can induce a temporary menopausal state with such side effects as hot flashes, vaginal dryness, and mood swings.

Microsurgery

Candidates: Women with small fibroids—less than 1.5 centimeters—or who suffer from severe, uncontrolled bleeding.

What it is: A doctor may use an instrument called a hysteroscope to remove fibroids on the inside of the uterus. In this procedure, the fibroids are either burned away with a laser or shaved. She or he can also use a hysteroscope to stop excessive bleeding in a procedure called *endometrial ablation.* These procedures are generally done on an outpatient basis, and there is no scar or severe pain. For small fibroids on the outside of the uterus, doctors can remove them with a laparoscope, a telescopic instrument inserted through an incision in the abdomen.

Drawbacks: Some surgeons don't have this equipment or know how to properly perform the procedures. Can only be used with small fibroids, and new fibroids may grow after the procedure.

Natural Healing

Candidates: Women with small fibroids that aren't growing rapidly.

What it is: Some folks believe that conditions such as fibroids are simply a signal that the body is toxic and needs cleansing. Some naturopathic professionals recommend treating gynecological problems naturally by cleansing the body with a strict diet of fruits and vegetables, in conjunction with vitamins and herbs. But don't rush out to the health-food store without consulting a health professional first: Each person's body is unique.

Drawbacks: This method calls for radical dietary changes. Women with severe fibroids that are growing rapidly and/or causing major health problems should use this option in conjunction with other forms of treatment.

Making the Decision

When you're sick and in pain, deciding whether or not to have a hysterectomy can be overwhelming. It's hard not to be intimidated by a doctor who may be urging you to go ahead with the surgery. Keep in mind that there are doctors who are overly eager to operate. *Always* insist on a second opinion before agreeing to any operation. Remember: It's your body, and you are the one who will have to live with the effects of the hysterectomy. Many women have both physical and emotional side effects after undergoing hysterectomy. The degree varies. For example, some women are so relieved to end the problem that led to the hysterectomy that the aftereffects of surgery seem minor. Other women, however, suffer complications after the operation—side effects that physicians often don't mention before surgery. Many are hesitant to discuss what they're going through.

Women who have oophorectomy (removal of the ovaries) go through menopause. They often experience menopausal symptoms such as hot flashes, insomnia, mood swings, and vaginal and urinary-tract changes. These side effects can be eased with estrogen-replacement therapy. You must discuss this option carefully with your doctor. (For more information on estrogen replacement, see chapter 17, "Menopause: Going Through the Change.")

Women who have hysterectomies without having the ovaries removed may occasionally notice menopausal symptoms. Some changes that have been reported by women are:

- Changes in sexual desire and response, including vaginal dryness and weakened orgasm
- Hair loss
- Breast changes
- Urine leakage
- Weight gain and bloating
- Chronic yeast infections

As with all kinds of surgery, a hysterectomy has its risks. You should know what kinds of complications exist:

Hemorrhaging. Sometimes bleeding is so heavy that you will need a blood transfusion. In most cases, the bleeding is caught before a serious problem results.

Anesthesia. Whenever surgery requires anesthesia, there is always a risk. Brain damage, stroke, respiratory arrest, and cardiac arrest are all possibilities. It's best to have a talk with your anesthesiologist before you go under.

Surgical mistakes. During surgery, the bladder or the ureter, the tube connecting the bladder and kidney, can be damaged. The ureter may be severed. Sometimes these mistakes may be caught during surgery; often, however, a second operation is needed to repair the ureter. That's why it's key to make sure the surgeon is experienced.

If a hysterectomy is starting to look like a real option for you, sit down with your doctor and ask some serious questions. You may want to take a friend or family member along for support. Here are some questions you should ask:

Why do I need a hysterectomy? Will the surgery treat my condition, or can I expect to have a recurrence of my symptoms?

What are the alternatives available to me? Can my condition be treated through medication, rather than surgery? Are there less invasive surgical procedures that I can choose?

Exactly what kind of surgery are you performing? Will you remove my uterus or both the uterus and my ovaries? If you are removing the ovaries, what is the reason?

What happens if I don't have the surgery? Will my condition improve with age, after I've reached menopause?

What can I expect from my recovery? What can I expect before, during, and after the surgery? How long will I stay in the hospital? Will there be any side effects from the surgery? Will they be permanent? Will I need a catheter after the surgery? A blood transfusion?

What can I do to prepare for the surgery? Will I need to take iron supplements if I am already anemic? Will I need to stop taking other medications?

Should I have blood drawn and stored in case I need a transfusion?

What will my life be like after the surgery?

It's also very important to talk to other women who have been through what you're going through. Ask friends and relatives the questions above. Ask a sister friend how she made her decision, who performed her operation, and how she felt afterward.

Choosing a Surgeon

Picking a doctor who is both skilled and sensitive can be a daunting prospect. Most of us were brought up to look at doctors with awe. But when choosing a doctor, it helps to remember that you are hiring her or him to do a job. Interview your doctor. Make sure you're comfortable and can talk frankly. You *are* paying her or him, so you should expect good service. "Some patients don't know where to turn and they think of the doctor as an adversary," says Ann B. Ward, M.D., an African-American OB-GYN who practices in Chicago. "But most doctors are there to help you. Choose a good doctor, someone who has a reasonably busy practice so that you know they don't need the money to survive. . . . And always, when a diagnosis is made, ask for as much information as possible." For more information see chapter 19, "Dealing with Doctors and Hospitals."

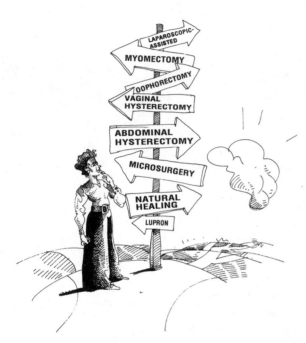

Making the difficult decision about hysterectomy.
((Drawing: Yvonne Buchanan)

Here are some tips for choosing a good surgeon:

Get a referral from someone who's already had the surgery. Most gynecological referrals come from satisfied patients. Or ask your family doctor or one of the organizations in this chapter's resource list to recommend someone.

Get a second opinion.

Visit the surgical suite of the hospital, and speak to the surgical nurses. Say, "I'm having a hysterectomy, and I've narrowed down my choice of a doctor. Who would you pick as a second or third choice?" Also, ask hospital employees which doctors they use.

Once you've chosen a doctor, call her or his office. Ask whether she or he is board-eligible or certified. If the doctor is not board-certified, it doesn't mean she or he is incompetent. But it is a gauge. Ask the doctor whether she or he has performed the type of surgery you need—and how many times.

Spend some time talking to your doctor. Ask questions until all of your concerns are addressed. Ask for booklets or informational videos so you understand exactly what the procedure will be like.

From a 1981 journal, Columbia Women's Hospital, Washington, D.C.:

I'm in the hospital for a hysterectomy. Endometriosis and fibroids have produced a personal pain management plan of four Percodan per day. I cannot trust my highly suspect doctor. He has refused to hear me or help me search out surgical alternatives. He has prescribed surgery; insists on it. He has not prescribed my three times per day brandies for washing Percodan down and taking me up into the land of numb and nod.

Sunday evening ushers in the long march of bloodletting technicians, vital sign monitors, nurses with final instructions. Monday morning arrives and so does the army of attendants to usher me into the surgical wing. They shoot me up to calm me down, dry up my saliva and guarantee no further resistance to this wrenching out of my one and only womb.

I am strapped down on the gurney and parked outside the operating suite for an hour, my eyes recording the chalkboard's list of hysterectomies scheduled for the day. Masked men and women, mainly white, swish past on sneakery soles. Some come to kindly hold my hand, talking me into confidence in this procedure some say they've done hundreds of times. They share sanitized stories about sons and daughters, surreptitiously inquiring into the number of children I have. They all know I am the Black hysterectomy. Besides every 31-year-old Black woman certainly has enough children—real or potential.

I wait. There is no ceremony. There ought to be. This womb has housed, hugged into being my only child, Imani Aisha, and temporarily sheltered two that lined up but did not march. This womb has served me up regular periods since 1959. It's mine, my own. It ought to be placed in a splendiferous dish, hand-thrown and hammered from gold.

But only for a little while.

Later they will tell me how short, precise and efficient a procedure it was, reveling in their self-proclaimed surgical proficiency. Even as they work to bring down my temperature caused by the stubborn infection that "some of you patients sometimes get after this procedure."

I search for days for comforts, ceremonies, for righteous rituals to consign my womb to its final resting place. Having held on for two pain-plagued years of periods that reduced me to infantile whimpers and a slim sex life, I thought myself ready to strike a bargain with God for a new woman, pain-free and repositioned in the world with strength and vigor. I knew I'd do anything.

I did.

> *"This womb has served me up regular periods since 1959. . . . It ought to be placed in a splendiferous dish, hand-thrown and hammered from gold."*
>
> —AMA R. SARAN,
> CONSULTANT FOR
> NONPROFIT MANAGEMENT,
> OAKLAND, CALIFORNIA

After the Operation

After surgery, some women experience the side effects mentioned above. Some women also suffer from depression after having hysterectomies. Because our society values women as vessels for reproduction, losing the uterus can make some women feel not just sad, but useless. Some women feel depressed because of the bodily changes the surgery causes. To ease the sadness, talk about how you feel with other women who have had hysterectomies or with understanding friends or family members. To find a support group, contact the HERS (Hysterectomy Educational Resources and Services) Foundation at (215) 667-7757.

You can lessen both the physical and emotional aftereffects by treating yourself right. Avoid fat, sugar, alcohol, salt, and caffeine, and nurture your body with fruit juices, vegetables, whole grains, and other foods that are good for you. Once you're up and about, try some exercise. Walking, swimming, skating, and yoga can help strengthen your body after surgery and ward off depression.

For More Information

ORGANIZATIONS

THE HYSTERECTOMY EDUCATIONAL RESOURCES AND SERVICES (HERS) FOUNDATION, 422 Bryn Mawr Ave., Bala Cynwyd, PA 19004; (215) 667-7757. HERS has a wide range of information on hysterectomy, how to avoid it, and the consequences of and alternatives to surgery.

WOMEN'S REPRODUCTIVE HEALTH NETWORK, P.O. Box 301607, Portland, OR 97230-9607; (503) 252-9024. The organization provides free information and support for women who are contemplating hysterectomies and for women who have had hysterectomies and are suffering side effects.

BOOKS

Hysterectomy Before and After: A Comprehensive Guide to Preventing, Preparing for, and Maximizing Health After Hysterectomy, Winnifred B. Cutler, Harper & Row, 1988.

Hysterectomy: Learning the Facts, Coping with the Feelings, Facing the Future, Wanda Wigfall-Williams, Michael Kesend Publishers, 1986.

Hysterectomy: Making a Choice, Martin D. Greenberg, M.D., Perigee Books, 1993.

How to Avoid a Hysterectomy: An Indispensible Guide to Exploring All Your Options—Before You Consent to a Hysterectomy, Lynn Payer, Pantheon, 1987.

The New Our Bodies, Ourselves: A Book By and For Women, The Boston Women's Health Book Collective, Touchstone Books, Simon & Schuster, 1992.

The No-Hysterectomy Option, Herbert A. Goldfarb, M.D., with Judith Greif, Wiley, 1990.

No More Hysterectomies, Vicki Hufnagel, M.D., and Susan K. Golant, New American Library, 1989.

Ourselves Growing Older: Women Aging with Knowledge and Power, Paula Brown Doress, Diana Laskin Siegal, and the Midlife and Older Women Book Project, Simon & Schuster, 1987.

The Well-Informed Patient's Guide to Hysterectomy, *Kathryn Cox, M.D., Dell Publishing, 1992.*

Women Talk About Gynecological Surgery: From Diagnosis to Recovery, Amy Gross and Dee Ito, HarperPerennial, 1992.

You Don't Need a Hysterectomy: New and Effective Ways of Avoiding Major Surgery, Ivan K. Strausz, M.D., Addison-Wesley, 1993.

17

Menopause: Going Through the Change

Menopause is one of the most written about, talked about, and least understood women's health issues of the decade. It's become hot news now, because an estimated 40 million of the most educated, outspoken, determined, and tenacious women of all time—the female Baby Boomers—will go through "the change" within the next decade.

This new interest in menopause is a far cry from the past, especially before the turn of the century, when talk of menopause was taboo. Our society has long regarded the aging woman negatively, and menopause has always been looked at as a disease, something unnatural, unpleasant, and frightening. We have been brainwashed into believing that once a woman's childbearing years are over, she's old, mad, and sexually unappealing.

Part of the reason for our society's negative, cruel, and shame-instilling attitudes about a natural part of our femaleness is that until the early 1900s, due to disease, physically hard work, and complications relating to childbirth, many women did not live long enough to experience menopause. Since the average life span of a woman in the early 1900s was forty-five years, women who lived beyond that age into their fifties and beyond were considered old—hags, even. "Menopause has long been kept in the closet," says Dr. Irma Mebane-Sims of the National Institutes of Health.

That is finally changing. Dr. Mebane-Sims, who is an African-American, is the program director of a landmark study of 875 post-menopausal women. Known as PEPI (Postmenopausal Estrogen/Progestin Interventions trials), this study will look at how hormone-replacement therapies affect cardiovascular-disease risk factors. It will also examine a variety of other factors, including quality of life and menopausal symptoms. Though the majority of respondents are white, 10 to 15 percent are women of color.

Though there is much speculation, little if any scientific data describes how "the change" affects us differently than it affects white women. "There well may be differences between Black and white women, but there is no hard data," confirms Dr. Mebane-Sims.

Anecdotal reports suggest that Black women are not as anxious about aging or menopause as our white counterparts are. Our feelings about menopause may be more similar to those of some of our African sisters and of some women of color in other parts of the world. In many societies in Asia, South Africa, South America, and Arabic countries, where

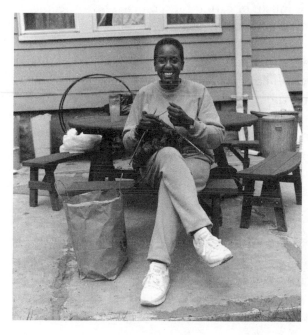

Black women seem to be more likely than white women to take aging in stride. *(Photo: Lisa Ross)*

aging friends and relatives are respected and revered, women reportedly have much more positive feelings about menopause and welcome the end of their childbearing years. Many women of African descent view "the change" as a natural part of life—not a medical problem to be cured. Many of us use home remedies (herbs and tonics used and recommended by our ancestors and friends), vitamins, and spirituality for comfort and relaxation as the primary means for managing or coping with discomforts related to the change.

Physical differences between Black and white women may also explain some of these differences in response. Fat cells produce estrogen, so women who are heavier may not feel dramatic symptoms that come with menopause's estrogen decrease. "Because Black women in the U.S. tend to be heavier, the internal production of estrogen may convey some benefit," says Dr. Mebane-Sims.

Racial differences aside, most women are not informed about "the change" and the health consequences it brings. It also appears that Black women may be even less informed than white women. Even if we are having symptoms similar to those white women experience, we may not be recognizing them. Some sisters are too used to having medical problems; menopausal symptoms may be just another thing. Stress is so high among Black women that some sisters may be assuming that hot flashes and other signs of menopause are just another signal that they're working too hard, worrying too much, or caring for too many other people.

That's how Anita Moore, a Washington, D.C., computer specialist, felt. She says she experienced dramatic changes, both physical and emotional, as she began to go through menopause. "Like most Black women, I had many responsibilities. In addition to being a wife, mother, and homemaker with a full-time professional career outside of the home, I was also caring for my father, who was very ill when I began the change. So for a long time I didn't even notice what was happening to me. I attributed all ailments to stress and fatigue. It was only after my father died that I realized I was in the midst of the change. In addition to having hot flashes that would wake me in the middle of the night, drenched in perspiration, I also developed a very short fuse. Sometimes, after a trying day at work, if my husband said one wrong word to me I'd go off. 'Damn it,' I'd say, 'I'm tired. Don't ask me for a thing.' And he wasn't the only person I was short and irritable with. I began being short with people at work. I also became extremely claustrophobic and had problems staying at my work station, which was rather confining. After a while I went to my physician for help. 'You've got to help me,' I pleaded. 'You've got to do something because I'm not myself anymore, and I cannot go on like this.' He put me on estrogen, and it has worked well for me. I've been on it for five years now."

We must not be caught off guard by menopausal symptoms. The change can be an important, challenging life transition and can signal the beginning of what can be the most carefree, exciting, creative, fulfilling, and powerful time of our lives. But only if we do three things: learn about it, plan for it, and make health care and lifestyle choices that will not only ease our passage through, but also protect our future health.

What Is Menopause?

Menopause is a gradual process. It starts when menstrual periods become irregular and ends with the final period. Doctors recognize it as twelve months of no menstrual period in a woman between the ages of forty-five and fifty-five who still has her uterus. Menopause can begin as early as age thirty-five or as late as sixty, although the average age is estimated to be fifty-one. Because our hormones fluctuate throughout the complex biological process during which our ovaries stop producing them, health-care providers advise women to continue using reliable birth control measures for twenty-four months following their last period.

No one fully understands why the ovaries stop producing estrogen or why that time varies among women. Interestingly, there has been no connection found between the age you had your first period and the age you'll arrive at your last period. So whether you started your period early or late has no bearing on when your menopause will occur. In a small study but one of the few involving menopausal Black women, Beryl Jackson, Ph.D., found that 36 percent of respondents reported going through the change between ages forty-six and forty-nine; 29 percent went through it between ages forty and forty-five; 25 percent between ages fifty and fifty-three; and 10 percent between ages fifty-four and fifty-eight.

Going through menopause later than average may be natural for some women, but prolonged menstrual bleeding, especially after periods have begun to diminish, may also be a signal of abnormal growths in the uterus or an overgrowth of the uterine lining, the endometrium. In some instances, these problems lead to cancer. For these reasons, you must have regular gynecological checkups (at least yearly) so that any such problems may be identified and treated as early as possible.

It is also important to note that women who experience late

menopause have a greater risk of developing breast cancer. All women in their fifties should take special care to do monthly breast self-exams and to have annual mammograms.

Women who have both ovaries completely removed will go through menopause immediately regardless of their age. This operation is called an oophorectomy. If the ovaries are left intact, or even if a portion of the ovaries remains, menopausal symptoms will not occur right away. One ovary or a portion of an ovary produces enough estrogen to prevent menopausal symptoms from occurring prematurely. For more on hysterectomy, see chapter 16, "The Hysterectomy Decision."

Signs and Symptoms of the Change

Experts estimate that 75 to 80 percent of women experience one or more symptoms in addition to irregularities of their menstrual cycles as they go through the change. However, it is estimated that only 10 to 35 percent are bothered by the symptoms enough to seek professional help. Among Dr. Jackson's Black female respondents, over 40 percent indicated that menopause brought very little change in their social lives.

Nonetheless, there's no shame in acknowledging the signs of menopause and asking for help. Women have found relief through all kinds of methods—from medication to herbs to support groups. According to "Menopause and More," a 1992 national survey conducted by the Midlife Women's Network, these are the most commonly reported menopausal and postmenopausal symptoms:

- Fatigue
- Weight gain
- Depression
- Irritability/mood swings
- Stress incontinence
- Anxiety
- Poor memory
- Hot flashes
- Night sweats
- Insomnia
- Vaginal dryness
- Irregular periods
- Urinary/vaginal infection

Hot Flashes

Hot flashes, caused by decreases in the hormones estrogen and progesterone, are the most common menopausal symptom reported by women
who go through the change naturally or surgically. In Beryl Jackson's
study, nearly half of the women reported they
had from fair to considerable difficulties with
hot flashes.

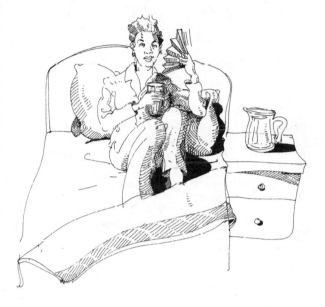

Although no one knows exactly how and
why hot flashes are triggered, they are a real
physical event. Just before a hot flash, some
women report they have a feeling that it's going
to happen. Then suddenly their hearts begin to
race, the skin temperature heats up, and they
begin to perspire, sometimes heavily. Some
women merely glow and become mildly moist,
while others burn and drip buckets. During a
hot flash a woman is literally engulfed with an
intense shock of heat, although no internal
fever occurs with it. "Most women report that
the flash begins in their chest area and moves
upward," says Sharon Byrd, M.D., a Virginia
Beach, Virginia, gynecologist who has conducted workshops on menopause for Black
women. "White women and light-skinned,

Many women find ways to stay cool during a hot flash.
(Drawing: Yvonne Buchanan)

thin Black women can actually see reddening of the skin in the chest,
neck, and face areas as the blood vessels near the skin dilate and cause
blood to rush into the pathway. In darker-skinned women, you don't see
the flush, but you see the sweating."

Some women experience mild flashes a few times a week, while others
may have as many as six in an hour. Some women have flashes at night
only. They are awakened to find themselves drenched and burning up.
While some women report being affected for only a few months to a
year, others report having hot flashes from one to ten years after their
last menstrual period. While hot flashes are not physically harmful, they
can be uncomfortable and embarrassing because they can happen at any
time and often in front of others.

Insomnia

Jackson found that 25 percent of menopausal Black women report trouble sleeping, and insomnia is the second most distressing symptom that

"Sometimes I lie down in the sand, breathing deeply to relax, and say that it's all right to feel crazy, or just let the tears flow."

—Peggy Dammond Preacely, civil rights activist, writer, and natural-health practitioner, San Pedro, California

During the past six months I have often found myself with a profound sense of sadness and tears completely unexpectedly. Those times are contrasted with complete euphoria at other times. I thought it was just me, until I read a couple of books about menopause, like Women of the 14th Moon, *and* talked to my friends. Now I realize that what's going on has a pattern to it.

Some days I'm the master conductor, and I can handle my daughter's crises, my husband's stress, what's going on at the three jobs I'm working, and I'm just fine. I feel like I'm on top of the world. Other days I can't even handle one thing.

Fortunately, I have studied and practiced natural-healing arts for nearly twenty years. So on days when my hormones are going crazy and my whole body just aches and aches—every single thing—I take dong quai, yam root, and uva ursi, which are all especially good for female problems and for maintaining a healthy bladder. Evening primrose oil helps me, too.

Some remedies and renewals that my friends and I have shared with each other are very effective for relieving the stress and strains brought on by the change. Every morning I drink a hot lemon drink to keep the bowels loose and prevent any sluggishness. The key foods that sustain me are brown rice, sweet potatoes, fish, yams, red beans, broccoli, cauliflower, carrots, and cabbage. When I can, I like to make a good batch of spinach soup, because it's rich in iron and other nutrients; when you're going through the change, the body needs more nutrients. My daily vitamins include B-6, Vitamin E for the hot flashes and dryness, and calcium.

Along with eating nutritious foods to restore energy and vigor, and to fortify you during this time, it's very important to be sure to reconnect your spiritual batteries. My lifeline is prayer and meditation. I also take myself to the beach so I can feel the sand and water. I swim in the sun or under the stars and go hiking to commune with nature. Sometimes I lie down in the sand, breathing deeply to relax, and say that it's all right to feel crazy, or let the tears flow. Music, nature, massage, exercise, deep breathing of fresh outdoor air, and gardening all help me. Lighting candles, burning incense, and taking long lavender-oil baths are also very soothing and refreshing.

Finally, my husband is very key to this whole process, this roller coaster I'm on. He's wonderful and will massage me and be very tender—if I can allow myself to accept tenderness at that time. It really helps to have a mate, close girlfriend, or family member that you can feel comfortable enough with to pull off that mask and allow that person to see you when you're most vulnerable. It really allows them to get closer to you and helps you to feel better.

sends women to their physicians for care. Some women have difficulty falling asleep, while others awaken in the middle of the night and cannot go back to sleep. Some researchers think that the problems result from disturbances in the hypothalamus gland that controls sleep, temperature, and hormone production. They believe that whatever disturbances trigger hot flashes also interfere with sleep patterns and brain waves. Some women experience only mild sleep problems that last for just a short time during and after the change, while others have more severe difficulties that last for years.

Mood Swings

Researchers disagree about whether the decline in estrogen during menopause causes women emotional difficulties. Some say moods may change due to the combination of physiological changes that affect a woman's overall well-being. Others say that while menopause is not in itself *the* cause of mood disorders, fluctuations in the hormone levels can intensify whatever feelings a woman is having due to her life circumstances. While scientists are busy debating mood swings, many women are saying they experience them. Fluctuating emotional states are the third most common symptom among menopausal women. Many women say they're feeling fine one minute and the next they feel extremely sad and burst into tears over nothing. Others say they are much more sensitive than ever before, that the slightest criticism hurts their feelings or makes them angry.

Growing older can be a crisis for a woman, depending upon how she feels about herself in general. Some experts say that if a woman has high self-esteem—feels good about herself, is confident, in control, and satisfied with her accomplishments and her life situation and has a loved one and/or a close circle of family and friends—menopause is not likely to cause her any psychological problems. If, however, she suffers from low self-esteem or is stressed out, then she may feel devalued and depressed when signs of aging appear and her fertility ends. Menopause may well exacerbate an already unhappy and/or stress-filled life. Poor diet and stress can also make mood swings worse.

Once menopause is over—when your periods have stopped completely—hot flashes, insomnia, and mood swings should go away. However, other changes that are caused by a lack of estrogen—vaginal changes, urinary tract/bladder problems, changes in sex drive, and bone thinning—begin during the change but continue as a woman gets older. For details on these conditions, see chapter 8, "Our Bodies Growing Older."

Sorting Out the Hormone Controversy

Considering whether or not to take hormones is one of the most diffi-cult decisions menopausal women have to make. Taking hormones—either estrogen-replacement therapy (ERT) or hormone-replacement therapy (HRT)—can protect older women against serious illness (such as heart disease and osteoporosis), and many sisters who replace lost estrogen are happy and relieved not to be bothered by problems like hot flashes. In fact, a study reported by Johns Hopkins University Hospital researchers found that women who used replacement therapy were less likely to die *for any reason* by age sixty-nine than women who didn't use it.

Many women dismiss ERT and HRT without having enough infor-mation to make an informed choice. Some also feel suspicious, because doctors have been quick to prescribe both ERT and HRT to women who complain of hot flashes and other symptoms of the change. Because so many of us don't trust our doctors and because we don't ask doctors enough questions (and they often don't take the time to explain things to us), we are wary of pursuing this option. What's more, women's health activists have accused doctors of "medicalizing" menopause, a nat-ural part of a woman's life, pushing hormones whose consequences haven't been well documented and ignoring the many self-help remedies that some women swear by. But beyond these social and political issues, there are real reasons to be hesitant about hormonal remedies to menopausal symptoms. They sometimes have serious side effects, includ-ing uterine and breast cancer and fibroid tumors—none of which have been well studied.

In 1991, the National Institutes of Health completed recruitment for a three-year clinical trial on the risks and benefits of hormone-replacement therapies. The researchers hope this study will provide some answers about the use of postmenopausal hormones. In the meantime, you'll need to weigh the pros and cons of replacement therapies with your doc-tor to decide whether ERT or HRT are right for you. To help, here are answers to some of your questions.

Why do menopausal women use replacement hormones?

Both ERT and HRT relieve menopausal symptoms. Estrogen proba-bly can play a role in preventing osteoporosis, a thinning of the bones that can lead to fractures in older women. Osteoporosis is a common reason women are advised to begin long-term use of hormones. Although Black women tend to have less osteoporosis than white women, fractures can be very debilitating for many Black women.

About two years ago, I began waking up in the middle of the night. The hair on the back of my head was soaking wet, and I couldn't fall back to sleep. I thought it was my job because I was going through a stressful situation there at the time. Then my menses became unpredictable. I'd have two cycles, then skip four. Sometimes I only had spotting, and it was a different color and carried a funny smell.

Of course I went to the doctor, two different ones, in fact. One thought I might have an ovarian cyst, but I took every appropriate test, and nothing unusual was detected. That's when I realized that at age forty-three I was beginning to go though the change. Knowing this upset me, because my mom had a terrible time with menopause, and I feared I would, too.

I then went almost six months without having a period. Around the time when it was due, my breasts would become very sore, and I'd get jittery. I also began to have insomnia. Then I started getting hot flashes all of the time, sometimes several times an hour. I could feel them coming. One came while I was lecturing a class. It began in my neck and then traveled upward. It felt like something was on the inside trying to get out. And the heat was horrible, like someone was holding a hot iron very close to my skin. I had always perspired heavily but nothing like now. My underarms poured water. And I also noticed that during the hot flashes my mood changed drastically. At times I felt irritable, angry, and beside myself with discomfort. And on top of the hot flashes, insomnia, and irritability, I also had lower back pain, dry skin, and vaginal dryness.

So I went to my family nurse-practitioner and told her she had to do something for me. Thankfully she understood because she is menopausal, too. She gave me a synthetic form of the female hormone progesterone, and I also now take vitamin E. Now I feel like myself again; no more hot flashes or insomnia.

It's funny; I used to hate my period, but now that it's stopping, I don't know. But the good part of it is sex. I have much more sexual desire than I've ever had. That's a real plus to me. I find myself thinking about it, about my lover, and I get embarrassed. Lovemaking is better for me, too. I solved my vaginal dryness problem with K-Y jelly, and now everything is fine.

I've learned a lot since beginning the change. I now know that what's happening to me is normal. When you realize that, it's a big comfort, because it means you're not losing your mind. I'm going to keep on learning and sharing my knowledge about menopause with women—my family, my friends, and once I finish my training to be a family nurse-practitioner, my patients. When you know about menopause it's not so scary. It's great when you realize you have options and you're not alone.

"When you know about menopause, it's not so scary."

—ELLEN KING, REGISTERED NURSE, CLINTON, MARYLAND

Estrogen may also be effective in preventing heart disease, the major killer of older women—Black and white. Estrogen can also prevent vaginal dryness, which plagues many menopausal women and continues even after the change is over. (It is generally applied directly in cream form.)

What is the difference between ERT and HRT?

ERT refers to the use of estrogen only; it can be administered as a pill, cream, or skin patch to raise estrogen levels after menopause. Because estrogen can cause changes in the uterus (including cancer), women who have not had hysterectomies are either monitored very carefully or given HRT. HRT is a combination of estrogen and progestin, the synthetic form of the hormone progesterone. The addition of progestin removes the risk of uterine cancer. However, the risks associated with progestins have not been fully evaluated.

How is estrogen linked to breast cancer?

The link between estrogen and breast cancer is controversial and confusing. Studies differ over how high the risk is, but it is a fact that estrogen is associated with breast cancer, and the addition of progesterone to HRT may raise the risk even further. A Harvard University study showed that women who take ERT have a 35 percent higher risk of breast cancer than women who do not. But many women are willing to take that risk because of the benefits of hormonal treatments. To compensate, they reduce other cancer risk factors by eating a low-fat diet with plenty of fruits and vegetables, not smoking, checking their breasts monthly, and getting yearly mammograms.

Women who have a family history of breast cancer should weigh the risks and benefits of taking hormones very carefully. And any woman who has or has had breast cancer should not take ERT or HRT.

How does HRT affect fibroids?

The connection between fibroid tumors and estrogen has not been well studied, but many experts see a link. This information is vital to Black women, because we are much more likely than white women to have fibroids in our uteruses. In the past, doctors have steered women who have or have had fibroids away from taking hormones. But the dose of estrogen in today's replacement therapy is much lower, even lower than the low-dose birth control pill. Still, women who have or have had them should probably not use HRT.

Are there other women who should not use ERT and HRT?

Women who have their uteruses intact should consider ERT carefully and talk it over with their health-care providers because of the risk of uterine cancer. If you have a history of cervical cancer, heart disease, stroke, liver disease, or unexplained vaginal bleeding, you must discuss your particular case with your physician. Because of our high rates of hypertension, many Black women who have high blood pressure wonder whether replacement therapy is okay for them. Dr. Byrd advises, "Being hypertensive does not preclude a Black woman from using HRT. If her blood pressure is controlled, she deserves a trial."

What happens when replacement therapy is discontinued?

Never discontinue any medication without discussing it with your doctor first. If you stop taking the hormones, either all or some of your symptoms will return. You will also lose the protective effects from heart disease (in the case of ERT), osteoporosis, and vaginal dryness.

This question-and-answer section was prepared with the help of the National Women's Health Network. For a detailed, thirty-five-page booklet summarizing the latest studies on ERT and HRT ($7.50), write to the Network at 1325 G St. NW, Washington, D.C. 20005. There are also several books available on ERT and HRT. See the resource list at the end of the chapter.

Natural Treatment

For many women, hormone-replacement therapy is not an option. Some have health problems and/or family medical histories that make it inadvisable. Others fear they may develop breast or uterine cancer. Still others just plain object to taking medication every day for years when they are not ill. Thankfully, many natural-treatment options exist.

Even though only limited research has been done on natural remedies—diet, exercise, biofeedback, vitamin and herb therapy—some findings indicate, and many women testify, that they are effective in eliminating or at least alleviating bothersome menopausal signs and symptoms.

Diet

Eating right has helped some women reduce menopausal symptoms. Choose foods that are loaded with vitamins and minerals and that are closest to the way nature created them—fresh, unprocessed, raw or lightly cooked, and without unnecessary additives. Also limit fat intake to 30 percent or preferably less of total calories, and make sure you're getting five servings of fruit and/or vegetables per day. Eat foods high in fiber such as vegetables and grains.

Avoid foods and drinks that contain caffeine, such as coffee, tea, colas, chocolate, and alcohol. They may trigger hot flashes, aggravate incontinence, and worsen moodiness. Sugar, spicy foods, hot soups, and hot drinks also trigger hot flashes in some women.

Make sure you're eating plenty of these foods:

Fresh, deeply colored vegetables: Beets, broccoli, cabbage, carrots, cauliflower, collards, cucumbers, kale, peas, turnip greens, and yams.

Grains and seeds: Black beans, red beans, brown rice, baked corn chips, trail mixes, whole-grain muffins.

Fruits: Bananas, watermelon, cantaloupe, oranges, and tomatoes.

Supplements

Vitamin E reportedly reduces the frequency and severity of hot flashes and increases energy and an overall sense of well-being when taken in daily doses of about 400 to 600 international units (IU's). When taken over a long time, women say it relieves vaginal dryness and related genital or urinary-tract problems, and it helps dry skin. It is also a well-known cancer fighter. While it is considered safe when taken in the recommended dose, women on anticlotting medication and those with a history of high blood pressure, diabetes, or rheumatoid heart condition should not take it without a doctor's recommendation. Because so many Black women have hypertension, diabetes, and heart disease, taking Vitamin E may not be a safe option for *all* of us.

When taken in doses of 50 to 200 milligrams a day, *vitamin B-6* has been reported to be effective in alleviating depression, emotional instability, fatigue, loss of libido, and the inability to concentrate. Caution: Don't overdo it. Large doses can cause serious neurological problems.

Calcium is important for the body. It makes possible muscle contraction (including heartbeat), brain function, and blood clotting. Menopausal women should consume 1,500 milligrams a day. If you are taking estrogen, limit calcium intake to 1,000 milligrams per day. While experts agree that it's best to get it from foods, that may be difficult or impossible for some people, so supplement if necessary. For maximum absorption, experts recommend spreading the dosage throughout the day. Good food sources of calcium include almonds, broccoli, dairy products, sardines and salmon with the bones, dark green vegetables like collards, turnip and mustard greens, and raw oysters. If it's necessary to use a supplement, take calcium carbonate or calcium gluconate. Both are easy to absorb.

Herbs

Dong quai is a Chinese herb that works like estrogen. Available in health-food stores, it has been termed "miraculous" by some women who say it helps reduce hot flashes and relieves vaginal dryness. However, you must remember that herbs are very powerful, so use this and all herbs under the supervision of a nutritionist or naturopath.

Widely acclaimed as an effective remedy for menopausal symptoms, *ginseng* is a Chinese herb that contains a hormonelike compound that mimics estrogen. Foods that contain plantlike estrogen include alfalfa, apples, carrots, garlic, green beans, oats, parsley, peas, pomegranates, potatoes, red beans, rice, sesame seeds, soybeans, sprouts, wheat, and yeast.

Evening primrose oil has proven to be effective for alleviating symptoms such as fatigue, depression, insomnia, and headaches, all of which are characteristic of premenstrual syndrome (PMS) and menopause. Some women report that it has also helped them with hot flashes.

Exercise

Physical activity improves life at any age and can relieve many symptoms of the change. It lessens hot flashes, night sweats, depression, insomnia, emotional problems, and sexual problems. Although no scientific studies have been done to absolutely prove the benefits of fitness, some experts theorize that exercise makes the body more tolerant of temperature extremes and better able to cool down fast.

Aerobic activities such as swimming, walking, biking, and running also relieve stress. This may help calm mood swings and lessen sleeping problems. Most importantly, exercise helps fight off chronic illness such as heart disease and bone loss. For best results, work out at least three times a week, for at least twenty minutes per session.

Stress Reduction

Most menopausal women report that when they are able to control stress, their symptoms are less intense and noticeable. And a study reported in a 1992 issue of *American Journal of Obstetrics and Gynecology* notes that slow, deep breathing reduced hot flashes by nearly half. So along with doing deep-breathing exercises, reduce stress with yoga, meditation, exercise, psychotherapy, and support groups. Frequent sex also alleviates stress and can help keep the vagina lubricated and fight insomnia.

For More Information

ORGANIZATIONS

MIDLIFE WOMEN'S NETWORK, 5129 Logan Ave. S., Minneapolis, MN 55419; (800) 886-4354 or (612) 925-0020. In addition to publishing the bimonthly newsletter *Midlife Woman,* the Network supplies information on new findings in medicine for the midlife woman.

NORTH AMERICAN MENOPAUSE SOCIETY, c/o University Hospitals, Dept. of OB/GYN, 2074 Abington Rd., Cleveland, OH 44106; (216) 844-3334. The Society offers a referral list for women looking for physicians who specialize in menopause.

NATIONAL INSTITUTE ON AGING, 9000 Rockville Pike, Bethesda, MD 20892; (800) 222-2225 or (301) 496-1752. The Institute also has many other publications on women and aging, including the booklet *Menopause.*

THE WOMEN'S MEDICAL AND DIAGNOSTIC CENTER, 222 SW 36th Terrace, Gainesville, FL 32607; (904) 372-5600. Studies menopause and menopause-related conditions and issues and offers a newsletter called *Transitions,* which covers medical information on midlife health and aging including nutrition and exercise.

BOOKS

The Change: Women, Aging and the Menopause, Germaine Greer, Alfred A. Knopf, 1993.

Estrogen: A Complete Guide to Reversing the Effects of Menopause Using Hormone Replacement Therapy, Lila E. Nachtigall, M.D., and Joan Rattner Heilman, HarperCollins, 1991.

The Estrogen Decision, Susan M. Lark, M.D., Westchester Publishing Co. (Los Altos, Calif.), 1994.

Estrogen: Is it Right for You? A Thorough, Factual Guide to Help You Decide, Paula Dranov, Simon & Schuster, 1993.

Hormones: The Woman's Answer Book, Lois Jovanovic, M.D., Fawcett Columbine, 1992.

Making the Estrogen Decision, Gretchen Henkel, Fawcett Columbine, 1994.

Managing Your Menopause, Wulf H. Utian, M.D., and Ruth S. Jacobowitz, Prentice-Hall, 1991.

Menopause: A Guide for Women and the Men Who Love Them,

Winnifred Berg Cutler, Celso-Ramon Garcia, M.D., and David A. Edwards, W. W. Norton, 1993.

Menopause: All Your Questions Answered, Raymond G. Burnett, M.D., Contemporary Books, 1987.

Menopause: A Midlife Passage, Joan Callahan, ed., Indiana University Press, 1993.

Menopause: A Self-Help Book: A Woman's Guide to Feeling Wonderful for the Second Half of Her Life, Susan Larkin, M.D., Celestial Arts (Berkeley, Calif.), 1990.

Menopause and Hormone Replacement Therapy: Facts and Controversies, Regine Sitruk-Ware, ed., Dekker, 1991.

Menopause and Midlife Health, Morris Notelovitz, M.D., and Diana Tonnessen, St. Martin's Press, 1993.

Menopause and the Years Ahead, Mary Beard, M.D., and Lindsay Curtis, M.D., Fisher Books (Tucson, Ariz.), 1991.

Menopause Naturally: Preparing for the Second Half of Life, Updated Edition, Sadja Greenwood, M.D., Volcano Press (Volcano, Calif.), 1992.

Menopause Without Medicine, Linda Ojeda, Hunter House (Alameda, Calif.), 1992.

No More Hot Flashes and Other Good News, Penny Wise Budoff, M.D., Warner Books, 1989.

Natural Menopause: The Complete Guide to a Woman's Most Misunderstood Passage, Susan Perry and Katherine O'Hanlon, M.D., Addison-Wesley, 1993.

150 Most Asked Questions About Menopause: What Women Really Want to Know, Ruth S. Jacobowitz, Hearst Books, 1993.

Ourselves, Growing Older: Women Aging with Knowledge and Power, Paula Brown Doress, Diana Laskin Siegal, and the Midlife and Older Women Book Project, Simon & Schuster/Touchstone, 1987 (an excellent book with lots of information on menopause by the women who produced *Our Bodies, Ourselves*).

The Silent Passage, Gail Sheehy, Fawcett Columbine, 1992.

Staying Cool Through Menopause: Answers to Your Most-Asked Questions, Melvin Frisch, M.D., The Body Press/Perigee Books, 1993.

A Woman Doctor's Guide to Menopause, Lois Jovanovic, M.D., with Suzanne Levert, Hyperion, 1993.

Women of the 14th Moon: Writings on Menopause, Dena Taylor and Amber Coverdale Sumrall, eds., The Crossing Press, 1991.

Women on Menopause: A Practical Guide to Positive Transition, Anne Dickson and Nikki Henriques, Healing Arts Press (Rochester, Vt.), 1989.

NEWSLETTERS

HOT FLASH: Newsletter for Midlife & Older Women, Jane Porcino, ed. Write Health Technology Management, P.O. Box 816, Stony Brook, NY 11790-0609. Subscriptions are $25 per year (published quarterly), $6 for back issues.

Midlife Wellness, The Women's Medical and Diagnostic Center, 222 SW 36th Terrace, Gainesville, FL 32607; (904) 372-5600.

Midlife Woman, Midlife Women's Network, 5129 Logan Ave. S., Minneapolis, MN 55419; (612) 925-0020 or (800) 886-4354.

PART III

OUR HEALTH CARE

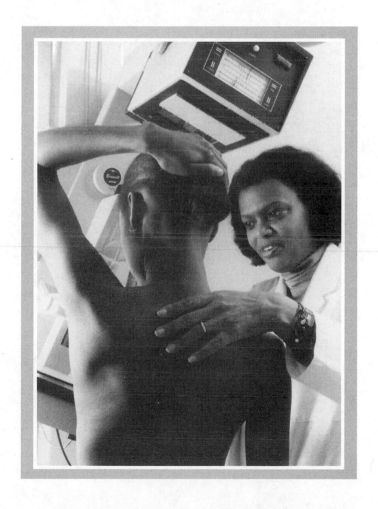

18

Checkups and Tests
We Can't Live Without

Going to a doctor or a clinic may be the last thing you want to do. Even though you know you *should* have a checkup, visit the gynecologist, or make a trip to a clinic for a mammogram, if you're like other Black women, you already have too much to do—work, family, children, and a thousand other responsibilities you don't have time for. Maybe you don't think you have enough money to pay for a doctor visit; you simply can't afford to be sick. Or you may simply be scared, afraid that you'll have *something* terrible, and you know your family can't cope without you. So you put off getting tested, unable to deal with the unthinkable "maybe."

If that's what's going through your mind, it's time to change your attitude. In the case of several serious diseases, including breast cancer, Black women have higher rates of death than white women because we don't seek medical care until the problem is in a later stage and therefore less curable.

Getting checkups and other kinds of medical tests is something all women have to *make* time for. Testing doesn't prevent you from getting sick, nor does it make you sick. Chances are you're just fine, but if you do have something, not knowing can allow a minor problem to turn into a serious one. In the case of cancer, the earlier a woman finds out that she has it, the more likely she is to survive and thrive. Equally important, getting screening exams and tests is an act of love. Your life and good health are the best things you can give to your family, friends, and yourself.

Here are some of the tests you can't live without.

Mammogram

At age thirty-five, a woman should get her first mammogram. Once you turn forty, you'll need a mammogram every one to two years, and then yearly after age fifty. If you have a family history of breast cancer, you may need mammograms more frequently.

Breast cancer is the most common form of cancer in American women, and frighteningly, experts estimate that one in every eight U.S. women will develop it in their lifetimes. For Black women, breast cancer is the leading cause of cancer death, and we are more likely than our white counterparts to seek the help of a physician only when the cancer is in later, more dangerous stages.

But no woman has to die of breast cancer; though it is dangerous, having it isn't usually a death sentence. Treatment exists and is highly successful when the cancer is detected early on. But a woman can't get treated for breast cancer unless she knows she has it, and that's what mammography is all about. For women who get regular mammograms, if a lump is found, it is likely to be about the size of a BB. On the other hand, in women who don't get mammograms (and don't do breast self-exams), the average lump is much larger, bigger than a silver dollar—and no woman wants that amount of cancer anywhere in her body.

Unfortunately, all too often Black women don't take advantage of the saving power of mammography. Only 58 percent of African-American women forty and older have ever had a mammogram to detect breast cancer, compared with 65 percent of all white women in that age group. That is one reason why our death rate from the disease is so high.

Although a yearly test is critical for women fifty and older, there's been some debate about the usefulness of screening women between forty and fifty. Nonetheless, we continue to recommend a baseline mammogram for thirty-five-year-old women and mammography every year or two for Black women between forty and fifty. Compared with white women, breast cancer strikes Black women at earlier ages, and we are less

After a routine mammogram, the radiologist came back and told me he had found a little hardening in my left breast and needed to do a biopsy. At first I thought, "Oh, no," but then I convinced myself that it was nothing. Like all of the women in my family, my breasts are cystic (lumpy), and I had also had a harmless cyst aspirated several years before. That lump hadn't been a problem, so I figured this one would be okay, too.

Before the biopsy, my husband and I spoke to the doctor. My husband asked, "What if it's cancer?" and the surgeon answered that we shouldn't talk about anything prematurely. I just sat there stunned. Hearing the word cancer caught me off guard. I just kept telling myself to trust in God and believe that everything is okay.

Sure enough, the surgeon found a small amount of cancer in my left breast. During the biopsy, he removed the cancer, taking out tissue about the size of an orange. He removed the same amount of tissue from the other breast, too, to make them even.

I went through seven weeks of radiation treatment but didn't have to have chemotherapy. I also have to take a drug called tamoxifen twice a day for the next five years. But I am grateful to have my life. I think God put it into my heart for me to have a mammogram. It was a blessing that I didn't need a mastectomy. That cancer was getting ready to get busy, but I didn't give it a chance.

It's funny too, that when I first called the diagnostic clinic to make the appointment for the mammogram, they told me it would cost $150. That seemed too high, so I found another hospital that would do it for half the price, except they couldn't give me an appointment for two months. But I thought about a woman at work whose grandmother had died of breast cancer and of a friend whose sister had it, and I paid the $150 and went in right away. And that early detection really paid off.

"Early detection really paid off."

—BRENDA J. CASTEEL-BELL, LEGAL SECRETARY, LOS ANGELES

likely to discover the cancer early on, which leads to more deaths. So mammography remains crucial for all Black women forty and older.

What Is a Mammogram?

Mammography is an X ray of the breast that is taken by a qualified radiologist or technician. She or he takes two pictures of each breast, from the top and from each side. The breasts are placed between plastic plates and flattened slightly to get a clear picture. Though some women com-

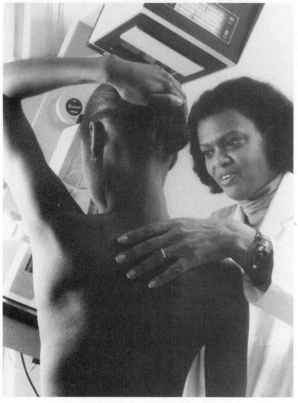

A patient gets positioned for her mammogram. *(Photo: Diane Allford/Allford Trotman Associates)*

plain of slight discomfort (which generally lasts no longer than thirty seconds), getting a mammogram doesn't hurt. And it's not dangerous. Though it does involve radiation, the dose is extremely low. It's much more dangerous *not* to have one than to have them regularly.

After the procedure (which should take about fifteen minutes), the radiologist will read the mammogram, looking for a lump or group of abnormal cells. Mammography can detect a lump up to two years before it can be felt. The vast majority of all mammograms turn up negative, and even when there is a lump, more than 80 percent of all lumps found in premenopausal women are *not* cancerous.

Where to Get a Mammogram and How to Pay for It

Your physician should be able to recommend a mammography facility, or you can check with your public-health department, local hospital, or women's clinic. In addition, mobile vans operated by city or county health departments offer free or low-cost mammography, and you can check your local media for special mammogram screenings every October, which is National Breast Cancer Awareness Month, or in April during Minority Cancer Awareness Week. A North Carolina program called Save Our Sisters (SOS) is an excellent example of how we Black women can help one another take care of ourselves. SOS uses community leaders to promote the need for mammography and has also coordinated "Adopt-A-Sister" to get local churches to sponsor low-income women who need mammograms. The National Cancer Institute (NCI) Information Service—(800) 4-CANCER—and the American Cancer Society (ACS)—(800) 227-2345—can let you know whether your community has a similar program and can recommend mammography facilities in your area.

When choosing a facility, it is very important to take both quality and cost into consideration. The American College of Radiology (ACR) has a voluntary accreditation program that is a sign of a quality facility. To find out whether your facility is part of this program, call the ACR—(703) 648-8900—or the ACS.

Since the accreditation program is voluntary, not all facilities take part. A nonprogram facility may be fine, but it's up to you to ask. Here are five important questions:

Do you use "dedicated" machines (which are specially designed for mammography)?

Is the person who takes the mammograms a registered technologist?

Is the radiologist who reads the mammograms trained to do so?

Does the facility perform at least ten mammograms per week?

Is the mammography machine calibrated (checked to make sure measurements and doses are correct) at least once a year?

The Breast Self-Examination

Once each month and at the same time each month, check your breasts for a lump, hard knot, thickening, or discharge, using this three-step process. It's best to check the week after menstrual bleeding has ended—rather than when you're premenstrual or menstruating, because the breasts tend to be lumpier or more tender than usual at those times. If you find something unusual, see a doctor right away.

In the shower: *Raise your arm above your head, and with fingers flat, move them over the breast (including the armpit) in a circular motion. Use your left hand for the right breast, right hand for the left breast.*

In front of a mirror: *Look for any changes in shape or contour of the breasts. Note any swelling, dimpling of skin, or changes in the skin or nipple. First inspect your breasts with your arms at your sides, then raise your arms high overhead.*

Then rest your palms on your hips and press down firmly to flex chest muscles. Left and right breasts will not match exactly—few women's breasts do.

Lying down (Current opinion is that this is the best way to examine your breasts, especially if they are large): *Put a pillow under your right shoulder and your arm behind your head. With your fingers flat, use your left hand to press gently in a circular motion. Include the armpit from the collarbone to below the breast. Repeat, using firm pressure, and gently squeeze the nipple for discharge. Repeat (and switch pillow and opposite arm) for the left breast.*

We must examine our breasts every month. (Drawing: Yvonne Buchanan)

A mammogram should cost between $50 and $150 (sometimes it costs more), and some health-insurance plans cover the charges. You can also call the NCI Information Service or the ACS for low-cost programs in your area. If you are sixty-five or older, Medicare will cover part of the cost of your mammogram every other year at some facilities, depending on your age. You'll need to contact your Medicare carrier for more information. Medicaid coverage varies state by state, so check with your local office.

Pelvic Examination and Pap Smear

Yearly for all women eighteen years or older and younger women who are sexually active.

Black women are approximately three times more likely to develop cervical cancer and more than twice as likely to die from it than white women. Plus, we are at particular risk for sexually transmitted infections (STI's) of all kinds, which, left untreated, can cause a variety of problems including infertility.

There is no good reason to skip getting a yearly gynecological checkup. If you do have cervical cancer, an STI, or other problems, your doctor can detect it early and save your life and ability to reproduce. The gynecologist may also examine your breasts, which along with your own monthly checks (and mammography, if you are older) helps detect breast cancer.

Pelvic Examination

During this exam, your doctor will look for the presence of any infection, abnormal growths, cysts, malformation of organs, or organs in the wrong position. You will need to lie on your back with your legs spread, knees bent, and your feet in metal stirrups. (Thoughtful doctors will cover the stirrups with cloth so that your feet won't be cold. Or you can wear socks.) She or he will cover you from the waist down with a sheet, but you can ask that it be removed if modesty isn't a problem and you want to see what's going on.

Wearing gloves, the doctor will examine your vulva, the opening to the vagina, in search of infection, vaginal discharge, and any lesions, growths, or sores. Then, using a speculum, she or he will look at the walls of your vagina and your cervix. This metal or plastic instrument may be cold and uncomfortable, but inserting it shouldn't trigger pain. She or he checks the shape of the cervix and looks for infection before taking a Pap smear by swabbing the cervix with a brush, wooden spatula, or cotton-tipped stick.

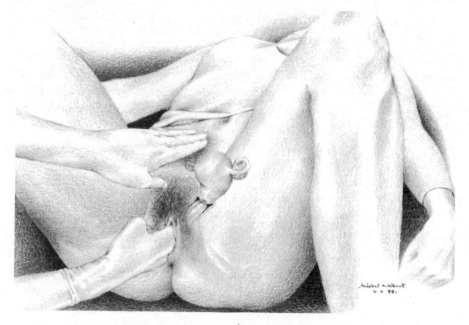

A manual inspection of
the uterus during a
gynecological exam.
*(Drawing: Michel Hebert;
courtesy of Montreal
Health Press, Montreal)*

The doctor should then gently remove the speculum and begin a manual examination of the pelvic region. She or he inserts two (gloved) fingers into the vagina and presses the opposite hand against the midsection of the lower abdomen to feel for any abnormalities of the uterus, ovaries, and fallopian tubes. The doctor then removes one finger from the vagina (the discharge may also be examined) and inserts it into the rectum to check for abnormal growths and blood in the stool. You may find this painful and unpleasant, but remember that it'll be over quickly.

No part of this examination should be sexual, although you may feel some stimulation, which is normal. The pelvic examination may be uncomfortable and distressing if you have not had sexual intercourse or used tampons, and you should mention this to the physician. Women who have been sexually abused may feel disturbed by this examination when it is conducted by a male physician. (In many cases, a male doctor will have a female assistant present during the examination.) In this instance, don't forgo the exam; find a woman doctor.

Pap Smear

The Pap smear is given to test for cancerous and precancerous cells. It can also detect many kinds of infections—viral (herpes, vaginal warts), fungal (yeast), bacterial (bacterial vaginosis), and protozoan (trichomoniasis or "trich")—as well as other STI's. (For some infections such as chlamydia, you will need additional testing, and the virus that causes AIDS cannot be detected by a Pap smear.)

After your physician has taken a sample of tissue from your cervix during the pelvic exam, she or he may take a look at it under the microscope to check for infection, but the bulk of the analysis is done in a lab. You should receive the results in one to four weeks (depending on the lab), and your physician is responsible for calling you if something is amiss. But if you haven't heard from your doctor, call her or him yourself. Your doctor receives a detailed report from the lab and should go over it with you.

Where to Get a Pelvic Exam and Pap Smear and How to Pay for It

Your family physician or gynecologist can take care of your gynecological checkup, or you can visit a clinic or your local health department. This exam may not be covered by health insurance unless you come in with a complaint, but many doctors will provide a diagnosis so that you won't have to pick up the charges. The examination, including the Pap smear, can range from over $200 (for a private physician in a city like New York) to less than $50 (in a clinic), and you may have to pay extra (about $20) to cover lab fees.

Depending on where you live, Medicaid may pay for pelvic examinations and Pap smears; it's best to check with your local officer. For women over sixty-five, Medicare will cover the cost every three years.

Routine Physical Examination
At least every two years depending on health and age.

This is an important procedure and gets more important as we grow older. Below are the tests that are generally part of a medical examination:

A physician or other health-care practitioner will generally check your height and weight, looking for changes since your last examination. Next she or he will test your vital signs—pulse, blood pressure, respiration, and (sometimes) temperature. Your eyes, ears, nose, and throat will also be examined.

Pulse. Your pulse is a measure of the heart contracting and pushing blood through the arteries. The health-care practitioner generally checks the pulse in your wrist or neck. The normal range is about sixty to eighty beats per minute for an adult (it may be less in people who exercise consistently) and faster for children. The pulse should be regular and strong, without skipped beats.

Blood pressure. High blood pressure or hypertension is very common among Black folks and more likely to be present in older people. It can lead to a number of serious ailments—such as heart disease and stroke—and every year 300,000 Americans die of diseases linked to hypertension. Since it has no symptoms, all too often people don't know they have it—which makes getting it checked all the more important.

The health-care practitioner will take a reading with a blood pressure cuff. She or he records the systolic pressure, which measures the heart as it contracts, and the diastolic pressure, which measures the heart at rest. The systolic pressure is the top reading; the diastolic, the bottom reading. The systolic number is more affected by stress; some people who are extremely stressed out show systolic readings that go off the chart. A typical normal reading would be 120/80. Here's how a doctor might look at your result:

SYSTOLIC (TOP NUMBER)	DIASTOLIC (BOTTOM NUMBER)	WHAT TO DO
Less than 130	Less than 85	Have blood pressure checked again in two years.
130–139	85–89	Have blood pressure checked again in one year. Modify your lifestyle by sticking to a low-fat, low-salt, low cholesterol diet, exercising at least three times per week, and working to control stress.
140–159	90–99	Have blood pressure checked again within two months; modify lifestyle.
160–179	100–109	Have medical evaluation or treatment within one month.
180–209	110–119	Have medical evaluation or treatment within one week.
210 or higher	120 or higher	Have medical evaluation or treatment right away.

From the National High Blood Pressure Education Program. These recommendations don't apply to everyone, because people differ in risk factors, medical history, and current health status. Only your doctor can provide advice for your particular situation.

If your reading shows that you have high blood pressure, your health-care practitioner may check your blood pressure more than once over several office visits because of what is called "white-coat hypertension." For us it might be better termed "white man in white coat hypertension," or anxiety brought on by the medical setting that causes the blood pressure to rise.

Respiration. Normal adults breathe about twelve to twenty times per minute (people in good physical condition may breathe more slowly), and respiration should be steady and neither very shallow nor very deep.

Temperature (not always taken). Elevated temperature may mean that your body is fighting infection. Normal temperature is 98.6 degrees F., slightly higher after ovulation.

Urinalysis. Urine tests detect the presence of sugar, blood, abnormal protein or acids and are used to diagnose kidney, bladder, and liver infections. These tests can also show the presence of drugs such as crack and cocaine.

You should wipe yourself clean before taking the sample, and try to catch the urine midstream rather than at the beginning or the end.

Your analysis may be done in the office or clinic or it may be sent to a lab. Your doctor should have the results within about forty-eight hours. Urine tests also detect pregnancy, but you shouldn't assume that a pregnancy test will be done. Ask about this specifically.

Blood tests. Your health-care practitioner may prick your finger and take a little bit of blood to measure the level of red blood cells. She or he may also draw two to three test tubes of blood from a vein in your arm to be analyzed in a lab. These tests can detect anemia, infection, cholesterol, sickle-cell disease or trait, and thyroid conditions. Your blood will not be tested for HIV unless you request it.

Your results should be ready in about a week. Always request a copy, and ask your doctor to explain anything you don't understand.

Immunizations. Most of us were vaccinated against a number of childhood diseases during our younger years, but several vaccinations require boosters later in life. You will need a tetanus-diphtheria booster to protect against tetanus, an infectious disease that is also known as lockjaw, and diphtheria, a viral infection that attacks the nose, throat, and tonsils. You should have a booster at about age twenty-five and then every ten years. Folks who are sixty-five or older should also have a yearly flu shot.

A routine physical examination shouldn't just be about testing. You should talk to your doctor about how you're feeling, what you're eating, exercise, and any other health concerns that come to mind. You should be able to talk openly and honestly with your doctor; remember that this person is doing you a service. If your doctor won't listen to your concerns, find another physician. For more information see chapter 19, "Dealing with Doctors and Hospitals."

If your doctor runs across something abnormal, you may need other kinds of tests. It's important to remember that medicine in this country

Twenty five years ago when I was twenty-five years old and in college, I was constantly bleeding; three weeks out of the month I was bleeding. I remember going to the doctor and lying on the table waiting to be examined. The doctor asked me to wait a minute while he took a phone call. I heard him say into the phone about another patient, "She has cancer, and I told her six months ago to come in and have that hysterectomy. But now it's too late. She's going to die."

After my biopsy, I was told that I, too, had cervical cancer and would need a hysterectomy. Normally I would have argued and asked questions, but I thought of what happened to that other woman. Right away, I told the doctor to go ahead and do the hysterectomy, because I didn't want to die.

Fifteen years after that first scare with cancer, I was looking in the mirror at my body and noticed that my left nipple had sunken in. I didn't know what it was or who to turn to, so I went to my supervisor, an older white woman who was like a maternal figure to me. I showed her my breast and she gave me the name and phone number of a doctor to see. Sure enough, I had cancer again and ended up in the hospital.

When I woke up out of surgery, I wasn't sure what had happened. A bandage covered my breasts, so I didn't know what I had left. When I finally looked, my entire left breast had been removed, and only a scar was left. I am a strong woman, so I didn't let my emotions run. A doctor in the hospital would come in every day and ask me, "Consuelo, is it getting to you yet?" and I'd always answer no. Then one day it did, and I started grieving. That doctor patted my leg and told me something that I'd never forget: "When God takes away one thing, he replaces it with another."

Through my recovery, through chemotherapy when I was sick and nauseated all the time for ten months and watching my hair come out in clumps, I never forgot what he said. When I wondered if a man would ever love me and touch me, I never forgot those words.

Now I realize that he was right. God took away my breast, but he gave me my life. After the cancer, I went through a spiritual transformation. As I opened up, gifts started coming to me. I started making clothes for cancer patients, staging fashion shows, writing poetry, and composing songs. I have thirty-seven gifts and talents; I realize that I can do anything now.

I also do public speaking. Before the cancer, I was a person who didn't like the limelight. I didn't like speaking out and preferred to be in the background. But now I speak to women in churches, women's organizations, schools, work groups—anywhere and everywhere I can. I tell them my story

"I am a person who survived cancer twice."

—CONSUELO JACKSON, CLERICAL REPRESENTATIVE, EVANGELIST, AND SPOKESPERSON FOR THE AMERICAN CANCER SOCIETY, ATLANTA

without hiding anything or sugarcoating anything and encourage them to check their breasts and get mammograms and Pap smears. I am a person who survived cancer twice. I believe that I survived to be a living witness to help somebody else.

is a business motivated by profit and that doctors are sometimes extremely cautious, recommending tests to establish a record in the case of a future lawsuit. So don't blindly agree to tests that seem excessive. Ask lots of questions so that you understand what's being done to you and why, and if something seems strange, get a second opinion.

For detailed information on medical tests, read *The Patient's Guide to Medical Tests* by Cathey and Edward R. Pinckney, M.D.

Where to Get a Physical and How to Pay for It

Physical examinations are often not covered by private health-insurance companies, which unfortunately aren't in the business of prevention. In some cases, a doctor will jot down a condition so that the insurance will pick up the charge. (Most health maintenance organizations do cover preventive care.) Your examination should cost from over $200 (for a private physician in a large city) to less than $50 (for a clinic visit). Neither Medicaid nor Medicare covers routine physical examinations.

Dental Care

Checkup every six months.

Along with brushing and flossing, a visit to the dentist every six months should be a regular part of taking care of your teeth. For more information on caring for your teeth, see chapter 2, "Our Skin, Hair, Eyes, and Teeth."

For More Information

ORGANIZATIONS: Breast Care

BLUE CROSS AND BLUE SHIELD ASSOCIATION, P.O. Box 527, Glenview, IL 60025-0527. Send $2 for a plastic breast self-examination card to hang on your shower and a ten-page brochure on early detection of breast cancer.

THE NATIONAL ALLIANCE OF BREAST CANCER ORGANIZATIONS (NABCO), 1180 Avenue of the Americas, 2nd floor, New York, NY 10036. Write for information about detection, treatment, and legislation.

NATIONAL CANCER INSTITUTE'S CANCER INFORMATION SERVICE, Office of Cancer Communications, National Cancer Institute, Bldg. 31, room 10A24, Bethesda, MD 20892; (800) 4-CANCER.

SUSAN G. KOMEN BREAST CANCER FOUNDATION, 5005 LBJ Freeway, suite 370, Dallas, TX 75244; (800) I'M-AWARE. Offers an information help line and a plastic shower card that explains breast self-examination.

ORGANIZATIONS: Cancer

THE AMERICAN CANCER SOCIETY, (800) ACS-2345, or contact your local office. Provides information on testing for and preventing all kinds of cancer. Also referrals to mammography centers accredited by the American College of Radiology.

AMERICAN HEART ASSOCIATION, 7272 Greenville Ave., Dallas, TX 75231-4596; (800) 242-1793; or contact your local office.

NATIONAL BLACK LEADERSHIP INITIATIVE ON CANCER, National Cancer Institute, Executive Plaza N. room 240, Bethesda, MD 20892; (301) 496-8589. Offers information on preventing and detecting all kinds of cancers.

NATIONAL CANCER INSTITUTE'S CANCER INFORMATION SERVICE, Office of Cancer Communications, National Cancer Institute, Bldg. 31, room 10A24, Bethesda, MD 20892; (800) 4-CANCER. Offers general information on testing for and preventing all kinds of cancer.

NATIONAL HEART, LUNG AND BLOOD INSTITUTE, P.O. Box 30105, Bethesda, MD 20824-0105; (301) 951-3260.

NATIONAL HEALTH INFORMATION CENTER, (800) 336-4797. Offers referrals and free pamphlets.

U.S. DEPARTMENT OF HEALTH AND HUMAN SERVICES, Office of Minority Health Resource Center, P.O. Box 37337, Washington, DC 20013-7337; (800) 444-6472. The staff can provide information and free or low-cost services and experts in your area.

19

Dealing with Doctors and Hospitals

D r. Martin Luther King, Jr., once said that "of all forms of inequality, injustice in health is the most shocking and inhumane." And that is exactly what many Black people are experiencing. Our lack of access to health care can be illustrated simply with one startling fact: A white American born in 1991 could expect to live to be seventy-six years of age, while a Black baby's life expectancy was seven years less. Worse, in the past several years white life expectancy has increased while ours—despite rapid advances in medical technology—has declined.

Our collective health problem can be blamed on many causes, and combined, these factors can be deadly. The stress of being Black in America, poverty, and poor eating and exercise habits all contribute to serious illnesses such as heart disease, cancer, stroke, and diabetes.

Our unfair health-care system makes the problem worse. Study after study shows that a person with Black skin has less access to health care and receives worse treatment than a comparable white person. The facts are:

The National Medical Association has found that 25 percent of Blacks have no medical insurance and 23 percent have no consistent source of health care.

A 1989 study found that although African-Americans had 75 percent more heart attacks, we were 50 percent less likely to have coronary angiography and 33 percent less likely to have coronary-bypass surgery—two lifesaving treatments. Other studies have reported similar findings. One of the researchers of a 1993 study noted: "Our study shows there is a clear race-related difference in the care received by blacks and whites."

Though we suffer more kidney disease than whites, Blacks are less likely to receive long-term hemodialysis, a treatment for severe kidney problems. The most favored recipients are white men ages twenty-five through forty-four, one study concluded. In a study of patients with end-stage renal disease who were covered by Medicare benefits, Blacks accounted for 33 percent of patients with the disease but for only 21 percent of patients who received kidney transplants.

The list of studies that illustrate how the health-care system discriminates against Blacks could go on and on. But where does that leave us? How do we deal with a medical system that can be unhelpful if not openly hostile? To get the most out of the health-care system, we must be educated consumers. We must learn to recognize and stand up to unfair treatment and demand to be treated with respect and dignity.

We must also *not* avoid the health-care system, despite its problems. While it's okay to be afraid if you're not feeling well or if you know that something's wrong, it's not okay to be so scared that you don't go to the doctor for diagnosis and treatment. With most health problems, the longer you wait, the worse off you'll end up. We must also understand how our bodies work and know as much about health and medicine as possible. And we must demand as much information as we can from our health-care providers by asking detailed questions.

The best way to avoid the medical-care system is to stay healthy by eating right, exercising, getting plenty of rest, and avoiding cigarettes, drugs, and too much alcohol. At best we only have to visit a doctor once or twice a year for a checkup and tests such as a Pap smear, pelvic exam, and mammogram (every year or two for women forty and over and yearly for women over fifty). For healthy people that minimum visit (or visits) can also be the maximum.

Choosing a Doctor

Every person should be able to choose her own doctor, but many can't because a lack of financial resources limits the options. If you are fortunate enough to be able to select your own physician, understand that it can be a tricky process. It's best to get a recommendation from someone you trust. Your doctor should be someone you can talk to, a person who listens to you and respects you as a human being. If she or he doesn't pay attention to your complaints and opinions or seems rude, find another doctor.

You should find out whether the doctor has been in trouble. The National Practitioner Data Bank has that information, but it's not available to the public. Instead check *10,289 Questionable Doctors,* a 1993 book that lists doctors who have been disciplined by the state or federal government. Look for it in the library, or order it from Public Citizen, 2000 P St. NW, Washington, DC 20036.

As you're shopping for a doctor, ask these questions:

What is your fee for a basic office visit?
Do you have a specialty or area of interest?
How long does it take to get an appointment?
Do you handle routine matters or do nurse practitioners, physician's assistants, or other staff deal with them?
Can I call you between appointments? How do I reach you if there's an emergency?
Will I have access to my medical records?
Which hospital are you affiliated with? (This is a very important question to ask since some hospitals provide better care than others.)

Doctor Visits

Many of us find it hard to go the doctor. It can be embarrassing to have to take off all of our clothes and be poked and probed by a physician. It's uncomfortable to have to talk about our "personal business," and it's also frightening to have to worry that something might be wrong. This universal problem has even been measured. Studies show that many patients suffer from "white-coat hypertension," a rise in blood pressure that's been blamed on anxiety caused by the doctor and the health-care setting.

For us the problem is worse. A telephone survey conducted a few years ago found that Blacks are less likely than whites to be satisfied with the way their physicians treat them. Black respondents were also more likely to report that physicians did not inquire sufficiently about their pain, did not tell them how long it would take for prescribed medicine to work, did not explain the seriousness of their illness or injury, and did not discuss test and examination findings.

Most of us don't feel at ease talking to doctors. Too often we are

On November 10, 1990, my car was hit head-on by a drunk driver in Seattle. The accident was only the beginning of my nightmare. I didn't know that I had broken my neck. And neither, apparently, did my doctors.

I was taken from the scene of the accident, x-rayed, and released within five hours, armed with pain pills and one of those soft collars wrapped around my neck. The emergency-room doctors told me I had a sprained ankle and a little bit of whiplash. I was told to go see my own doctor the next day for a follow-up. I was in so much pain I couldn't walk or move. I don't know how I got out of the hospital. I stayed with a friend who helped me get around. I couldn't even brush my teeth, the pain was so horrific.

The next day, I went to my HMO clinic. That's when my hell all started. At the clinic, my doctor took more X rays. He said he couldn't find anything wrong with me except whiplash. He told me that I had to start moving around right away or I would build up scar tissue in my neck. I told him that I couldn't move at all. If I moved my head, I would get this excruciating pain that traveled down to my hand. The doctor told me it was because I wasn't moving enough. His whole attitude was of total indifference, like "I'm the medical professional here, I know what I'm talking about, you don't." He told me, "You need to go back to work. If you don't go back, you'll never work again."

But work was out of the question. I couldn't exercise. Walking was impossible. Pain medication didn't help one bit. I couldn't sit or lie down, so I had to kind of stretch out with pillows propping me up. And two or three times every week, I would go back to the same doctor who told me the same thing: "There's nothing wrong with you." This went on for four weeks. By that point, I was totally traumatized. I thought I was crazy. I began to seriously question my reality. I could no longer do what I once was able to do.

Finally, my doctor ordered new X rays. As soon as the X-ray technicians saw how much pain I was in, they put me on a stretcher and called in a neurologist. I was put in a hospital room. My head was taped to the bed. I was crying. I said, "But I walked in here." They told me, "You walked in here, but you won't be walking out." After looking at my X rays, the specialist told me, "God was with you. I don't know how anybody could have missed this." Not only had I broken my neck, the doctor said, but I had also ripped all the ligaments that held my neck up, and I had a head injury. I would have to have surgery right away. And because of the delay in treatment, recovery would take that much longer.

I'm still recovering from my accident. I still have pain. Because of the head injury, my attention span is gone. Even today, I can't remember certain

"This wasn't just a misdiagnosis. I was the victim of racism, sexism, and white male arrogance."

—JEANETTE GIBSON AGU, SCHOOLTEACHER, SEATTLE

words. I can't spell anymore, even though I used to be a good speller. I'm working with a neuropsychologist so that I won't feel so victimized. I'm working on my anger. I'm trying to rebuild my confidence. My independence. My trust.

This year, I filed a complaint against my group health-insurance people. As far as I'm concerned, this wasn't just a misdiagnosis. I was undertreated. I was the victim of racism, sexism, and white male arrogance. I'm thinking about suing, but my lawyer warns me that I have to be emotionally strong so that I can deal with the rigors of a trial. I don't think I'm there yet. I can't believe that I still get so emotional about my accident two years after the fact.

But I'm working on it. I read a lot about peace and love and healing. I get inspiration from books detailing how other people have recovered from injury and illness. And every day, I recite an affirmation: All is well. All is well.

---

intimidated by them. Too many of us make the mistake of thinking of them as godlike—highly educated authority figures who know all there is to know about medicine and our bodies. We see them as miracle-working white men in white coats. And the fact that most doctors *are* white men adds to the distance between doctor and patient.

Most doctor visits are short and hurried. A study sponsored by *Medical Advertising News* found that doctors spend only eleven minutes on average talking with their patients. We generally spend longer than that in the waiting room! Private doctors have little incentive to spend time with patients. In our capitalist medical system, time is money, so the more patients doctors can rush through, the more money they make. Clinics and emergency rooms are generally overcrowded, so that some doctors are too harried to spend much time with patients or explain things thoroughly.

Most doctors are also not trained to communicate. Until very recently, most medical schools didn't teach future physicians how to talk to their patients. Too often doctors use big words and complicated terms; in fact, the *Medical Advertising News* study found that 90 percent of patients have trouble understanding what their doctors are saying. Some physicians prefer to be in complete control and don't want their patients to ask questions or challenge them.

No one should be dissatisfied with health care. Remember that you are paying your doctor for a service. You have a right to demand the kind of care that meets your needs and to control what happens to your body.

Talking to your doctor and getting him or her to explain things should not be a trial. You should also tell the doctor how you're feeling, because it's your body and you understand it best. Here's how you can make the most of your doctor visits.

Keep a brief and concise written record of how you're feeling, and document any symptoms or changes your body is going through. This way you'll have that information on hand when it's time to go to the doctor.

Write down any questions you may have for your physician. This will make it easier to address the concerns once you're face-to-face. Bring along medical records.

Ask questions until you are satisfied that you understand everything you're being told. Make sure you understand why you have to have certain tests and what they mean. Ask about alternatives to any treatment the doctor suggests. Inquire about medication you're given—how long you have to take it, what side effects it has. Ask how to prevent a problem from recurring.

Be honest, rather than saying things just to please your doctor. Tell the truth about eating habits, stress, sexual activity, alcohol intake, and other habits that may affect your health.

Be specific. Don't assume the physician can read your mind. Say everything that's bothering you—and make sure she or he is really listening to you.

Ask how much tests, exams, and treatment cost. Call the insurance company to find out whether what you need is covered.

Take a friend or relative with you, especially if you're uneasy. Plus, another pair of ears will help you recall later what was said.

Follow your doctor's instructions. Listen carefully, ask questions, and take notes if you need to. Before you leave, review what you've been told to make sure you understand it. If you don't intend to do what the doctor tells you, be honest, and maybe she or he can come up with a plan that works better for you.

Seek assistance from other members of the health-care staff. Talk to the nurse or physician's assistant who generally works closely with the doctor.

Before you leave the office or clinic, make sure you know when you have to come back. If you need another appointment, schedule it before leaving if you can.

Find out as much as you can about your condition. Some studies have

shown that physicians aren't always up on the latest research and sometimes offer outdated advice. Go to the library and look through books
and journals. Call specific organizations to request information. Get a
second opinion. Then phone the doctor and discuss your research if you
need to.

The Black-Doctor Dilemma

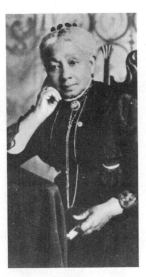

Dr. Susan Smith
McKinney Steward, one
of America's first Black
female physicians,
graduated from medical
school in 1870.
(*Photo: Brooklyn
Historical Society*)

In 1864, one year before the end of the Civil War, Rebecca Lee
Crumpler graduated from the New England Female Medical College,
becoming the first African-American woman to receive a medical degree.
Rebecca J. Cole and Susan Smith McKinney Steward were also early
Black women medical pioneers. Cole received her M.D. from the
Women's Medical College of Pennsylvania in 1867 and practiced for
fifty years in Philadelphia, South Carolina, and Washington, D.C.
Steward graduated from the New York Medical College and Hospital for
Women in 1870 and was class valedictorian. Though she was often
greeted by her male colleagues at Bellevue Hospital in New York with
"hisses, indecent language, paper balls and other missiles," Steward had a
successful family practice in Brooklyn and later in Ohio. She was the
cofounder of the Women's Hospital and Dispensary in Brooklyn (1881)
and the official physician to the Brooklyn Home for Aged Colored
People.

Despite this illustrious history of Black female doctors, these days few
Black women practice medicine. When we go to the doctor, chances are
high that we won't be treated by someone who looks like we do. Only
18 percent of all physicians are women of any color, 3 percent are Black
of either gender, and a scant 1.2 percent are Black women.

Still, we can be proud of the sisters who have broken through. As the
director of the Office of Research on Women's Health, Dr. Vivian Pinn
is the highest-ranking Black woman at the National Institutes of Health.
Her office was developed in 1990 to make sure that federally funded
research includes women's health issues, that women are included in federal research projects, and that more women are brought into medical
careers. In 1993, Dr. Joycelyn Elders became the Surgeon General, the
nation's top doctor. And although the proportions are low, the 1990
bureau of census reports that just more than seven thousand Black
women are practicing medicine.

We can look forward to gains in the future. In the last several years,
the number of Black women entering medical school has risen slowly
but steadily. The Association of American Medical Colleges notes that in

1991 Black women comprised just over 9 percent of women graduating from medical school, up from 7 percent in 1987.

We must encourage young people as well as Black women of all ages to become doctors and other kinds of health-care providers. The costs can be high—students of color who graduated from medical school in 1990 owed an average of about $51,000 in student loans—but so can the rewards, especially for those who work with Black patients. "We need physicians and health-care workers who are sensitive to the problems and will go back to the community," Dr. Pinn has said.

There are also many other health-care positions available. Laurell Lasenburg entered the health-care field in 1987 as an HIV counselor. She now counsels female prisoners at Rikers Island in New York about preventing HIV and AIDS and living with the virus. "I feel I have something special to offer people," says Laurell, who is working on her master's degree in social work. "I'm a compassionate and caring person, and whatever a patient needs, I'm going to fight for."

Here is information on health-care professions (when you contact these organizations, be sure to ask about financial aid).

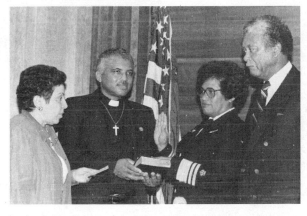

Dr. Joycelyn Elders, the country's first African-American Surgeon General, at her official swearing-in ceremony.

What it takes to become a physician: A college degree that includes premed course work in the sciences, followed by four years of medical school and a three-to five-year postgraduate hospital residency.

What it takes to become a nurse: Practicing nurses come in two categories. Licensed practical nurses receive approximately a year of training at a vocational school, while registered nurses study for two, three, or four years in programs run by colleges or hospitals.

What it takes to be a nurse practitioner or certified nurse-midwife: Because of a shortage of health-care providers, nurse practitioners and nurse-midwives have taken a visible and growing role. They now perform many of the tasks that were once done by physicians. Nurse practitioners and certified nurse-midwives are licensed registered nurses with advanced training. They can make diagnosis, prescription, and treatment decisions. Nurse practitioners work in a variety of settings, while midwives specialize in providing prenatal, delivery, and postpartum care for women and also offer family-planning counseling and gynecological services.

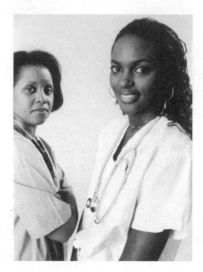

Nursing is a rewarding career, and nurses are in high demand.
(Photo: Diane Allford/Allford Trotman Associates)

What it takes to be a physician assistant: Under the supervision of a doctor, physician assistants (PA's) treat people for common illnesses, diagnose problems, and perform diagnostic tests and minor surgical procedures. Before entering a two-year PA program, you'll need a minimum of two years in college. A college degree and some health-care experience are increasingly expected.

Hospital Care

No one looks forward to going to the hospital. But checking in may be worse for us than for our white counterparts. A Johns Hopkins University study found that though Black patients come into hospitals with more serious problems, we spend fewer days there than white patients with the same degree of illness. Another study reported that Black patients are much less satisfied with the quality of hospital care than white patients are.

However, there are many ways to make a hospital stay more bearable. We must ask plenty of questions, demand quality care, and know whom to speak to in case of a problem.

Getting the Best Care

In most cases, if something is seriously wrong, your primary-care physician (the family practitioner or internist) will refer you to a specialist. Following are descriptions of the most common specialists.

Anesthesiologist: Dispenses anesthetics and monitors the conditions and vital signs of patients undergoing surgery.

Cardiologist: Diagnoses and treats heart disease.

Dermatologist: Diagnoses and treats skin problems.

Ear, Nose, and Throat (ENT): Diagnoses and treats problems of the ear, nose, and throat; also called an otolaryngologist.

Endocrinologist: Diagnoses and treats disorders of the endocrine glands, which regulate the hormones, such as the thyroid.

Family Practitioner: Deals with and oversees the total health care of the individual and her family, including children.

Gastroenterologist: Diagnoses and treats problems of the gastrointestinal tract (stomach, intestines, and other parts of the digestive system).

Geriatrician: Deals with diseases of the elderly and problems associated with aging.

Hematologist/Oncologist: Diagnoses and treats cancers and diseases and disorders of the blood and blood-forming parts of the body.

Immunologist: Studies and treats problems of the body's immune system, including allergies, infections, and life-threatening illnesses such as AIDS.

Internist: Diagnoses and treats diseases, especially those of adults. They may subspecialize in another area.

Nephrologist: Deals with diseases of the kidney.

Neurologist: Diagnoses and treats nervous-system disorders such as multiple sclerosis.

Obstetrician/Gynecologist: Diagnoses and treats problems associated with the female reproductive organs and deals with the medical aspects of and intervention in pregnancy and labor.

Ophthalmologist: Diagnoses and treats diseases and injuries of the eye.

Optometrist: Examines the eyes and diagnoses and treats visual problems, but is an O.D., not an M.D.

Orthopedist: Treats and corrects deformities or damage to the bones, muscles, and ligaments.

Osteopath: These doctors complete four years of study to earn a degree of doctor of osteopathy (D.O.) rather than an M.D. They practice a system of medicine that emphasizes the body's natural ability to defend itself against disease and heal if it is intact physically and psychologically. When necessary, D.O.'s correct disorders by manipulating parts of the body.

Pathologist: Diagnoses and monitors disease by means of information gathered by lab tests and microscopic examination of tissue, cells, and bodily fluids. Pathologists also do autopsies.

Pediatrician: Diagnoses and treats diseases of childhood and monitors growth, development, and wellness of children.

Plastic Surgeon: Restores and improves body parts.

Podiatrist: Diagnoses and treats diseases, injuries, deformities, and other conditions of the foot. Earns a D.P. (doctor of podiatry) rather than an M.D.

Preventive-Medicine Specialist: Assists in making lifestyle changes that improve health and prevent disease.

Psychiatrist: Treats mental illness and emotional problems; some work with psychologists who also treat mental illness but can't prescribe medicine. (For more information see chapter 21, "Emotional Pain, Stress, and Healing with Therapy.")

Pulmonologist: Diagnoses and treats diseases of the lungs and chest tissue.

Radiologist: Studies and uses various types of radiation, including X rays, to diagnose and treat disease.

Reproductive Endocrinologist: Deals with problems related to reproduction and infertility.

Rheumatologist: Diagnoses and treats inflammation, deterioration, and other problems (such as arthritis) having to do with the joints and connective tissue.

Urologist: Diagnoses and treats diseases of the urinary system.

(From *The Consumer's Guide to Medical Lingo* by Charles B. Inlander and Paula Brisco. For information on alternative-medicine providers see chapter 20, "Alternative Healing.")

You must choose a specialist carefully to make sure that person is qualified. If you require a certain medical procedure, ask how many times the doctor has performed it; as the saying goes, practice makes perfect. You should also ask whether she or he is board-certified or board-eligible and what board did the certifying. Board certification is not required, but a doctor who is board-certified or board-eligible in a particular specialty has been trained in that area.

For more information on board certification or to see whether a doctor is board-certified, contact the American Board of Medical Specialties, 1007 Church St., suite 404, Evanston, IL 60201-5913; (708) 491-9091.

You must also ask which hospital the physician is affiliated with. This is an important consideration, because depending on how complicated your procedure is, it may be better to choose the hospital first and then find a good surgeon who's affiliated with it. Here are some things to think about:

If you need treatment that is fairly complex, consider a hospital or center that specializes in that field. For example, a cancer patient who lives in New York City may want to be treated at Memorial Sloan-Kettering Cancer Center or in Boston at the Dana-Farber Cancer Institute. To find out about specialty health centers, contact the organizations that deal with specific diseases such as the American Cancer Society, the American Heart Association, and so on.

In the case of a serious problem, a university-affiliated hospital may also be a good bet. They generally have state-of-the-art equipment and top doctors, and many have clinics that specialize in certain areas such as the Comprehensive Sickle Cell Centers at the Howard

University College of Medicine and at the Wayne State University School of Medicine. (One note of caution: Because university hospitals are training centers, some have been accused of performing too many and unnecessary procedures.) Again, check with specific organizations or read *Health Care U.S.A.* by Jean Carper, which provides listings of clinics, physicians, hospitals, research centers, organizations, and so on.

If you need treatment that is more common and less complicated—such as having tonsils removed—you have more hospital options. Here are questions to be asked:

Is the hospital conveniently located? Can my family and I get there easily?

What are the visiting hours, and can children visit?

Does the hospital have a patient advocate? Patient advocates can assist with problems.

Does the hospital explain the patient's rights and responsibilities?

What is the hospital's (and your physician's) success record in the specific procedure I need?

Who is responsible for maintaining my personal-care plan? Can my family and I be kept up-to-date on my medical care?

Does the hospital have social workers? What services do they provide?

Will a discharge plan be developed before I leave the hospital?

Will the hospital staff, including the physician, explain how I must continue my care at home after discharge? Will I get written instructions about medication or medical devices?

Does the hospital have a written description of its services and fees? What resources does the hospital provide to help me if I need financial assistance?

Is the hospital clean?

Is the hospital accredited? Accreditation means the hospital is meeting national standards. To check on a hospital call the Joint Commission on Accreditation of Healthcare Organizations at (708) 916-5800.

Decisions to Make Before You Check In

If you are told that you need surgery, get a second opinion. A Rand Corporation study found that some 25 percent of all surgical procedures performed in the U.S. are unnecessary. Besides, in many cases, if you don't get a second opinion, health insurance won't cover the procedure. This isn't an insult to the doctor; it's standard procedure and common sense. You may also have to have the surgical procedure preapproved. Check your insurance policy to be sure. The U.S. Department of Health and Human Services runs a toll-free second-surgical-opinion hotline: (800) 638-6833.

Other questions to ask the doctor:

What is wrong with me? What is my illness or condition?
How many of these procedures have you done?
How often do you do this procedure?
How often is this procedure done in this hospital?
What is your success rate with this operation and that of the hospital?
What is your rate of complications?
(In the case of a new procedure) What are the advantages over the old way?
What happens if I don't have this operation?
What are the alternatives to this treatment?
What are the side effects and risks of this procedure?
What is the probability that the problem will recur?
How much will it cost?

You will also need to know as much as possible about your hospital stay before you check in. Ask your doctor these questions:

How long will my stay be?
What are the risks involved?
Will I be given anesthesia? What kind?
Will I need a transfusion?
How long can I expect to be in the recovery room?
Will I have a special diet when I wake up? Before I'm admitted? After I'm released?
Will I need special care after I've been discharged? For how long?
Will follow-up visits be necessary?
How long before I'm back to normal?
Will I be on any medication after I get home? Are there side effects?
Will there be any restrictions to my physical activities?

The American Hospitals Association recommends that you bring the following items to make your stay comfortable:

Nightgowns or pajamas, slippers, and socks
Books and magazines
Your address book to call loved ones
A schedule of visiting hours for friends and family

A roll of quarters in case you can't afford the fees for hospital phones
African cloth, photographs, art, and dolls to spruce up your room and make
  you feel more at home

During Your Stay

Get a copy of the patient's bill of rights as soon as you get to the hospital—and read it. Many hospitals have them posted. Here is a sample patient's bill of rights from the University Hospital of Brooklyn:

As a patient in a hospital you have the right, consistent with law, to:
1. Understand and use these rights. If for any reason you do not understand or you need help, the hospital must provide assistance, including an interpreter.
2. Receive treatment without discrimination as to race, color, religion, sex, national origin, disability, sexual orientation or source of payment.
3. Receive considerate and respectful care in a clean and safe environment free of unnecessary restraints.
4. Receive emergency care if you need it.
5. Be informed of the name and position of the doctor who will be in charge of your care in the hospital.
6. Know the names, positions, and functions of any hospital staff involved in your care and refuse their treatment, examination or observation.
7. A no-smoking room.
8. Receive complete information about your diagnosis, treatment and prognosis.
9. Receive all the information you need to give informed consent for any proposed procedure or treatment. This information shall include the possible risks and benefits of the procedure or treatment.
10. Receive all the information you need to give informed consent for an order not to resuscitate you. Also have the right to designate an individual to give this consent for you if you are too ill to do so.
11. Refuse treatment and be told what effect this may have on your health.
12. Refuse to take part in research. In deciding whether or not to participate, you have the right to full explanation.
13. Privacy while in the hospital and confidentiality of all information and records regarding your care.

14. Participate in all decisions about your treatment and discharge from the hospital. The hospital must provide you with a written discharge plan and written description of how you can appeal your discharge.
15. Review your medical record without charge and obtain a copy of your medical record, for which the hospital can charge a reasonable fee. You cannot be denied a copy solely because you cannot afford to pay.
16. Receive an itemized bill and explanation of all charges.
17. Complain without fear of reprisals about the care and services you are receiving and to have the hospital respond to you.

(Provided courtesy of Edison Bond, Jr.)

If you have a problem or don't understand something, ask to speak to the patient advocate (also called the patient representative). That person is there to assist you during your stay. Don't consent to any procedure that you're unclear about. Too often as Black women we have had our right to informed consent violated. It has been documented that some Black women have had to undergo procedures even though they didn't understand what was being done to them. In some cases, they were sterilized. Some of these women were unable to read the consent forms that they signed; others were coerced and threatened.

Informed consent means that you have the right to know what is being planned, the risks and benefits of the treatment plan, and the alternative forms of treatment, including the option of no treatment.

You must fully understand what you're being told. Don't sign anything that you don't understand.

The night before your surgery (or before), try to meet all of the people who will work with you—internists, nurses, aides, anesthesiologists. Ask as many questions as you like. Also, get a good night's sleep. Surgery tends to go more smoothly when the patient is relaxed.

If You Need Blood

Hundreds of Americans, including the late Arthur Ashe, contracted AIDS from bad blood they received through transfusions. However, since 1985, every unit of donated blood has to undergo a series of tests that indicate HIV. (Blood donated before 1985 is not part of the current supply, and frozen blood has been tested or thrown out.) In the summer of 1993, the FDA imposed even more stringent guidelines on blood centers to insure safety of the blood supply.

Despite assurances by government officials, there is still a very small

When I got pregnant, nearly two years ago, I decided that I needed to be well prepared and educated. I didn't want to leave everything in my obstetricians' hands. I read and reread childbirth books, gathering information as far as what is likely to happen during labor, birth, and delivery.

You'd think that health-care professionals would want to work with women who are knowledgeable and can ask the right questions. I realized, however, that the conservative mainstream medical profession would rather have a more passive patient, someone who does as she's told and doesn't ask questions. As I reflect back, I remember feeling like being in a five o'clock rush hour during my prenatal visits, especially when I attempted to ask my doctors questions. Although it's easy to be intimidated by people in white uniforms, I'm not. I see them as human beings like myself, not demigods.

About four weeks before my due date, one of my obstetricians insisted that I have a pelvic X ray. She wanted to be certain my uterus could accommodate a twin vaginal delivery. I had no family history of small uteruses, plus I was in excellent health. I didn't want this procedure. I pleaded with her. It was to no avail. She threatened that she would have to give me a C-section if I didn't agree to a pelvic X ray. I was totally stressed out because I read in one of my many books about how most doctors question the potentially harmful risk of radiation to the fetus. (What was my doctor's problem?)

Once my labor started, I had to battle verbally with the nurses to be allowed to walk around in the hospital room. They wanted to confine me to the fetal heart monitors, where I'd have to lie flat all the time despite the brutal contractions. I didn't agree with them. Books, other mothers, and the midwives told me labor is shortened, the cervix dilates more efficiently, uterine activity is increased, and, most important, pain and discomfort is lessened by walking during labor. Even my doctor later confirmed that walking helped to speed up my labor.

After my doctor examined me and decided it was "showtime," before I knew it an entire team came into the room—doctors and anesthesiologists. There were at least five other people besides Norman, the dad-to-be, and myself. I didn't want to appear like an overgriping patient, and I knew I had probably annoyed the staff already by insisting on walking. But I was aggravated when one of the anesthesiologists turned off my soothing ocean-sounds cassette tape.

As the anesthesiologist administered the epidural in my spine, he nonchalantly said to his colleague, "Check her legs for paralysis." I was horrified. "Excuse me," I said, "Why are you acting like I'm a slab of meat?" At least he apologized. But I was in labor. Where was the sensitivity and comfort?

"'Excuse me,' I said, 'Why are you acting like I'm a slab of meat?'"

—KAREN HALLIBURTON, WRITER, HACKENSACK, NEW JERSEY

Happily, seven and a half hours later, I vaginally delivered two healthy baby boys, Sean and Kyle (luckily, just a few days before the scheduled pelvic X ray).

Perhaps the health-care professionals thought I was a difficult person. Maybe. But I see my challenging certain routines and procedures as the actions of a person who is not intimidated by authority, who knows her rights and speaks up when she feels she's being taken for granted or underestimated.

It's the expectant mother's responsibility to empower herself and not rely totally on the doctor, but seek other sources of information. Most importantly, there should be an open communication with your obstetrician to let her or him know what you want during labor and delivery.

---

risk that donated blood is infected with HIV. It can take up to sixteen weeks after HIV infection for the body to produce antibodies to the virus. Because the current screening tests detect antibodies to the virus rather than the virus itself, infected blood donated during this period could theoretically slip through the screening process.

If you're worried, you can donate your own blood or get a relative to do it. (These are only options for elective procedures; in the case of emergency, there is no time to spare.) There are other reasons to use your own blood. Some rare types of blood such as U-negative are found in Blacks but not whites. Also, about 20 percent of Blacks have type B, compared to 11 percent of whites. This means that twice as many Blacks require that type or type O when they need a transfusion.

Here's what you need to know:

Autologous donations: This means that you donate your own blood for your own use. You'll need to do it at least two times, usually a week apart, during the month before your surgery. Blood keeps for forty-two days, but in some cases it can be frozen for later use. However, freezing and storing blood can be very costly.

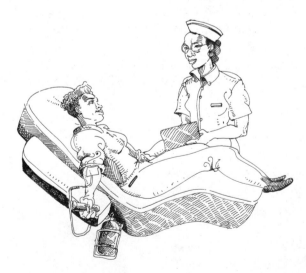

Donating blood is safe and virtually painless. *(Drawing: Yvonne Buchanan)*

Directed donations: Friends or relatives can donate blood for you. However, it's important to note that more directed donations test positive for HIV than do random donations.

Intraoperative blood salvage: In this procedure, doctors recover blood lost during surgery, clean it, and transfuse it back into the patient. Blood salvage can cost several hundred dollars, and it can't be used if the body part being operated on is infected or cancerous.

Our rare blood types make it imperative that we donate blood for one another. The American Association of Blood Banks (AABB) and the American Red Cross compile rare-donor files so that if you need a transfusion and require rare blood, your hospital can locate it for you. But it's up to us to keep the pool well stocked.

There's absolutely no risk of contracting HIV by giving blood. All blood-collection centers use a brand-new, sterile, prepackaged needle for each donation. A needle is used one time and then thrown away.

For more information, contact AABB, 1901 Glenbrook Rd., Bethesda, MD 20814; (301) 907-6977; or the American Red Cross, 17th and D Sts. NW, Washington, DC 20006; (202) 737-8300.

Before You Check Out

When you're ready to leave the hospital, make sure you have everything you need to get you through the recovery process—equipment, nursing care, diet, and exercise. Get it in writing. Also ask for an itemized bill from the cashier. *Mother Jones* magazine reported that more than 90 percent of all hospital bills contain errors—and 75 percent are errors in favor of the hospital. So check your bill carefully to make sure you aren't being charged for services you did not receive. If there's something on the bill that isn't clear, ask to speak to the patient advocate.

If you think you're being billed for something you never authorized or received, ask the hospital to show proof that the item or service was provided. Don't pay a disputed charge until the situation is rectified. If your insurance company is paying the bill and you suspect a problem, contact its fraud division.

In Case of Emergency

Sudden death from heart attack is the leading medical emergency in the country. But according to a study conducted by the University of Chicago and the Chicago Fire Department, about half of "sudden deaths" from heart attacks could have been prevented if bystanders had taken action. And compared to whites, Blacks were less likely to receive cardiopulmonary resuscitation (CPR) from a bystander. Although some white people refuse to help one of us, too many of us just don't know how to perform CPR.

Until Help Arrives

It's important that we all know how to respond in an emergency situation. It could save the life of a friend, relative, neighbor, or stranger. In the excitement of an emergency you may be frightened or confused, but try to stay calm. Follow these steps recommended by the American Red Cross:

1. Check the scene for safety, and check the victim for level of consciousness, breathing, pulse, and bleeding.
2. Call 911 or the local emergency number.
3. Care for the victim.

If the victim is unable to speak, cough, or breathe, give abdominal thrusts: Place your fist just above the navel, and give quick upward thrusts until the object is removed.

If the victim isn't breathing, give rescue breathing: Tilt the head back and lift the chin. Pinch the victim's nose shut. Give one slow breath about every five seconds.

If air won't go in, give abdominal thrusts: Give up to five abdominal thrusts. Look for and clear any objects from the mouth. Tilt the head back and reattempt breaths. Repeat these steps until breaths go in.

If the victim is not breathing and has no pulse, give CPR: Place your hand on the center of the victim's breastbone. Compress the chest fifteen times. Perform rescue breathing, giving two slow breaths. Repeat sets of compressions and breaths until the ambulance arrives.

For more information, contact your local chapter of the American Red Cross; request a copy of the free booklet "Til Help Arrives," or ask for information about first aid and CPR classes. You can also read *The American Medical Association Guide to Emergency First Aid* or the *American Red Cross First Aid and Safety Handbook* by the American Red Cross and Kathleen A. Handal, M.D.

The next step is the emergency room. Remember that it is against the law for hospitals to deny treatment to emergency-room patients or women in active labor. The practice of denying treatment, known as patient dumping, is used to avoid caring for people who are uninsured and have no money to pay for health care, who have an "undesirable" illness (such as AIDS), or belong to an ethnic "minority" group.

If hospital employees try to deny emergency care to you or a loved one or try to transfer you to another facility against your wishes, let them know that you know the law.

According to the Emergency Medical Treatment and Active Labor Act, which was passed in 1986, hospitals must provide an appropriate screening examination to all persons who present themselves for emergency treatment to determine whether the patient is in an emergency medical condition or active labor. If an emergency condition or active labor exists, the hospital must provide, within its capability, whatever treatment is necessary to stabilize the patient's condition. A patient in unstabilized condition may not be transferred to another facility unless

How to Complain

You might be mad as hell at your doctor or at something that happened to you in the hospital, but don't think "malpractice suit" right away. They are expensive, time-consuming, and hard to win. There are steps to take first:

Talk to the doctor or nurse. Be very clear about what's bothering you.

In the hospital, ask to speak to the patient advocate or patient representative. Their job is to be on your side. However, because they are employed by the hospital, there's a limit to what they can do for you.

Call the local or state medical society. They can sometimes help resolve doctor-patient disputes. Contact the American Medical Association (312-464-5000) or check the phone book for the number.

Report your doctor to the state department of health and the state licensing authority.

Doctors can be disciplined for things such as:

- Refusing to provide care because of race, color, or ethnic origin
- Performing services not authorized by the patient
- Practicing while drunk or on drugs
- Ordering excessive or unnecessary tests or treatments
- Failing to make patient records available

Contact your state department of health for more information.

she or he requests the transfer or unless certain criteria have been met, including a physician's certification that the benefits of the transfer outweigh the risks, acceptance by the hospital that is to receive the patient, and transportation provided with appropriate equipment and personnel.

Hospitals can be fined up to $50,000 for each violation of the law. If you have a medical emergency and someone tries to deny you entry, insist on seeing a doctor or the hospital's patient advocate.

This law applies to emergency medical care only. Far too many of us think of the emergency room as a clinic. It's not. Care is hurried; emergency-room doctors specialize in emergencies, not in primary care; and your care will be inconsistent because you'll be treated by a different doctor each time. Even if you don't have insurance, there are other ways to pay for medical care, such as Medicaid and Medicare, or you can seek out a low-cost clinic in your area.

Advance Directives

If you go into the hospital, you will be asked to fill out an advance directive. This is a legal form that you complete to express your preferences for medical treatment *before* you are unable to do so.

Basically, you'll have two options:

Living will. This document states how you wish to be cared for in the event of a terminal illness (this generally means six months to live) if you cannot communicate for yourself. The wills vary, but, for example, you may choose a do-not-resuscitate (DNR) order. This means that physicians, nurses, and others will not try to revive you if your heart has stopped or you aren't breathing.

Health-care proxy. This is a form you sign to allow someone you trust to decide about treatment if you lose the ability to decide for yourself. This health-care agent can have as little or as much authority as you choose.

Advance directives should be noted on your medical records. You can get either a health-care proxy or a living will from your patient advocate if one isn't offered.

For More Information

ON BECOMING A PHYSICIAN

Contact the NATIONAL MEDICAL ASSOCIATION, 1012 10th St. NW, Washington, DC 20007; (202) 347-1895.

ASSOCIATION OF AMERICAN MEDICAL COLLEGES, Section for Minority Affairs, 2450 N St. NW, Washington, DC 20037-1126; (202) 828-0400.

ON BECOMING A NURSE

Contact the NATIONAL COMMISSION ON NURSING IMPLEMENTATION PROJECT, 3401 S. 39th St., Milwaukee, WI 53215; (414) 382-6191.

NATIONAL BLACK NURSES ASSOCIATION, INC., 1012 10th St. NW, Washington, DC 20001; (202) 393-6870.

ON BECOMING A NURSE PRACTITIONER

Contact the NATIONAL ALLIANCE OF NURSE PRACTITIONERS, P.O. Box 44707, L'Enfant Plaza SW, Washington, DC 20026; (202) 675-6350.

AMERICAN COLLEGE OF NURSE-MIDWIVES, 818 Connecticut Ave., Suite 900, Washington, D.C. 20006; (202) 289-0171.

ON BECOMING A PHYSICIAN ASSISTANT

Contact the AMERICAN ACADEMY OF PHYSICIAN ASSISTANTS, 950 N. Washington St., Alexandria, VA 22314-1552; (703) 836-2272.

ON FINANCING MEDICAL EDUCATION

Read *Financial Aid for Minorities in Health Fields*, published and distributed by Garrett Park Press, P.O. Box 190B, Garrett Park, MD 20896; (301) 946-2553. For information on precollege programs to help prepare students for health professions, contact Science Service, Inc., 1719 N St. NW, Washington, DC 20036; (202) 785-2255.

ORGANIZATIONS

AMERICAN HOSPITAL ASSOCIATION, 840 N. Lake Shore Dr., Chicago, IL 60611; (312) 280-6000. Publishes a directory of hospitals in the United States and offers other literature.

AMERICAN MEDICAL ASSOCIATION, 515 N. State St., Chicago, IL 60610; (312) 464-5000. The professional association for physicians.

AMERICAN MEDICAL WOMEN'S ASSOCIATION, 801 N. Fairfax St., suite 400, Alexandria, VA 22314; (703) 838-0500. Association for women health-care practitioners.

JOINT COMMISSION ON ACCREDITATION OF HEALTHCARE ORGANIZA-TIONS, 1 Renaissance Blvd., Oakbrook Terrace, IL 60181; (708) 916-5600. Request the brochure "Helping You Choose Quality Hospital Care."

NATIONAL HEALTH LAW PROGRAM, 2639 S. La Cienega Blvd., Los Angeles, CA 90034; (310) 204-6010. For information on legal issues in medicine.

NATIONAL MEDICAL ASSOCIATION, 1012 10th St. NW, Washington, DC 20001; (202) 347-1895. Professional association for Black physicians.

NATIONAL WOMEN'S HEALTH NETWORK, 1325 G St. NW, Washington, DC 20005; (202) 347-1140. An advocacy organization that deals with women's health issues.

THE PEOPLE'S MEDICAL SOCIETY, 462 Walnut St., Allentown, PA 18102; (215) 770-1670. A nonprofit health-advocacy organization that provides consumers with information about medical rights under the law. Membership is $20 a year and includes the *People's Medical Society Newsletter*. The group has also published several books that are listed below.

PATIENTS RIGHTS HOTLINE, 215 W. 125th St., room 400, New York, NY 10027-4426; (212) 316-9393. Provides information on patients' rights and how to resolve problems with hospitals.

WOMEN'S HEALTH ACTION MOBILIZATION (WHAM), P.O. Box 733, New York, NY 10009; (212) 713-5966. Activist women's health organization.

BOOKS

The Consumer's Legal Guide to Today's Health Care: Your Medical Rights and How to Assert Them, Stephen L. Isaacs and Ava C. Swartz, Houghton Mifflin, 1992.

The Fight Back Guide to General Hospital Care, David Horowitz and Dana Shilling, Dell Publishing, 1993.

Mama Might Be Better Off Dead: The Failure of Health Care in Urban America, Laurie K. Abraham, The University of Chicago Press, 1993.

150 Ways to Be a Savvy Medical Consumer, the staff of the People's Medical Society (Allentown, Penn.), 1993.

Patient Power: Solving America's Health Care Crisis, John B. Goodman and Gerald Musgrade, Cato Institute (Washington, D.C.), 1992.

Take This Book to the Hospital with You, Charles B. Inlander and Ed Weiner, People's Medical Society (Allentown, Penn.), 1993.

Your Medical Rights, Charles Inlander and Eugene I. Pavalon, People's Medical Society (Allentown, Penn.), 1994.

20

Alternative Healing

When it comes to health care, many sisters have turned away from mainstream medicine, literally returning to their roots. "Root women" practiced and continue to practice "alternative" medicine in the Motherland, and when Africans were enslaved they brought their caretaking traditions with them to the United States, the Caribbean, and Brazil. Some actually cornrowed seeds of medicinal herbs into their hair so that part of home would always be with them. They planted these seeds and thus were able to continue using many of their old herbal remedies. Their wisdom, passed down through the generations, still inspires Black women healers today, particularly herbalists and midwives in the rural American South and other areas of the African diaspora.

Chances are, almost everyone has experienced some form of natural healing—tea, honey, and lemon your mother gave you at night to send a cold packing, or your mate's kneading hands when you've had a rough day. You probably don't even have to reach back very far in your family tree to find a grandmother or a great grandmother who used clove oil to soothe a throbbing tooth, soaked her aching feet in a tub of Epsom salts or knew of some herbal concoction to ease a variety of ailments.

Acceptance of the various types of alternative healing is growing, even among those who were once thoroughly skeptical. Holistic healing often focuses on prevention and costs less than mainstream medicine in the long run. Many practitioners believe they can help some patients avoid surgery. Since these methods are less invasive, they are gentler on the body and thus not as likely to cause side effects.

However, alternative medicine remains controversial. Few studies have been done on its effectiveness, so clashing opinions abound. But in 1992 the National Institutes of Health finally established an Office of Alternative Medicine. Now research can be conducted to evaluate and validate some of the so-called folk remedies our foremothers swore by for generations. Scientists can now explore new approaches for tackling AIDS, herpes, cancer, and other disorders conventional medicine has failed to defeat. Many sufferers of these illnesses already rely on alternative remedies.

What Is Holistic Healing?

What chiropractors, herbalists, acupuncturists, and other practitioners of natural healing have in common is that they take a holistic approach: They view the patient as a physical, emotional, and spiritual whole, not as a collection of ailing body parts to be treated separately. This kind of medicine has a long history among our people. In some of the world's oldest known medical documents, Imhotep, the ancient Egyptian scientist, wrote about holistic treatments, diets, and food. Mind you, this was *centuries* before the birth of Hippocrates, the Greek physician who is known as "the father of medicine."

Contemporary Western medicine treats "the mind in a psychiatric clinic, the spirit in a church, and the body in a hospital," Dr. Llaila O. Afrika writes in his book, *African Holistic Health*. We visit a gynecologist, a cardiologist, a dermatologist—a different specialist for each complaint. In contrast, traditional African cultures see the body, mind, and spirit as inextricably linked not only to one another, but also to their surroundings. By taking the whole person into account, alternative healers today attempt to deal with the *causes* of a disease.

Mainstream synthetic drugs and surgery, on the other hand, often simply suppress the *symptoms*. Natural healers believe that illness may stem from the patient's diet, emotional state, or environment. These conditions must be changed for the patient to be truly well, not just temporarily symptom-free. For example, if you have an operation to remove fibroids from your uterus but you don't change your eating habits or lifestyle, these benign tumors are more likely to return.

Many of us practice religious rituals, meditation, or visualization of

"Acupuncture and any other holistic medicine means not giving my body over to the doctor."

—REGINA JONES,
PUBLIC RELATIONS
EXECUTIVE AND WRITER,
LOS ANGELES

Fifteen years ago when I was in my midthirties, I weighed over 250 pounds, was running a newspaper and raising five kids. Needless to say, I was under a lot of stress. I went to the doctor, and he warned me that my high blood pressure was dangerous. I realized that I needed to reduce the stress because I was a real candidate for a stroke, since my family had that history.

About the same time, I had been thinking about taking yoga classes. My yoga teacher was a vegetarian who was into natural, holistic things. We became close friends, and I began to incorporate many of those things into my life. My diet started to change. I gave up fat, sugar, and alcohol. I went to a nutritionist and it changed more. I was still under a lot of stress, and yoga helped cool me out. I started feeling better. I lost weight—not a lot—but I lost it. I felt great.

About ten years ago, my cousin gave me a gift: her acupuncturist. That's when I started using acupuncture as a stress reducer and as my form of medicine. My body responded very well to it. If I was stressed and hysterical, a treatment would calm me down. If I had a cold, I would go to the acupuncturist to help clear it up.

A few years ago, a gynecologist found a cyst on my ovary. When I went for tests, I heard a couple of doctors arguing about what was wrong with me. They wanted to do exploratory surgery to see what was wrong. I refused. I left and went straight to my acupuncturist and then to the nutritionist. In three months, the doctors couldn't find the cyst, couldn't find anything wrong.

Later, when I went for a routine mammogram, they found a shadow on my breast. Once again, they wanted to do surgery. Once again, I refused. This time I also went to a hypnotist for relaxation. I grew a garden of organic vegetables and ate all raw, healthy foods. And again, in three months, my breast was healthy. The doctor told me to do whatever it was I was doing.

Don't get me wrong: I still think there's a need for regular medicine. I go for my regular Pap smear and mammograms. I see my dentist and have my teeth cleaned. But that form of medicine is there for crisis. But I do not believe in turning over my body or my life to a physician and letting him play God. Doctors are there to assist us in our healing process.

For me, acupuncture and any other holistic medicine means not giving my body over to the doctor. It means working with them to heal myself.

ourselves in positive situations to find peace with ourselves and our environment. These are forms of the spirituality our ancestors believed was so essential to the well-being of their communities. Such practices are also an important component of a holistic approach to wellness.

Does Holistic Healing Work?

Holistic techniques can prevent and treat a variety of ailments such as back problems, chronic pain, addictions, fibroids, headaches, allergies, colds and other viruses, sleep disorders—the list goes on and on. Alternative medicine can also be used to treat serious illness such as cancer, diabetes, and heart disease. In fact, for the first time ever, in 1993 a form of treatment for heart patients that relies on dietary changes, meditation, visualization, and exercise was endorsed by the health-insurance industry.

Holistic treatments also worked for Nailah Beraki. Now a massage therapist, Beraki was in law school in California when she was hit by a car in 1984. Her brain hemorrhaged and she remained in a coma for a week. The doctors said she would be a vegetable. But when she woke up, paralyzed on her left side, she began the painstaking process of regaining her memory and the movement of her limbs. Then she started having blackout seizures.

"I was in constant pain," Beraki recalls. "To control the seizures, they put me on medication they said I'd have to take for the rest of my life." She went off that medication in 1988 and hasn't had a seizure since; she is fully recovered today. Though physical therapy certainly helped her, she is convinced that her remarkable restoration was largely due to massage, visualization (to control the pain), and herbal remedies.

Beraki would be the first to admit that there's nothing magical about natural healing. It doesn't mean going to someone, lying down, and saying, "Okay, make me better." Alternative healers urge their patients to take responsibility for their own health and to draw on their bodies' natural resources for getting well. "Being a patient isn't about giving up power to someone who's going to fix it,'" says Loretta Mears, a chiropractor in New York. "It's about empowering yourself. I can't fix much if you aren't going to be an active participant. You have to figure out how to read your body and how to pay attention to symptoms so that we as a team can work together."

Making It Work for You

The most important thing you should know about natural medicine is this: It should never be an absolute substitute for conventional medicine.

Some Black folks rely too heavily on folk remedies because they don't trust the country's white-male–dominated medical establishment. However, most alternative practitioners believe that there is room in the health field for both natural healing and Western medicine. They realize that some conditions require surgery, CAT scans, or the setting of broken bones, for instance. And women must have yearly gynecological exams including Pap smears, and women forty and older must have mammograms every year or two, and yearly after age fifty.

It is important that you see your medical doctor or health-care practitioner before embarking on a course of natural healing. While you may meet with skepticism about the form of natural treatment you'd like to try, at least you will be better informed about any health condition you may have that could put you at risk. Also, never go off prescription drugs without first discussing it with the physician who prescribed them.

Conventional medicine and alternative healing often work well together. There's nothing wrong with taking advantage of the wisdom and experience of both. Besides, if you follow a healthy, natural diet, drink medicinal teas, practice yoga and t'ai chi, get frequent massages, and so on, chances are you won't need to be visiting your doctor or clinic very often.

Finding a Good Healer

Healers vary in their educational backgrounds. Some have formal training, including degrees in medicine (such as naturopaths), while others are self-taught. Laws determining whether or not a holistic practitioner must be certified or licensed vary from state to state. One of the best ways to find a good natural health practitioner is by word of mouth. You can also consult holistic publications available in health-food stores across the country and call the appropriate professional organization. You'll feel most comfortable with a practitioner who takes the time to answer all your questions and whose manner you find warm and pleasant. If you don't get a good vibe in your initial conversation or meeting, you may want to try someone else.

Here's an alphabetical look at the main areas of alternative healing in our community.

Acupuncture

Originating in China some five thousand years ago, acupuncture involves putting fine needles in specific parts of the body to deaden pain or promote healing. Other groups of people are believed to have devel-

oped similar methods of treating illness. Some
rural Africans are said to cure by scratching
particular points on the body, and some
Alaskan natives stimulate specific areas with
stones.

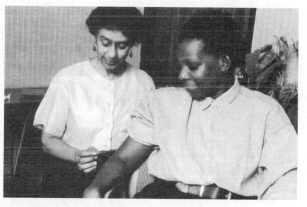

How It Works

The Chinese believe that chi—our life
force—must circulate unhampered throughout the body to maintain good health. When
the flow of this vital energy is blocked, sickness or pain results. Located just beneath the
skin all over the body, groups of acupuncture
points are said to correspond to internal
organs. The points that affect a particular

Acupuncturist (left) placing needles in a patient's
forearm to unblock specific body points and allow
energy to flow. *(Photo: Sheila A. Mason)*

organ become tender when that organ is involved in illness.

Once the points are sufficiently stimulated by the needles, the energy
is unblocked and the balance between the body's yin and yang (opposing
forces) is restored and pain or illness is often healed.

What It Does

Acupuncture works especially well for treating pain, such as headaches,
migraines, arthritis, and sprains or similar injuries. Among the conditions it also can help are menstrual and other gynecological problems,
skin disorders, asthma and other allergies, drug and smoking addictions,
obesity, depression, and weakened immune systems.

Most acupuncturists now use disposable needles, so there's no need to
worry about contracting AIDS or other infectious diseases. Since the
needles are very thin and sharp, patients usually feel no more than a
slight prick when they are inserted. It looks more painful than it feels.
When a needle reaches the proper spot, though, it occasionally causes a
mild ache or feeling of heaviness. The needles are left in for anywhere
from a few seconds to twenty to thirty minutes. Sometimes they are gently rotated before being painlessly removed. The number of needles used
during a treatment ranges from about six to twenty.

How often you visit an acupuncturist will depend on the nature of
your problem. Some people feel relief right away, while others need four
or five weekly treatments before they see any change. Still others are
treated once or twice a week for a few months or longer. Drinking coffee
or taking prescription drugs can stall or prevent success.

In nearly half the states in the country, only M.D.'s can legally prac-tice acupuncture. Whether an acupuncturist is a physician or not, make sure that she or he has had extensive training in acupuncture and has a comfortable knowledge of Western medicine as well. Plan to spend about $60 to $80 for the first treatment, which includes a lengthy con-sultation, and $25 to $50 for additional visits. Some insurance compa-nies cover acupuncture, most often when performed by an M.D.

Aromatherapy

Thousands of years ago, while the Chinese were developing acupunc-ture, Egyptians were using aromatherapy to combat sickness. In this method of healing, a plant's essential oil—its concentrated healing prop-erty—is extracted from its leaves, flowers, stem, root, or bark. This isn't so far-fetched when you keep in mind that plants are the basis for mod-ern drugs today, either as actual ingredients or as models for synthetic duplication.

How It Works

In aromatherapy, the plant oil is usually massaged into the skin or occa-sionally put on the tongue and is absorbed into the body. It can also be inhaled when worn as perfume, dropped in the bath, burned as incense, steamed, or diffused into the air of a room. Since the fragrance and heal-ing property of a plant go hand in hand, the Egyptians used the same oils for perfume as they did for medicinal purposes.

What It Does

Aromatherapy is believed to be most beneficial in reducing premenstrual symptoms, improving circulation, healing wounds, treating acne, and fading stretch marks from pregnancy.

Psychological aromatherapy is a growing field. It works because the part of the brain that controls our sense of smell is close to the part that controls our feelings. Abena Asantewaa, a Michigan psychologist, has begun helping her patients alter their moods through aromatherapy so that they are more open to uncovering and exploring the root causes of their troubles. She blends essential oils to elicit various calming, mind-stimulating, or antidepressant effects. After consultation with patients, she recommends that they use particular oils or combinations on their own. She has found that for some, the effects of these oils are almost immediate. When a depressed woman dabs on some sandalwood, for example, she'll start to feel better right away. Then she can more easily

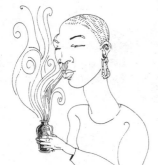

Aromatherapy uses fragrance to promote healing and well-being. (Drawing: Yvonne Buchanan)

Ten years ago I became committed to improving my health. I started changing my diet by weaning myself away from red meat. I continued by eliminating chicken, then fish, and then refined sugar. To play wise, a nutritionist, herbalist, and a naturopathic doctor guided me through this cleansing process. During this serious withdrawal period, my body would feel achy on more than one occasion, and I would get compelling headaches. I didn't realize how addictive certain foods could be.

About the same time, I began exploring the world of aromatherapy. Prior to receiving formal training and education on the subject, I read everything I could find about essential oils and their healing properties.

My father became seriously ill in the last few years. Two years ago he had another stroke, and it looked like this was it. I could not handle the idea of him leaving me. I knew I had to get grounded and address this whole issue of death. So every night I began my evening by sprinkling a few drops of undiluted lavender, neroli, and rose oils in my warm bath water. I then immersed my body into this pool of aromas, closed my eyes, and thought of happy memories.

After two weeks had passed, the universe opened up to me. I was able to accept whatever was to come. It was the night before my father's operation that I went to his hospital room, sat on the chair adjacent to his right arm and looked at him with a new pair of eyes. All at once, all the emotions and feelings that I had held in my heart for years came rushing out. My father overtly cried, I gazed into his face and calmly said, "Dad, whatever happens, it is okay. You did the best you could." I knew he could not talk after his most recent stroke, but when he half-smiled, it all came together for the both of us from that point on.

My challenge was to learn to let go of the fear of losing him. The essential-oil therapy aided me tremendously with that lesson by helping to unify my mind/physical/emotional connection.

In my opinion, aromatherapy should not be viewed as a cure-all for every problem but rather as a fragrant helper with therapeutic properties that can help disperse the stress that builds up in your body. I take care of myself with the understanding that there is a holistic approach to this. Aromatherapy is part of it.

> *"I'm taking care of myself with the understanding that there is a holistic approach to this. Aromatherapy is part of it."*
>
> —MARCIA WHITE, HOLISTIC AESTHETICIAN, ROSLYN, NEW YORK

examine the underlying reasons for her depression. Like other holistic practitioners, Dr. Asantewaa realizes that a combination of factors leads to good mental and physical health. After using her relaxation oils as well as modifying their diets, some patients have gotten relief from high blood pressure.

A consultation with an aromatherapist runs from $75 to 150. Buying essential oils themselves can be expensive, depending on the plant. (With many plants, the amount of oil that is so painstakingly extracted is minute.) The cost can vary from $7 to more than $300 an ounce. However, the oils are very potent, so you only need to use a little. They must be carefully stored to retain their power. To stretch them and to use them more easily for massage, essential oils are often blended with other vegetable oils, such as almond, sesame, grape-seed, and avocado.

Here's a sample of aromatherapy oils and some of the benefits they are said to have. An aromatherapist can advise you on whether to use them topically, in massage, in your bath, or to inhale them:

African peach: An antidepressant; opens up the emotions.
Cinnamon: Fights colds and flu.
Frankincense: Relaxing; heightens the spiritual consciousness; also helps clear up respiratory congestion.
Juniper: Good for bladder infections.
Geranium: Helps heal facial herpes and athlete's foot; repels insects.
Lavender: Very relaxing; soothes burns and heals wounds; used to treat vaginitis and cystitis.
Peppermint: A stimulant; gets rid of headaches, fever, chills.
Rose oil: An antidepressant; helps people cope with grief.
Rosemary: Stimulates the brain and helps improve memory; can also calm; eases headaches; heightens sex drive.
Sandalwood: An antidepressant.

Chiropractic

In 1895 when a Canadian immigrant in Iowa made his deaf janitor hear again by manipulating his spine, contemporary chiropractic was born. The ancient Egyptians, Chinese, Hindus, and Babylonians had all used similar techniques, but the practice had faded away. Once subject to imprisonment in the United States, chiropractors are now said to be the most widely accepted alternative healers in the world.

How It Works
Chiropractors believe that some health problems are caused by a misalignment of the vertebrae in the spine. Adjusting the spinal column

with the hands is thought to unblock nerve impulses and blood flow. The body is then able to use its own healing power, chiropractors say, without the aid of surgery or synthetic drugs.

What It Does

Slipped discs and pain in the low back, shoulder, arms, and neck are all said to be successfully treated by chiropractors. Pregnant women can also benefit. This is one of the least invasive ways of dealing with the back pain, knee problems, and headaches that expectant mothers often suffer.

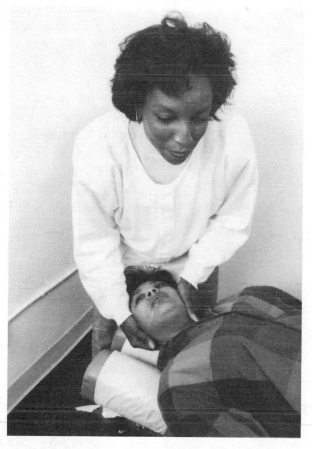

But because the nervous system is involved, chiropractors believe that all kinds of other surprising conditions can be relieved as well. "I've worked on women for low back pain who have later said they don't have menstrual cramps anymore," says chiropractor and herbalist Loretta Mears. "Or I work on someone who has a pain in his shoulder and his asthma gets better."

The theory behind this is that one part of the central nervous system may control two very different parts of the body. Chiropractors can't say, though, that adjusting the same vertebrae in two different people will always have the same results. "It's a very individual thing," explains Dr. Mears. "Just like not everyone can take Tylenol and get rid of a headache."

A chiropractor realigns the neck of a patient. *(Photo: Ray Bailey; courtesy of Desiree Williams)*

Chiropractic treatments aren't generally uncomfortable. While you may hear cracking sounds, such as when you crack your knuckles, this doesn't hurt. Counseling about nutrition and exercise are an important part of this healing art.

However, chiropractic is not without risks. Since chiropractors deal with the spine, one of the most delicate and important parts of your body, it is essential to find a practitioner who is highly experienced and highly recommended. A good chiropractor will refer a patient to medical specialists if necessary.

Chiropractors undergo extensive training similar to that of medical doctors, except that they concentrate on the spine. Instead of M.D., they have D.C. (doctor of chiropractic) after their names. In some states they can deliver babies and perform acupuncture. The initial consultation might range from $40 to $200, with additional chiropractic adjustments running from about $25 to $100 per visit. Most medical-insurance companies cover chiropractic to some degree.

Colonics

"Not having colonics is like keeping a garbage can in your house that you never empty," says Daya Oliver, a nutrition consultant and colon hygienist in Harlem. She explains that colonics cleanse the large intestine with water. This is necessary, she says, because all of us, from years of eating overly refined food with little roughage, get a thick mucous buildup on the walls of our intestines. Thus the theory is that the nutrients we consume can't be absorbed properly. She also believes that waste matter becomes impacted and toxins remain in our bodies.

How They Work

As with an enema, which cleans the lower intestine, water flows in and out of the rectum through a lubricated tube. However, while an enema uses only about 2 quarts of water, a colonic uses between 15 and 20 gallons. But during the twenty-minute procedure the flow is very gentle, and you're never holding more than a few ounces of fluid at a time.

Sometimes herbs are added to the water to help soften waste matter and wash out bacteria.

What They Do

Some people who have periodic colonics say they are surprised by how much better they feel. Oliver says that this is because they are eliminating the waste that otherwise would remain in their bodies too long. Some of her clients have reported that they stop having menstrual cramps after they begin colon hygiene. Oliver also recommends fasting—four times a year, with each change of season—as an additional way of detoxifying the body. "Colonics and fasting are wonderful tools not in and of themselves," she says, "but in conjunction with upgrading your diet and maintaining spiritual health."

Just as you should before beginning any form of alternative healing, see your medical doctor first. Make sure you do not have a medical condition that could be worsened by colonics or fasting. Both of these prac-

Fasting

"The minute we stop eating, the body starts housecleaning," says nutritionist Daya Oliver. "Fasting is one of nature's oldest tools."

Many people believe that periodically giving your digestive system a rest can do wonders in eliminating waste and toxins from the body. Through Yoruba religious traditions, Muslim Ramadan, and Christian Lent and Good Friday, fasting or giving up particular foods has been used for centuries among Black folks for purification, heightened spirituality, and healing.

There are several different kinds of fasts—fruit-juice, herbal-beverages, vegetable-juice, water. With some you eat solid food after sundown, while with others you consume only liquids for days at a time.

No matter which type you choose, be sure to conduct it under the guidance of someone who is experienced in nutrition and leading fasts. New York holistic-health consultant and fasting specialist Queen Afua has developed a nutritional liquid-fasting method that she believes cleanses, rejuvenates, and strengthens the body. She suggests fasting for twenty-four hours once a week on the day you were born, and a three-, seven-, or twenty-one-day fast four times a year, just before the change of each season. This can help stave off the colds and other illnesses that often accompany a change in weather, she says.

Queen Afua's regime is outlined in her book, Heal Thyself for Health and Longevity. Her fasts consist of freshly pressed juices of organic fruits and vegetables, purified or distilled water, herbs, enemas, natural laxatives, and colonics. Also essential are salt baths and exercise. As the body begins to detoxify itself, you may experience one or two symptoms such as headaches, dizziness, fatigue, depression, impatience, blurred vision, or vaginal discharge. Drinking only herbal teas and vegetable juices instead of fruit juices for a while, having enemas and massages, and getting plenty of rest can help stop these reactions. Some people say that being on a light vegetarian diet before fasting can prevent these symptoms. However, these reactions could also be signs of serious health problems, so your doctor's supervision is recommended.

tices have health risks if done too frequently, with improper guidance, or under certain circumstances. Some physicians believe, for instance, that colonics can be dangerous during pregnancy.

The initial colonics consultation might run $75 to $125, with follow-up treatments ranging from about $35 to $65 each. Occasionally medical insurance covers colonics if prescribed by a doctor. Be sure to choose a person who is qualified. Get a recommendation from someone you trust, and then ask the practitioner about her or his training and how long she or he has been practicing. Make sure you choose someone you're comfortable with.

Herbs

Herbs were used for healing at least as far back as 3000 B.C. in China and Egypt and probably long before. In parts of the Caribbean, Brazil, and the American South where doctors are scarce, Black women herbalists use skills passed down through their families.

Like the title character in Gloria Naylor's novel *Mama Day,* some of their foremothers served not only as healers but also as midwives, social workers, and marriage counselors. Living on a remote Georgia/South Carolina sea island, Mama Day prepares to treat a sick infant:

"She scalds the countertops before opening her canvas pouch and laying her dried herbs out on them. She don't use much: all together it's only a teaspoon of senna pods, coltsfoot, horehound, white cherry bark, and black cohosh set to steep into the third change of water. She weighs them out by touch—some the roots, some the leaves, some the whole plant."

How They Work

Herbs are widely believed to be good for treating many different complaints, including uterine fibroids, menstrual problems, menopausal symptoms, coughs, colds, flu, headaches, constipation, diarrhea, fatigue,

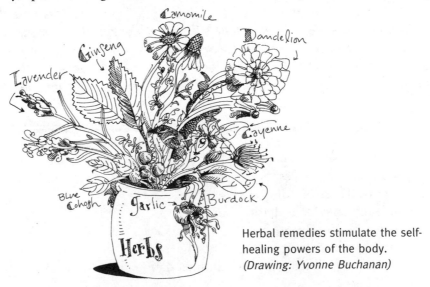

Herbal remedies stimulate the self-healing powers of the body.
(*Drawing: Yvonne Buchanan*)

burns, insect bites and stings, and toothaches. Instead of masking or suppressing symptoms as synthetic drugs do, herbal remedies should be used to stimulate the self-healing powers of the body by cleansing and rebalancing it. "They're not to be substituted for drugs," says chiropractor and herbalist Loretta Mears. "Some people go out and take white willow bark whenever they have a headache. Well, what's the difference between taking that and taking aspirin if you don't figure out why you're getting the headaches in the first place?"

What They Do

Be sure to consult an experienced herbalist before plunging in. Herbs are generally milder than modern drugs, so results aren't usually as immediate. Some do have side effects, though, especially if taken for long periods of time. Also remember that two people don't necessarily react the same way to the same herb or dosage.

Changes in your lifestyle and diet must often accompany herbal remedies. For instance, herbs may help get rid of a bladder infection. But if the infection is being caused because you're eating too much sugar, engaging in unprotected intercourse, or having sex in a position that is irritating your bladder, the problem will continue.

Herbal remedies are made from roots, leaves, flowers, stems, seeds, resin, fruit, or bark. Various parts may have different effects. Herbs generally come in (or are made into) the following forms and are sold in health-food stores:

Tea: Usually 1 teaspoon of the dried herb (roots, bark, or leaves and flowers) or 3 teaspoons of the freshly crumbled herb in 1 cup of boiling water, steeped for five to ten minutes.

Infusion: Similar to tea, but drunk cool or lukewarm.

Capsule: Contains the ground herb.

Tablet: Ground, compressed, and coated.

Tincture: A concentrated extract in liquid form that is put in tea or dropped in your mouth.

Extract: In liquid form, about ten times more potent than tincture.

Solid extract: Can be spread on toast.

Syrup: Herbs are boiled and mixed with honey.

Powdered: To be mixed with water (hot water brings fastest results).

Poultice: Herbs are mixed with water, spread on cloth, and applied to skin.

Salve: Herbs are baked with beeswax and vegetable oil.

Liniment: Powdered herbs are mixed with rubbing alcohol, for external use.

Here's a sampling of common herbs and some of the benefits they are thought to have:

Angelica, or dong quai (root): Nourishes the female reproductive system; used as a tonic for anemia (but never take when pregnant or if you have diabetes).

Blue cohosh (root): Regulates menstrual flow and aids in childbirth.

Burdock (root, leaves): The root is considered an excellent blood purifier, has been used to treat gynecological infections; tea made from the leaves heals skin disorders and canker sores.

Cayenne (fruit): This hot red pepper is said to be used by African women in a douche to cure and prevent vaginal infections; helps bolster body's immune system, and good for hay fever.

Camomile (flowers): Regulates menstruation and relieves cramps.

Coltsfoot (root, leaves): Helps you cough up phlegm.

Dandelion (root, leaves): Rich in nutrients, dandelion greens are good for female reproductive organs.

Echinacea (root): Commonly used as a cold remedy; also helps fight infections and cleans the blood of toxins.

Garlic: A natural antibiotic that supports the autoimmune system and rids the body of invasive organisms; also helps lower blood pressure.

Ginger (root): Brewed as a tea, can help relieve morning sickness.

Ginseng (root): Good for digestive problems.

Golden seal (root): Strengthens the immune system, used for colds, flu, stomach and liver problems (extended use may cause vaginal infections).

Lavender (whole plant): Relieves nausea.

Lemon grass (whole plant): Aids with kidney, liver, and spleen ailments.

Red raspberry: Helps heal canker sores.

Senna (leaves): A laxative.

Uva-ursi (leaves): Helps relieve urinary disorders and excessive menstruation.

Homeopathy

Dating back to the eighteenth century, homeopathy treats like with like. Patients are given minute doses of substances that produce symptoms similar to those of the diseases they suffer from. Homeopaths believe that in this way the body's vital force, or self-curing action, is stimulated. (A similar principle is used by mainstream medicine with immunization.)

How It Works

Here are a few homeopathic remedies for common ailments (have fun pronouncing the names!):

Antimonium Tartaricum: Bronchitis

Arsenicum album: Hay fever with violent sneezing

Belladonna: Colds with high fever

Bryonia alba: Splitting headaches

Caulophyllum Thalictroides: Severe menstrual cramps

Chamomilla: Earaches with buzzing in ears

Pulsatilla: Morning sickness during pregnancy

Oscillococcinum: The flu

Nux vomica: PMS (premenstrual syndrome)

Natrum muriaticum: Depression

What It Does

Always given in extremely diluted doses, homeopathic medications are usually made from herbs (such as poison ivy) or minerals (including sodium chloride) and occasionally from animal substances (snake venom, for instance). The medicine comes in liquid drops or in sugar pellets dissolved under the tongue. A number of different practitioners can advise you about homeopathic remedies. A number of medical doctors, naturopaths, chiropractors, nutritionists, nurses, and physician assistants have studied homeopathy, or you can contact a practitioner who specializes in homeopathic methods. You can get homeopathic remedies from health-food stores, but it's best to talk to a practitioner before taking them. Chronic fatigue, allergies, autoimmune conditions, and menstrual problems all seem to respond especially well.

Massage

We all know that a massage can feel *really* good. It relaxes us, relieves tension, and makes

Naturopathic Medicine

"Taking a holistic approach, we use treatments that will stimulate the body's own ability to heal itself," says Andrea Sullivan, Ph.D., N.D., a naturopathic physician who specializes in homeopathy, nutrition, and herbal medicine in Washington, D.C. "We look at patients' mental and emotional states as well, not just their physical health."

A true naturopathic doctor (N.D.) undergoes four years of premed, then four years of graduate-level medical studies. The first two years, like those of medical school for an M.D. (Doctor of Medicine), focus on the basic sciences. But this is where the similarity ends. For the N.D., the emphasis then shifts to clinical training in nutrition and alternative therapies including herbal medicine, homeopathy, natural childbirth, acupuncture, visualization, massage, chiropractic, and exercise therapy. N.D.'s often continue their studies to specialize in one or several of these areas. Some insurance companies cover treatment. While N.D.'s practice in all fifty states, they are licensed in only a few.

For additional information, contact the American Association of Naturopathic Physicians, 2366 Eastlake Ave. E., suite 322, Seattle, WA 98102; (206) 323-7610.

us think we're royalty. It helps us feel nurtured in a society where not enough nurturing goes on, especially for those of us of African descent. But done with experienced hands, massage can have a variety of physical benefits as well.

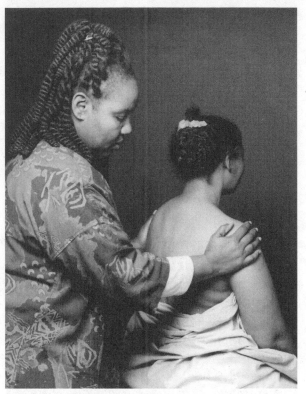

Massage therapist Nailah Beraki releases tension by unblocking the body's energy flow. *(Photo: Kim Weston)*

Common types of massage are Swedish, shiatsu, and foot reflexology. Swedish massage consists of long, flowing hand strokes aided by vegetable oil or powder. Shiatsu, which doesn't require lubrication, involves pushing acupressure points (those used in acupuncture) with the fingers. In reflexology, where deep pressure is applied to the feet only, specific parts of the feet are said to correspond to healing various organs in the body.

How It Works

The kneading of flesh has been found to improve lymph and blood circulation, help eliminate waste and toxins from your system, and alleviate pain by lessening the inflammation and swelling of joints. This can be particularly welcome for discomfort during and after pregnancy and is a good way of diminishing postpartum depression.

Studies have also shown that incubated premature babies who were massaged doubled their weight in half the time as those who weren't touched this way. Massage can also increase nutrition to muscles and improve muscle tone. It is especially successful in preventing or delaying the atrophy (weakening of muscles) that results from inactivity due to injury. Because it encourages the retention of the nutrients that aid in tissue repair, massaging areas near bone fractures can speed healing.

What It Does

In her ten-minute "stress breakers," head-neck-and-shoulder massages, New York holistic-health consultant Hafeezah Basir helps people convert the energy from stress into constructive energy. "If we don't let energy flow, it gets blocked, and that's what we experience as tension, anxiety, pressure, and fear," she says. Massage can help unblock this energy. Basir, who often works on clients in their offices right at their desks, also uses aromatherapy, visualization, and positive affirmation to help people be their best selves.

Massage therapists receive about two years of training at a certified school or institute. Expect to pay anywhere from $50 to $125 for a forty-five- or sixty-minute session. Foot reflexology begins at around $35. Insurance sometimes covers massage in part, particularly if prescribed by a physician.

Choose a therapist you're comfortable with. You have the right to tell the therapist if her or his touch hurts or if you want to stop the massage at any time. Drink plenty of water before your session, and it also helps to loosen your muscles with a hot shower or bath beforehand.

For More Information

ACUPUNCTURE

Contact the AMERICAN ASSOCIATION OF ACUPUNCTURE AND ORIENTAL MEDICINE, 4101 Lake Boone Trail, suite 201, Raleigh, NC 27607; (919) 787-5181; the National Commission for the Certification of Acupuncturists, 1424 16th Street NW, Washington, DC 20036; (202) 232-1404; or the Traditional Acupuncture Institute, the American City Bldg., 10227 Wincopin Circle, suite 100, Columbia, MD 21044; (301) 596-6006.

AROMATHERAPY

Contact the INSTITUTE OF NATURAL PSYCHOLOGY, 223 N. Rowland St., Cassopolis, MI 49031; (616) 445-5190.

CHIROPRACTIC

Contact the AMERICAN BLACK CHIROPRACTORS ASSOCIATION, 1918 E. Grand Blvd., St. Louis, MO 63107; (314) 531-0615; American Chiropractic Association, 1701 Clarendon Blvd., Arlington, VA 22209; (800) 986-4636 or (703) 276-8800; or the Association of Chiropractic Colleges, 2005 Via Barrett, P.O. Box 367, San Lorenzo, CA 94580.

COLONICS

Contact the AMERICAN COLON THERAPY ASSOCIATION, 11739 Washington Blvd., Los Angeles, CA 90066; (310) 390-5424.

HERBS

Contact the AMERICAN BOTANICAL COUNCIL, P.O. Box 201660, Austin, TX 78720; (800) 373-7105 or (512) 331-8868; or the Herb Society of America, 9019 Kirtland Chardon Rd., Mentor, OH 44060; (216) 256-0514.

HOMEOPATHY

Contact THE INTERNATIONAL FOUNDATION FOR HOMEOPATHY, 2366 Eastlake Ave. E., Seattle, WA 98102; (206) 324-8230; Homeopathic Educational Services, 2124 Kittredge St., Berkeley, CA 94704; (800) 359-9051; or the National Center for Homeopathy, 801 N. Fairfax St., suite 306, Alexandria, VA 22314; (703) 548-7790.

MASSAGE

Contact THE ASSOCIATED BODYWORK AND MASSAGE PROFESSIONALS, P.O. Box 1869, Evergreen, CO 80439-1869; (303) 674-8478; or the Swedish Institute, 226 West 26th St., New York, NY 10001; (212) 924-5900.

ORGANIZATIONS

AMERICAN HOLISTIC MEDICAL ASSOCIATION, 4101 Lake Boone Trail, suite 201, Raleigh, NC 27607; (919) 787-5146. Publishes a referral directory of association members.

HOLISTIC HEALTH HOTLINE, P.O. Box 25717, Seattle, WA 98125; (800) 994-4445 or (206) 486-4445. Offers referrals for holistic medicine in the Seattle area, provides some national resources, and publishes a newsletter called *Holistic Health News*.

OFFICE OF ALTERNATIVE MEDICINE, National Institutes of Health, Executive Plaza S., suite 450, 6120 Executive Blvd., Rockville, MD 20892-9904; (301) 402-2466. Helps patients with serious illnesses such as cancer and AIDS locate information on alternative forms of medical treatment.

BOOKS

African Holistic Health, Llaila O. Afrika, Sea Island Information Group (Silver Spring, Md.), 1989.

Aromatherapy: The Encyclopedia of Plants and Oils and How They Help You, Daniele Ryman, Bantam Books, 1993.

Back to Eden: The Classic Guide to Herbal Medicine, Natural Foods, and Home Remedies, Jethro Kloss, Back to Eden Books Publishing Co., (Loma Linda, Calif.), 1989.

Basic Herbs for Health and Healing, Rashan Abdul Hakim, Sundial Products (Bronx, N.Y.), 1989.

A Consumer's Guide to Alternative Medicine, Kurt Butler, Prometheus Books (Buffalo, N.Y.), 1992.

EveryWoman's Health: The Complete Guide to Body and Mind by Top Women Doctors, D. S. Thompson, M.D., ed., Simon & Schuster, 1993.

The Family Guide to Self-Medication: Homeopathic, Boericke & Tafel, Boericke & Tafel, Inc. (Santa Rosa, Calif.), 1988.

Forever Young, Paul Goss, N.D., M.T., self-published (Compton, Calif.), 1985.

Healing Herbs: The Ultimate Guide to the Curative Power of Nature's Medicines, Michael Castleman, Rodale Press, 1993.

Health Without Drugs: Alternatives to Prescription and Over-the-Counter Medicines, Arabella Melville and Colin Johnson, Simon & Schuster/Fireside, 1990.

Heal Thyself for Health and Longevity, Queen Afua, A&B Books Publishers (Brooklyn, N.Y.), 1992.

The Home Herbal Doctor, Howard H. Hirschhorn, Parker Publishing Company (West Nyack, N.Y.), 1982.

The Natural Family Doctor, Andrew Stanway and Richard Grossman, Simon & Schuster/Fireside, 1987.

The Women's Guide to Homeopathy, Andrew Lockie, M.D., and Nicola Geddes, M.D., St. Martin's Press, 1993.

PART IV

OUR EMOTIONAL WELL-BEING

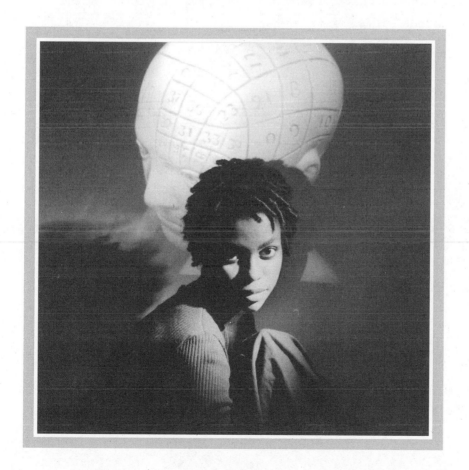

21

Emotional Pain, Stress, and Healing with Therapy

"Y ou better not never tell nobody but God. It'd kill your mammy."

In the opening sentence of her Pulitzer Prize–winning book *The Color Purple*, Alice Walker captures the essence of many Black women's lives with regard to our mental health. Like Celie, an incest survivor who is the main character of the novel, many of us have internalized the message that if we speak the truth about our lives, we will disappoint, hurt, anger, or indeed symbolically "kill" family members, friends, or colleagues.

Saddled with the heavy burden of being "strong" Black women, we have all too often sacrificed our physical, spiritual, and emotional health for the well-being of others. Deeply aware of the inequities Black people have suffered since being forcibly taken from African shores, Black women historically have taken care of our children, parents, spouses, lovers, elders, and friends before we have taken care of ourselves. As Black women we have put our needs on the back burner, not because we are innately selfless, but rather because of the deep love we carry for our people and our heritage.

Many of us have been praised, honored, and recognized for the enormous contributions we have made to the continued survival of Black people in a racist society—and rightly so. Yet while we appreciate the awards and accolades we as Black women receive from our community, they do not always compensate for the sacrifices we routinely make on behalf of others. The tributes do not completely soothe the deep psychological wounds we suffer because of both our gender and our race. As the Black scholar and publisher Barbara Smith has powerfully noted, "It is not something we have done that has heaped this psychic violence and material abuse upon us, but the very fact that because of who we are, we are multiply oppressed."

If we aim to live healthy, productive lives, to empower our people and to achieve our personal and professional goals, it is vital that we examine the impact racism, sexism, and homophobia can have on our emotional

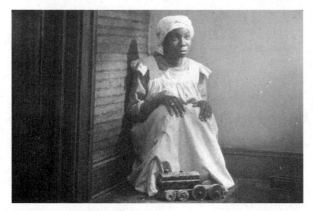

Whoopi Goldberg in the role of Celie from the movie *The Color Purple.* Celie was an incest survivor. *(Photo: Globe Photos, Inc.)*

health. Contrary to the messages we have received about staying silent or "carrying everything to the Lord in prayer," it can be enormously healing for us to share our problems (and our triumphs!) either with trained mental-health professionals or with others who can help us sift through and better understand the complexity of being Black and female. (For more on self-help support groups, see chapter 22, "The Self-Help Revolution.")

Too often Black folks avoid seeking help for emotional troubles. But it is important for Black women to reassess the notion that solutions such as psychotherapy are only for "crazy white people" or that it is shameful and a sign of weakness to experience emotional pain. Given the real stresses and strains in our lives, we would be "crazy" not to empty our hearts of the multitudes of hurts so many of us have suffered. We should learn to talk about our pain and what we're doing about it with those we trust so that family and friends can support the healing process.

The Price We Pay

Traditionally viewed as the "backbone" of our people while at the same time being negated daily in so many aspects of our lives, we Black women are under tremendous psychological pressures. The National Black Women's Health Project reports that over 50 percent of Black women live in emotional distress.

In fact, many health-care professionals believe that sisters are suffering from emotional pain in epidemic proportions. "My estimate is that 80 percent of Black women are deeply troubled," says Denese O. Shervington, M.D., a psychiatrist who practices in New Orleans. "Many of them are women who by all external appearances seem to be functioning well. They are holding down good jobs and taking care of their families. But after a short time in treatment, it becomes evident that they are severely depressed."

Common symptoms of depression include changes in appetite resulting in weight loss or gain, lack of energy, sleep disturbances such as insomnia or early morning waking, overwhelming feelings of inadequacy or worthlessness, heavy drinking or drug abuse, and frequent thoughts of suicide or death.

The general depression that many Black women suffer is often compounded by problems in our intimate relationships, notes Dr. Shervington. "In addition to dealing with racism, lots of Black women experience rejection in their relationships that takes a heavy toll on them," she says. "As a response to the rejection, the women will often engage in self-destructive behavior such as substance abuse or unsafe sex. They develop a hopelessness and very fatalistic attitude toward life because they don't feel good about themselves or believe they have anything to live for."

Stress and Anxiety

One of the best (and least expensive) ways for we sisters to improve our emotional health is to begin to look at stress and the role it plays in our lives.

As Opal Palmer Adisa, a writer who lives in Berkeley, California, puts it: "Did you ever wonder why so many sisters look so angry? Why we walk like we've got bricks in our bags and will slash and curse you at the drop of a hat? It's because stress is hemmed into our dresses, pressed into our hair, mixed into our perfume and painted on our fingers. Stress from the deferred dreams, the dreams not voiced; stress from the broken promises, the blatant lies; stress from always being at the bottom, from never being thought of as beau-

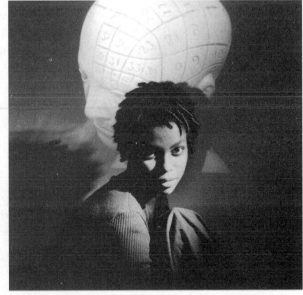

Self-examination helps heal emotional wounds.
(Photo: Debbie Egan-Chin)

"I've had to replace the self-hating messages our society feeds us with positive self-affirmations."

—TONI LONG, EXECUTIVE ASSISTANT IN INVESTMENT-BANKING FIRM, BROOKLYN

At the age of twenty-two, on the verge of graduating from college, I sat in my room crying, unable to go to classes. I remember being in so much pain. Not a physical pain but an unrecognizable pain that felt like a paralyzing weight. The world around me changed and became a dark, scary, gloomy place. It was as though someone dropped a veil over my eyes; like I was in mourning. I couldn't imagine a future where I didn't feel this way, but I knew I couldn't live like this.

Despite the severity of my feelings, I was still able to pretend nothing was wrong when in public. I still laughed and joked around. I was still able to carry on intelligent conversations.

I was still able to go to work, but as I began to feel worse, I found myself calling in sick with greater frequency. I would create stories about a physical illness, because I knew that my mental distress wouldn't be seen as valid. As a Black woman from a lower middle-class background, I knew that quitting my job was not a financial option. I also knew that I couldn't drop out of school during the last quarter of my senior year.

This only made my depression worse, and my feelings of hopelessness and helplessness grew. It was during one of those days, sitting in my room, that I decided I had to do something to change my situation. I could either kill myself to end this constant pain, or I could get help. I didn't believe in suicide, so I called the counseling center on campus and spoke to a psychologist. Within a few days I was seeing a therapist once a week.

While in therapy, I realized that I had felt this way as a child. I discovered that my depression was linked to the sometimes impossibly high standards I hold myself to. I don't allow myself room for "failure." For me, failure is an absolute weakness that must always be avoided. When something happens that I perceive as failure, I blame myself and become depressed.

To get a grip on my depression, I started to view it differently. It's an illness that needs treatment and attention like any other ailment. It's a disease that has to be monitored like diabetes or high blood pressure. I also learned that while I will not always be depressed, I have a greater tendency to become depressed if I do not apply what I've discovered about myself and how I react to my surroundings. I've had to replace the self-hating messages our society feeds us with positive self-affirmations.

To further my healing process, I also talked extensively to my mom about my feelings. At first she didn't understand what I was going through and was hurt by some of the things I said about her and about my childhood. But now she realizes how serious this is and wants me to get better. Being able to share with her how I've felt for years really made a difference in how I feel now. I no longer have to carry that weight alone. I've allowed someone close to me to be privy to my secrets, someone who has known me all my life.

Currently I am seeing a therapist and working on my depression. I'm learning not to hold myself to such high standards and not to treat life's little setbacks as major failures. It helps when I think about the great legacy of Black women—gay and straight, middle- and working-class, abled and disabled, formally educated and self-taught—of which I am a part. When I think about how my sisters have struggled and survived oppression in this country for hundreds of years, I know that I can and will live a full life, dealing with but never being consumed by my depression.

---

tiful; stress from being a Black woman in America. . . . We are stressed out!"

Stress can affect our bodies in many ways. It can cause or worsen emotional problems such as depression. Stress can also produce physical trouble. Studies show that stress weakens the body's immune system and makes us more vulnerable to diseases that Black women are already at risk for such as high blood pressure, diabetes, and heart problems. "If you don't take care of the stress in your life, your body will tell you about it," says Lorraine Bonner, M.D., a sister who practices in Oakland, California.

Stress manifests itself as frequent headaches, recurring colds, tight muscles, irritability, depression, and changes in eating habits and weight. Because of our conditioning to take care of everyone else before we take care of ourselves, sisters often respond to stress in ways that only make matters worse: by ignoring the symptoms, working harder to "get things under control," or by trying to escape through food, drugs, alcohol, or nicotine.

"I think that Black women need to begin to take a more global, non-Western health philosophy in terms of looking at how our mental, physical, and environmental status all interact and affect each other," says Sydney Perry, a certified massage therapist who lives in Oakland, California. Perry says that Black women can replenish themselves holistically by incorporating stress-reduction strategies into their lives. Here are ten ideas that can get you started. Remember that no one can follow all these suggestions all of the time. Be gentle with yourself!

Become more aware of stress and how your body responds to it. Rather than always thinking that something is wrong with you—you're naturally a high-strung sister or you're prone to getting colds—notice the way your mind and body react when you're under stress.

Learn how to calm your mind through meditation, deep breathing, yoga, or chanting.

Try to exercise regularly. Physical activity is a good antidote for sickness, depression, and fatigue.

Improve your diet. Cut down on sugar, salt, coffee, chocolate, red meat, alcohol, and refined carbohydrates. Consume more whole grains, vegetables, chicken, fish, soy products, and herbal drinks.

Pamper yourself. Get a massage, sleep late, take a warm bath, soak in a hot tub—especially when you are aware of extra stress in your life.

Develop a supportive group of friends with whom you don't have to "wear the mask."

Start keeping a journal in which you can document your mental, physical, and spiritual health.

Determine whether it's time to get a new job or to restructure your current position. If work pressures are the main cause of the stress in your life, you may want to move on.

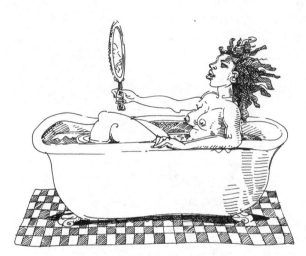

Pampering yourself relieves stress and helps you see your own beauty. *(Drawing: Yvonne Buchanan)*

Think positive and try to find the humor in life. Laughter can be the best medicine.

Look in the mirror and repeat these words, given to Black women by poet/playwright Ntozake Shange:

> *i found god in myself*
> *& i loved her*
> *i loved her fiercely*

Getting Help

As Black people we share a long legacy of keeping silent about our true feelings. During the slavery era our very survival often depended on our ability to "stay mum" and withstand the brutality we experienced every day. Generations of Blacks have bowed their heads and swallowed their pride rather than speak out about the indignities and oppression they have suffered at the hands of white racists. In short, masking our pain has helped us survive in a society that has done us great physical and emotional harm. Many of us grew up with the message that we should never let white people know what we are really thinking because they will use the knowledge against us. Moreover, Black women have historically kept emotional problems hidden from friends and family members so as not to be a "burden" to them.

Because you can still get up and go to work every morning or get the kids off to school, you may feel that you are coping well with the emotional difficulties in your life. And you should feel proud of yourself for being able to function in a society that gives us so many negative and distorted messages about Black women. But you should know that you can lay down your burdens if they get too heavy for you. There is nothing wrong with asking for help when you feel you can no longer cope with a bad relationship, work problems, family conflicts, et cetera.

Think about how you're *really* doing, and honestly assess whether you have any of these feelings or behavior:

- Inability to sleep
- Sadness
- Hopelessness
- Dejection
- Nervousness, anxiety
- Uncontrollable crying jags
- Thoughts of suicide
- Tiredness or other symptoms that have no medical explanation
- Excessive drinking or drug use
- Inability to make decisions or concentrate

If so, you many need to seek help. This does not mean that you are crazy or having a nervous breakdown. It simply means that you have been affected by the demands and pressures in your life. Therapy and other kinds of support services are nothing to be ashamed or afraid of. You owe it to yourself to get help.

What Therapy Can Do for You

Working with a trained mental-health professional can help alleviate some of the depression you may be feeling. Talking about your problems with an impartial person who does not hold any judgments about you or your behavior can lead you to understand yourself better and enable you to make the changes you'd like to make in your life.

For many Black women, therapy can be a stimulus for growth, change, and a reaffirmation of self-worth. Counseling creates a space for you to drop the mask of being a "strong Black woman" and gives you permission to express the truth about your fears, joys, worries, accomplishments, or frustrations.

Therapy can help you confront the emotional problems in your life and give you the tools to deal with them in a healthy, constructive manner. Sisters report that they have found counseling beneficial for a number of issues including eating disorders, substance abuse, incest, family conflicts, career decisions, skin-color concerns, grief, bad childhood experiences, rape, racism, struggles with sexuality, and relationship problems. If it is troubling *you,* there is no problem too big or too small to discuss with a trained mental-health expert.

Choosing a Therapist

Probably the best place to start your search for a caring, competent counselor is with other Black women. Ask friends and coworkers if they know a local therapist you might see. There are probably community mental-health agencies in your area that you can contact. Therapists affiliated with a nearby college or university should also be able to give you a referral.

Media images about psychotherapy have led many sisters to believe that the therapeutic process is one in which you pay a lot of money to lie on a couch and talk to a cold and distant white man. In fact, growing numbers of Black mental-health specialists are using therapeutic models based on the experience of African-descended people instead of those of the white establishment.

For instance, in Afrocentric therapy, the counselor seeks to help Black clients understand how our identity has been shaped by racism and then guides us toward alternative standards by which to measure our self-worth, according to Linda James Myers, Ph.D., an associate professor of Black Studies at Ohio State University and author of *Understanding of Afrocentric World View: Introduction to an Optimal Psychology.* "In a society that negates both Blackness and femaleness," Myers says, "Black women who adhere to the dominant cultural standards will always come up feeling inferior and deficient."

"In an Afrocentric approach to therapy, Black women are given tools to create a different frame of reference so they can see that they are intrinsically worthy," Dr. Myers explains, adding that for Black women, having the family involved is also an essential part of healing. "Primarily it's a spiritually based approach to counseling that teaches that all our experiences as Black women, both good and bad, are blessings that can lead us to greater understanding of ourselves. Your self-worth rises when you come to believe that you are being blessed in life instead of constantly beleaguered."

Most health-insurance plans cover some percentage of therapy costs, and many counselors offer a sliding scale based upon your income. You should check with your insurance provider to find out whether therapy is covered, what percentage, and what kind of therapists the company will pay for. In many companies employee-assistance programs provide counseling free of charge for workplace and other issues. For more information on therapy, especially Afrocentric therapy, see the articles "Healing with Therapy" (*Essence,* March 1992) and "A Guide to Psychotherapy" (*Essence,* June 1989).

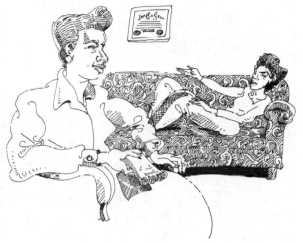

Talking to a qualified therapist can help solve problems. *(Drawing: Yvonne Buchanan)*

There is no best kind of therapist; you should choose based on who you feel comfortable with. Some sisters only feel comfortable talking to another Black woman. Others are okay with a Black person of either gender or a woman of any race. For others race and gender don't matter at all. You should consider how you feel about the race and gender of a therapist and choose according to your comfort level. Also, if you have a specific problem, you'll want to choose someone who specializes in that area, such as incest, relationships, or workplace issues.

There are several kinds of practitioners who specialize in emotional health. For a referral in your area, call the various professional organizations listed below.

Psychiatrists are licensed doctors who have completed medical school and undergone additional training in psychiatry. They are the only therapists who can legally prescribe drugs, and they are licensed by their state medical boards. It's important to note that some women steer clear of psychiatry because its tenets are based on a medical model and male orientation. Professional organizations: American Psychiatric Association, 1400 K St. NW, Washington, DC 20005; (202) 682-6000 (this group has a Committee of Black Psychiatrists that addresses issues concerning Black psychiatrists and patients; call 202-682-6096 for more information); and the Black Psychiatrists of America, 2730 Adeline St., Oakland, CA 94607; (510) 465-1800.

Psychologists hold graduate degrees from schools of psychology, education, and social science. Licensed psychologists must have a Ph.D., and they are licensed state by state. Many have expertise in the development and administration of psychological tests. Professional organizations: American Psychological Association, 750 First Street, NE, Washington, DC 20002-4242; (800) 374-2721 or (202) 336-5500; or the Association of Black Psychologists, P.O. Box 55999, Washington, DC 20040-5999; (202) 722-0808.

Social workers are trained in undergraduate programs and graduate schools of social work. They practice in a variety of settings including hospitals, clinics, schools, and community agencies. Many licensed clinical social workers set up their own private practices. Certified social workers are certified by state licensing services, but social workers can practice without certification. Professional organizations: National Association of Social Workers. You can call the national office located at 750 First St. NE, suite 700, Washington, DC 20002; 800-638-8799; or the National Association of Black Social Workers, 8436 W. McNichols Ave., Detroit, MI 48221; (313) 862-6700.

Certified psychoanalysts must have at least a master's degree and four years of training in an institute accredited by the National Association for the Advancement of Psychoanalysis (NAAP). But anyone can practice psychoanalysis without NAAP certification. Psychoanalysts provide intensive, long-term individual therapy that usually involves many sessions per week. Professional organization:

Your Absolute Rights As a Client

1. You have the right to expect complete confidentiality.

2. You have the right to report any therapist who abuses you sexually or otherwise to the agency in your state that regulates the profession. If you don't know whom to contact to report such abuse, ask a close friend or colleague to help you. Protect yourself and others by telling someone about your abuse.

3. You have the right to talk about your feelings without being ridiculed, put down, or patronized. Under no circumstances should you continue to see a therapist who criticizes or makes fun of the way you express yourself; who makes any inappropriate racial or sexual remarks; who forces you to try counseling techniques that make you uncomfortable; or who suggests that you use alcohol, drugs, or increased sexual activity to help you better cope with your emotional problems.

NAAP, 80 Eighth Ave., suite 1501, New York, NY 10011; (212) 741-0515.

Mental-health counselors must have at least a master's degree in mental health, clinical training, and several other requirements before they are eligible for membership in the National Academy of Certified Clinical Mental Health Counselors. Professional organization: American Mental Health Counselors' Association, 5999 Stevenson Ave., Alexandria, VA 22304; (800) 326-2642 or (703) 823-9800 ext. 383.

Marriage and family therapists have at least a master's degree in marriage and family therapy and two years' postgraduate training to belong to the American Association for Marriage and Family Therapy (AAMFT). Professional organization: AAMFT 1100 17th St. NW, Washington, DC 20036; (202) 452-0109. For referrals, call (800) 374-2638.

Certified pastoral counselors offer a spiritual angle to therapy and must have at least a master's of divinity degree and other qualifications before they can be certified by the American Association of Pastoral Counselors (AAPC). Professional organization: AAPC, 9504A Lee Highway, Fairfax, VA 22031; (703) 385-6967.

Questions to Ask

Once you determine which type of therapist you'd like to work with, you should prepare a checklist of questions before starting therapy. Here are some guidelines developed by Julia A. Boyd, a Black psychotherapist who practices in Seattle and author of *In the Company of My Sisters: Black Women and Self-Esteem:*

1. Interview, either by phone or in person, several therapists before making the choice. A counselor who declines or is reluctant to be interviewed is likely not to be sensitive to your needs.
2. Write down beforehand a list of questions to ask. Some examples of things you might want to find out include:
   Educational and professional background.
   Years of experience and practice.
   Knowledge of ethnic and cultural diversity and how the knowledge was obtained (for example, through schooling, living or working in communities of color, or working with people of color). You should ask these questions even if the person is Black.
   Professional fees.
   Cancellation policy.

Availability of a sliding scale.

Personal references.

Kinds of problems that person has treated. (Remember that you will be trusting this individual with private and personal information about yourself and that you have a right to know whom you are trusting.)

3. Evaluate your satisfaction with the counseling process. Trust your own feelings and comfort level with the therapist. If you are not pleased with your therapy or haven't met goals you've set for yourself, remember that you have the right to terminate therapy. Don't stay with someone who is not meeting your needs.

Psychiatric Disorders

Some emotional difficulties can be resolved with the support of a trusted friend or pastor or with the help of a competent psychotherapist. Participating in self-help support groups and practicing stress-reduction techniques can also ease emotional distress.

However, those who are suffering from the emotional pain that mental illnesses can cause require psychotherapy, appropriate medication, or a combination of both in order to feel good again.

The symptoms of mental disorders can be mild, moderate, or severe. Most people with mild or moderate degrees of depression, for example, can still fulfill their job and family responsibilities. But those whose illness is severe usually cannot work or socialize at all.

Scientific research is beginning to yield findings that certain mental disorders—such as depressive illnesses, panic disorder, and schizophrenia—run in families. This suggests a possible biological factor in these conditions. To further support the theory that mental disorders have a biological link, people suffering from these serious illnesses improve substantially or completely when they receive proper medication.

For the most part, mental disorders are equal-opportunity illnesses; they occur at the same rates in Blacks as whites. And just as mental disorders affect both groups equally, effective treatments are available for those who seek help, regardless of race or gender.

Many people, however, suffer needlessly because they fear that others would think of them as "crazy" if they were to seek out the help of a mental-health professional or take a prescribed medication for their condition. In fact, studies show that only one in three people with depression seek help for the illness. When not in treatment for their disorders, people with severe depressive illnesses or schizophrenia are at great risk of hurting themselves or killing others.

When properly diagnosed and treated, however, people almost always get better or become well again. With effective treatment, people with illnesses such as severe depression, bipolar affective disorder, or schizophrenia can lead relatively normal and rewarding lives.

Some of the most common psychiatric disorders follow.

Anxiety Disorders

These are the most common types of psychiatric disorders, affecting 10 percent of the population or 18 million people and striking women twice as often as men. Though everyone feels anxious from time to time, extreme, persistent worry is the core symptom in anxiety disorders. *Phobia* is the most common type, and some studies show that phobias are more common in Blacks than in non-Blacks. A phobia is an intense fear reaction to an object or an event that carries little or no danger. For example, some phobias include unwarranted fear of crowds, heights, tunnels, elevators, or public humiliation. *Agoraphobia* (officially defined as "fear of the marketplace") is the most disabling phobia; some people with this problem become so fearful and panic-stricken that they never leave their homes.

Though less common than phobias, another type of anxiety disorder—*panic disorder*—can be extremely debilitating, affecting every area of life. No one is quite sure what causes its hallmark symptom, known as a panic attack—a sudden feeling of extreme anxiety and the racing heartbeat and breathlessness that come with it. While some sufferers find that stress triggers a panic attack, others can't predict when it will happen. Some describe a panic attack as "the feeling that someone put a gun to my head." Others say it feels like a heart attack. In fact, many sufferers end up going from doctor to doctor in search of a cure for the physical symptoms that go along with an attack.

Panic disorder is diagnosed when four panic attacks occur in a four-week period (or one attack occurs with one month of sustained fear of having another). Panic-attack symptoms must include at least four of the following:

- Sweating
- Shortness of breath
- Heart palpitations
- Chest discomfort
- Unsteady feelings
- Choking or smothering sensations
- Tingling

- Hot or cold flashes
- Faintness
- Trembling
- Nausea or abdominal distress
- Feelings of unreality
- Fears of losing control, dying, or going insane

If you have a number of these symptoms and cannot find a medical explanation for them, you may be suffering from panic disorder—especially if you've been under a lot of stress. Seek the help of a qualified mental-health expert as soon as possible. Lifestyle changes and brief psychotherapy may be all you need. In some cases, people with panic disorder may need medication.

For more information, see "Is It Stress?" (*Essence,* April 1992), which offers helpful analysis from two African-American experts in panic disorder, Carl Bell, M.D., of Chicago and Freda C. Lewis-Hall, M.D., of Washington, D.C.; or contact Anxiety Disorders Association of America, 6000 Executive Blvd., suite 513, Rockville, MD 20852; (301) 231-9350. You can also call (800) 64-PANIC to receive a free brochure on panic disorder.

Two other kinds of anxiety disorders are worth mentioning. *Post-Traumatic stress disorder (PTSD)* is a recurrent reaction to a psychologically traumatic event. Though it is often linked to soldiers suffering the affects of war, PTSD is actually more common in women than in men. For example, women who have been raped, beaten, or abused (as either children or adults) sometimes complain of common PTSD symptoms—sleeplessness, anxiety, nightmares, reexperiencing of the traumatic event, and emotional numbness. PTSD may also develop after other emotional traumas, such as car accidents, earthquakes, and sudden loss of loved ones.

Obsessive-compulsive disorder (OCD) is an anxiety disorder marked by repetitive thoughts and behaviors that are difficult if not impossible to control. Though this problem affects Blacks and whites equally, some experts believe that the problem may go unrecognized and untreated in African-Americans. OCD sufferers often feel compelled to perform certain tasks or rituals over and over even though they know that the behavior makes no sense. Two of the most common OCD rituals are washing and checking the hands. A sufferer may have an excessive fear of contamination (the obsession) and wash her or his hands many, many times a day (the compulsion). Other typical compulsions in OCD suf-

We had seen it coming on since Christmas. It started with my grandmother's compulsive need to talk about God and death. Her eyes would soften, and a surrender would wash across her face. "Honey," she would confide, "God says it won't be long before I slip into darkness and become the next Christ."

This wasn't her first brush with mental illness. Grandma had long been on antipsychotic medications to help control her occasional delusions and trips in and out of reality. She visited a psychiatrist once a month and managed to be highly functional. She'd sometimes talk craziness, but usually we'd change the subject or refuse to speak about God, and she'd snap back.

But now something was different. The usual distractions didn't work, and she just didn't seem like my usual vivacious, sassy Grandma, who loved to talk about sex and celebrities. Now she was obsessed and livid when we refused to discuss her health complaints or her death. New psychiatrists and different medication were only somewhat effective.

In a few months, my parents were getting calls at all hours from my grandmother, who believed there was a drug conspiracy on her nice, middle-class block. My mother, father, and I were beginning to feel annoyed, frustrated, and angry. Why was this happening to her, and more personally, why was she doing this to us? I didn't even like visiting her or being around her at all. Finally she began a religious ceremony that involved lighting matches. We all feared she was losing ground and could put herself in serious danger so, reluctantly, we had her admitted to a hospital.

I went to visit her, and she would tell me that she feared for her life and was protecting the family with her feet. Listening to this gibberish, I felt such loss; I just wanted my grandmother back. Where was the woman who chastised her friends for hiding their age and put on her Reeboks to walk three miles in under an hour? Where was my sassy grandmother who had gently reminded me to have safe sex?

I asked myself over and over how this could happen to a woman whose strength had helped her fight her way through the humiliation of the racist South, and who always found humor in life, even through a divorce and the death of her second husband. As if being an African-American woman in this country wasn't enough, now she battled imagined demons.

It took her a month to recover, and after a series of tests she began to stabilize and then improve dramatically. With new medication and a new psychiatrist, she was released from the hospital. Though she still talks about God too much, she is much better, and I no longer feel annoyed and angry at her. I have vowed to be more patient and understanding, because she can't help what she feels. I'm just relieved to have Grandma back.

"I felt such loss; I just wanted my grandmother back."

—ALLISON ABNER, WRITER AND TV PRODUCER, NEW YORK CITY

ferers are to repeatedly check to make sure their doors are locked and to continuously arrange items such as folded clothes.

Affective Disorders

These disorders of mood strike 6.3 percent of the population or 11.6 million people. Two types of affective disorders are *major depression* and *bipolar disorder* (also known as *manic-depressive illness*). Major depression strikes women twice as often as men, and bipolar disorder affects women and men equally.

Though everyone feels down or blue from time to time, major depression is much more serious. It is a debilitating illness that can lead to suicide. The National Foundation for Depressive Illness offers this self-test to determine whether you or a loved one may be suffering from major depression:

I feel extremely sad all or most of the time.

I seem to have no energy.

I've lost interest in most of the activities I used to enjoy.

I sleep much more (or less) than usual.

I eat much more (or less) than usual.

I have trouble concentrating, remembering, and making decisions.

I feel hopeless about the future.

I feel worthless.

I feel anxious.

I think about death and suicide.

If you have symptoms like these and they have persisted for at least two weeks, seek therapeutic help.

People who suffer from bipolar disorder endure dramatic and unpredictable mood swings that can go from euphoric elation to deep depression. During manic episodes, the sufferer may experience delusions or hallucinations and may exhibit bizarre behavior. The plunge into depression can give sufferers such overwhelming feelings of despair and hopelessness that they may be at risk for suicide.

Schizophrenia

Sometimes called borderline personality disorder, this is a complex mental illness with a variety of symptoms including delusions (sometimes paranoid), auditory or visual hallucinations, rambling speech patterns, and increasingly erratic and incoherent behavior. People suffering from schizophrenia often report hearing "voices" that instruct them to behave in abnormal ways. In the most advanced stages of the disease, people with schizophrenia lose touch with reality and turn inward to a world of fantasies and obsessions that prevent them from carrying on a normal life.

If you or a loved one are experiencing symptoms of any of these psychiatric disorders, seek immediate treatment from a local mental health treatment center, private mental-health professional, or your family doctor. In the case of a severe mental illness, a psychiatrist's help may be necessary, because the patient may require medication.

For specific information about these disorders, contact the American Psychiatric Association, Public Affairs Office, 1400 K St. NW, Washington, DC 20005; (202) 682-6142. The group has very detailed pamphlets in its "Let's Talk Facts About . . ." series and will send sample copies free of charge.

For More Information

ORGANIZATIONS

DEPRESSION AWARENESS, RECOGNITION, AND TREATMENT PROGRAM, Department GL, room 10-85, 5600 Fishers Lane, Rockville, MD 20857; (800) 421-4211. The recording on the 800 number provides information on how to get help for clinical depression. Call (800) 64-PANIC for information on panic disorders. This organization is a part of the National Institute of Mental Health listed below.

NATIONAL ALLIANCE FOR THE MENTALLY ILL, 2101 Wilson Blvd., suite 302, Arlington, VA 22201; (703) 524-7600. First-time callers can reach volunteer-operated help line at (800) 950 NAMI.

NATIONAL FOUNDATION FOR DEPRESSIVE ILLNESS, INC., P.O. Box 2257, New York, NY 10116; (800) 248-4344 or (212) 268-4260. The 800 number has a recorded list of the symptoms of depression and information on how to get help.

NATIONAL INSTITUTE OF MENTAL HEALTH, INFORMATION, RESOURCES AND INQUIRIES BRANCH, Parklawn Bldg., room 7C-02, 5600 Fishers Lane, Rockville, MD 20857; (301) 443-4513. Contact this division for help with inquiries about any aspect of mental health.

NATIONAL MENTAL HEALTH ASSOCIATION, 1021 Prince St., 3rd floor, Alexandria, VA 22314-2971; (800) 969-6642 or (703) 684-7722. Call for referrals or free written materials on depression and the warning signs of mental illness.

BOOKS

Chain Chain Change: For Black Women Dealing with Physical and Emotional Abuse, Evelyn C. White, Seal Press, 1985.

The Consumer's Guide to Psychotherapy, Jack Engler and Daniel Goleman, Simon & Schuster, 1992.

The Dance of Anger, Harriet G. Lerner, Harper & Row, 1985.

Gender and Stress, Rosalind Barnett et al., eds., Free Press, 1987.

Getting Up When You're Feeling Down: A Woman's Guide to Overcoming and Preventing Depression, Harriet Braiker, G. P. Putnam, 1990.

Psychological Storms: The African American Struggle for Identity, Thomas A. Parham, African American Images (Chicago), 1993.

Silencing the Self: Women and Depression, Dana C. Jack, Harvard University Press, 1991.

Sisters of the Yam: Black Women and Self-Recovery, bell hooks, South End Press (Boston), 1993.

Too Good for Her Own Good: Breaking Free from the Burden of Female Responsibility, Claudia Bepko and Joann Krestan, HarperCollins, 1990.

Trusting Ourselves: The Sourcebook on Psychology for Women, Karen Johnson and Tom Ferguson, Atlantic Monthly Press, 1990.

Women, Race and Class, Angela Y. Davis, Random House, 1983.

Understanding of Afrocentric World View: Introduction to an Optimal Psychology, Linda James Myers, Kendall/Hunt Publishing Company (Dubuque, Iowa), 1988.

22

The Self-Help Revolution

I n living rooms, kitchens, community centers, and church basements, in cities such as Atlanta, New York, Detroit, Los Angeles, Philadelphia, Oakland, and Washington, sisters gather in small groups just to talk. What ties these women together is a common theme: They are all sick and tired of being sick and tired, and they come together to do something about it. In these self-help groups Black women learn how to cope with health issues in ways that are most valuable and meaningful— through the real-life experiences of their sisters.

Chances are you've heard about these meetings or others like them, because a lot of sisters have started going to self-help groups of all kinds. Women sit in circles and talk about a concern they have in common; the topic might be parenting, weight control, addiction, or depression. These meetings differ from the kind we usually attend; there is no president or real authority figure, no one takes minutes, and the business is very personal. Each person listens intently as another talks about her life predicament, to which everyone seems able to relate. Heads nod, murmured "uh-huhs" punctuate the testimony, and there's so much hugging. One hears over and over: "Sister, I know just how you feel!" At the end, members thank one another for sharing intimate details of their lives.

The National Black Women's Health Project's self-help network is part of a broader self-help movement, a spiritual revolution in America that is attracting larger and larger numbers of women of all colors. Self-help, or mutual support groups, as they are called, focus on how members cope with significant life predicaments and the wisdom gained in the process. Scholars estimate that today between seven and twelve million Americans, primarily women, participate in self-help support groups.

These groups provide one more option to check out when you need help coping with a problem or would like to enhance your support system. Given the complexity of modern living, professional services will never be adequate to take care of this enormous need. Some social scientists predict that by the turn of the century self-help groups will be the favored method of delivering mental-health services in America.

Working through tough interpersonal issues together in groups strengthens the social fabric of our communities. The group functions like a miniature mental-health democracy where free expression is encouraged, as long as it does not unfairly pain another. A good self-help group is easy to join, empowers members, and costs very little money.

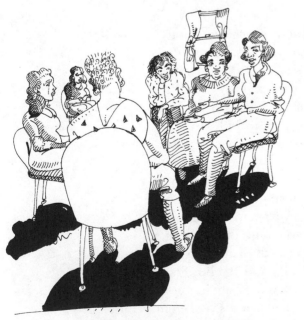

Self-help support groups provide a nonjudgmental forum for sharing feelings. *(Drawing: Yvonne Buchanan)*

Sisters in Self-Help

Talking about our health issues in groups provides a framework for understanding why Black women have poorer health status than other women. As we talk about lifestyles and confront the realities of being both Black and female in America, we bring personal awareness to impersonal statistical data.

In self-help groups we put our problems in perspective, so we can support one other to take responsibility for those parts of our lives that only we can change. Group members offer one another affirmations and encouragement to be healthier. We learn that it's okay to take care of ourselves first.

Whether in a formal self-help group like a chapter of the National Black Women's Health Project or in a tiny, informal mutual support trio, we can undertake the work to

I ran to Houston almost thirteen years ago when my marriage became unbearable. With two young daughters, I was determined to start a new life. I decided to open a travel agency. Things were going pretty good when a routine medical checkup ended with a recommendation that I have a hysterectomy.

My doctors assured me that I'd be in the hospital for three to four days and then recovering at home for another four to six weeks. It was hard to ask my mother to come and be with us at home, but I did and she agreed. We were all shocked when the surgery resulted in a thirty-day hospitalization, the first ten days of which were in intensive care. The physical recovery was much longer than anticipated, straining relations with my family. The emotional recovery was a lonely journey fraught with feelings of abandonment, blame, and guilt. I was barely back on my feet when my ten-year-old daughter was diagnosed with a tumor growing on her skull.

Putting my own needs aside, I sought a specialist in whom I had complete confidence. Three surgeries in an eighteen-month period were traumatic for my child and for me. After the second surgery, my daughter's teacher and I both noticed that her walking seemed awkward and difficult. The neurologist assured me her recovery was progressing as expected and I was probably "smothering her with too much attention." A third surgery was necessary to remove the rest of the tumor mass that was imbedded in her skull. This surgery took much longer than the previous ones. In the recovery room, I learned that my daughter was paralyzed from the waist down.

Angry, frightened, and confused, I again sought comfort from family members. My daughter's father heaped blame on me for proceeding with the surgery and refused to come to Houston to visit her. A kindly nurse in the hospital suggested another consultation with a different doctor. This new doctor examined my daughter, her X rays and medical records. He confirmed my earlier suspicions that she was not responding well to the treatments. He suspected the increased doses of anesthesia administered during the third surgery had caused the paralysis. He thought my earlier concerns with her walking should have been taken as a warning signal and treated more seriously. In time, he believed, she would return to normal.

As my daughter's physical condition improved, my emotional state worsened. Consumed with fear and self-blame and exhausted from the round-the-clock care a paralyzed child requires, I literally fell apart as soon as she was able to return to school. Each day I arose, got the children off to school, and returned to my darkened room, where I spent the day in seclusion. I got dressed in time to greet them when they returned in the afternoon. Knowing

"In my family asking for help was a sign of weakness. It never occurred to me that other people could help me with these serious problems."

—FLORETTA MORRIS, SELF-EMPLOYED, HOUSTON

I needed help but fearful that professional care would result in additional problems, I managed to get out one day and go to the library. There I found a flyer announcing a group that offered emotional well-being through a self-help method of "will training." Recovery Inc., I learned, was started by a psychiatrist back in the 1930s to help patients with mental illnesses who could not afford the time or the cost of psychoanalysis. He worked with lay people to perfect the methods and then, in the early fifties, turned the organization over to its members. Now, led by its members, the organization has hundreds of chapters.

At first I went several times a week. It was the commitment to the group that motivated me to get dressed and get out. Gradually, I noticed my spirits lifting, and I could accomplish more tasks each day. The Recovery method taught me how to spot the myriad daily frustrations in life and to deal with them. I stopped holding in all my feelings and learned that other people benefited when I talked about my success in handling a problem.

Recovery really worked for me. I still attend meetings in Houston, and whenever I travel I seek out meetings in other cities. In my family asking for help was a sign of weakness. It never occurred to me that other people could help me with these serious problems. But Recovery has given me the family I never had and taught me the value of emotional support in meeting the challenges of everyday life.

To find out more about Recovery Inc. or to find a chapter in your area, call (312) 337-5667.

improve our health. In groups we can learn how to meditate, stop smoking, exercise, relax, and even to find ways to be alone with ourselves and not be lonely. We can practice how to push away from the dinner table, sleep on an empty stomach, and tell people our true feelings without experiencing deprivation or fear. A caring sister from a support group will go with you for a mammogram more readily than to a bar for a drink. Many of us who grew up too fast have found unconditional acceptance in our self-help groups with other girlfriends who like to play. Instead of sucking up all that anger and repressing our joy, we learn how to exhale and allow our real selves a chance to come out.

In NBWHP self-help groups, Black women are encouraged to help one another take charge of their lives and support these changes once they occur. Activities/behaviors to facilitate control include:

Helping sisters see options that reflect taking control of their lives. This may mean suggesting alternatives that reflect an active, purposeful orientation.

Supporting sisters who make active, purposeful decisions and carry them through.

Supporting women who take healthy risks as they attempt to make changes in their lives.

Encouraging women to look at their lives and decisions critically so that they can make changes.

Appreciating and supporting women so that they believe they are worthy of taking charge of their lives and moving toward wellness.

Finding a Group That's Right for You

There is a self-help group for almost every human problem, especially emotional problems, physical disorders, and diseases. There are groups for the bereaved, for parents of children with head injuries, for children with cancer and for their families, for incest and child-abuse survivors, for adult children of alcoholics, for workaholics, and for people who have been victimized by the medical system. (To find a group in your community, see "For More Information" at the end of this chapter.) When facing a critical life situation, it's important to remember that you are not alone. Many others who have faced a similar predicament will provide emotional company on your journey.

Prospective members need to assess their reasons for joining a group and then do a little research to select the right one. Think about the kind of group to join, what you want to accomplish in a group, and how much time you have for meetings and related activities. Don't think that a self-help group is a place to go and unload all your concerns in one or two meetings and that's that. Mutual support and the willingness to share responsibility for the group with other members and to give back to the group are important self-help traditions. In order for groups to grow and thrive, they must rely on members who are willing to both give and get. If you only want information or short-term counseling, it might be more efficient to pursue another form of help. It is appropriate, however, to visit a group and observe how it works to help to decide whether the group is right for you.

Once you have a few groups to check out, make a list of questions you'd like answered. Call the group contact person or visit the group and get answers to those questions before agreeing to join. Some of the factors that help prospective members decide on a group include:

Time and place of meeting. Is it convenient and safe? Is the environment conducive to my personal needs?

Cost. Self-help groups are generally free, charge low dues, or rely on unregulated contributions of members. The group determines what the money collected is used for. If a fee for service is collected or the costs exceed $6 per meeting, the group may not be a real self-help group.

Meeting format. What are the opening and closing rituals of the group? What are the methods for exchanging information and supporting members? Are members required to speak, give testimony, present information? Make sure the meeting format matches your needs.

Traditions. What practices has the group developed to support members? Are there opportunities, special ceremonies, or ways of relating to group members that promote bonding? Is there hugging and touching? Are these traditions comfortable for you?

Leadership and decision making. Is one person responsible for the leadership duties, or are they shared among group members? How are decisions made and carried out? Do these practices seem reasonable to you?

Responsibilities of members. What do members do at each meeting? Set up the room? Bring refreshments? Lead the discussion? Collect the dues? Select the topics for discussion? Tell their stories? Find out what is really expected of each member.

A candid discussion with the group contact person or a couple of members will assist you in determining whether this is the right group for you. Be sure to think about and explain what you want to get from the group and identify any expectations that make you feel uncomfortable. It's okay to tell the group leader that you don't like to talk a lot or that you prefer not to be touched by strangers. A good group leader or facilitator, as they are often called, will be very explicit with you and help you get to know everything about the group.

Getting the Most from a Self-Help Group

A self-help group is more meaningful when we have the communication skills to help others and to get the help we're seeking. The peer-helper relationship challenges us to take risks, to be honest with ourselves and others, to trust and be trusted, and to take responsibility for making the group environment psychologically safe. Each person accepts responsibility to maintain an environment that is free of criticism, condemnation, and judgment that unfairly hurts others. The group members must outline what the acceptable behaviors are within group meetings and between group members.

Typical group guidelines are:

- Start on time and end on time.
- What gets said in the room stays in the room.
- One person at a time speaks.
- No cross talk.
- No blaming or judging.

For many of us, neither the families we come from, the jobs we work at, nor our relationships operate under these kinds of guidelines. The new ways of interacting and communicating in a self-help group may be overwhelming initially. Ask a seasoned member to help you, or form a buddy relationship with another member who is willing to show you the ropes. The same self-help centers that give information about groups often have workshops to introduce newcomers to self-help. In these experiential-learning settings, you will learn about the following concepts:

"I" Statements. Personal self-disclosure and ownership of the ideas that you bring to the group are more easily understood if you say "I think" or "I believe" or "I want" as opposed to "people think" or "everyone believes" or "we all want."

Active listening. The ability to focus all your attention on the speaker. To hear with your ears, your heart, and your mind. Try to put yourself in the speaker's place and feel her experience.

Helpful responding. Letting the person talking know you understand what she is saying, how she actually feels. Stay with the speaker until she has finished, without interrupting, preempting, or interpreting her remarks. A simple, "me too" disclosure is the most powerful form of support.

Wait time. Letting five seconds elapse before responding. Use the silence to stay focused on what you heard. It prevents crowding the speaker and interruptions.

Silence. Make good use of longer periods of silence. Do not push to verbalize every thought or feeling. Allow lots of open spaces in meetings.

Avoiding giving advice. In self-help groups, members talk about their experiences rather than telling others what they "should" do. The lessons learned by others inform our own decisions.

Self-help group meetings are bound to touch you in ways that produce powerful emotional responses. Regular attendance at meetings helps to modulate the emotional ups and downs that may accompany

> *"Finding Black women who offered me unconditional acceptance and a willingness to listen was like discovering gold."*
>
> —Joyce Jones Guinyard, chiropractor, Los Angeles

People look at me and think I have it all; nothing could possibly be missing in my life. I'm a successful professional, married with two sons and a happy family life. As a health-care professional, I have considerable information about maintaining my health and well-being, but as a Black woman I have a lot of pain about the losses in my life. It took me a long time to acknowledge that pain and to take the steps to recover from those losses.

I attended the National Black Women's Health Project conference in California in 1992. These wonderful women, whom I did not personally know, greeted me with open arms, firm hugs, affirmations, and joy. "Sister, welcome! I'm so glad you are here." Many times during the weekend that was said to me; people seemed to really care about my feelings. I wanted to keep that experience with me. When I found out there were no active self-help group meetings in my community, I decided to start one. Since my needs actually included getting more emotional support as well as physical exercise in my life, I ended up starting two groups.

Growing up in a family with five siblings, I realized, shaped my responses to many situations in later life. I was a quiet child who never got in trouble. I liked to read, had firm goals from my earliest years, and worked hard to do well in school. Consequently, my parents gave me less attention than my sisters and brother who always seemed to demand more. I watched in silence as they acted out. Even today my family calls on me for medical advice and other kinds of help, which I don't mind giving. But they never feel like I have needs, too. Rarely does anyone call and ask, "Can I do something for you today?" I know they care, but we didn't learn how to express appreciation and validate each other as children. Finding Black women who offered me unconditional acceptance and a willingness to listen was like discovering gold.

One group meets monthly. There are eight members, and we rotate meetings at each other's homes. Whoever's house the meeting is in is the facilitator for the meeting that night. Another member volunteers to be the group's secretary. So my role in the group is manageable; the last thing I want is to be totally responsible for a whole group of women. At our meetings we talk about our lives in real ways that we often don't do with our partners, family members, and colleagues.

One night, I only wanted to cry. My group understood and did not pressure me to talk. After the meeting, I was able to tell another sister what was making me sad. I was feeling a lot of guilt around my mother's death and also a lot of anger toward her. It took about an hour for me to wind my way back through the story of my mother's death and its effect on me. Being a *health professional, I felt like I should have been at her side in the hospital. I left to get a few hours' respite and to look after my family. She died while I was away, and that weighs very heavily on my heart. Also I had wanted to tell my mother about my feelings growing up. I wanted her to know how neglected I felt and how unfair it was for other children to get such a disproportionate share of the attention in our family. I felt stuck in our relationship and wanted to get those feelings out of the way so we could be closer before she died. Unfortunately, that didn't happen.*

In talking this through with another self-helper, I learned how the forgiveness I sought could still be attained. After listening intently to me for a long time, my new friend told me about similar feelings she had when her father died. Part of her grieving included writing him letters, having "long talks" as if he were there, and forgiving him for his neglect. She was able to put herself in her father's place and try to understand the situation from his point of view. They "agreed" to forgive each other. Knowing that my feelings weren't silly and that others had worked through similar difficulties provided some immediate relief. I'm learning to be more gentle with me, to stop being so hard on myself.

the experience of "feeling your feelings." Just like aerobics, the emotional exercise of mutual support requires certain preparation, active participation working at your own pace, and a cooldown before leaving the meeting. Breath work and relaxation are good preparation; arriving early and chatting with others before the meeting will help you make the transition into the group easily. Most group meetings have a quiet meditation, song, or closing ritual to help members get some closure before leaving.

Sometimes there are difficulties in groups. Here are some potential problems:

Breaking trust or confidentiality

Arguing

One member monopolizes the group

One member constantly judges or puts down others

The facilitator and other members must identify and work together to solve group problems such as these. Talking honestly to one another—with group guidelines and ground rules in mind—helps.

What happens when a sister feels it is time for her to leave the group and move on? For any number of reasons, members will eventually decide to leave because they have attained the goals they set for themselves or they are not getting what they want from the group. Leaving the group can be difficult for both the woman leaving and the other members. The following NBWHP guidelines can help members deal with departures:

Members need to accept what the leaving member perceives as real.

Members should not try to convince her that it is wrong to leave.

Each member needs to have equal time for response to the leaving member.

Leaving the group needs to be viewed as a positive, strengthening step and experienced by the entire group in an empowering way. Some groups may want to have a celebration, party, dinner, or ceremony to mark this event. This can be a time to let a sister know how special she is, how much she has enriched the lives of other members, and how much she will be missed.

If a group isn't right for you, that doesn't mean you should give up on the self-help process. Try seeking another group instead.

For More Information

ORGANIZATIONS

Throughout this book, we offer information about self-help groups that focus on particular areas.

A CIRCLE OF SISTERS, 405 W. 147th St., New York, NY 10031; (212) 459-4806. Ask for a copy of *Conscious Connections,* a directory of Black women's support circles.

THE NATIONAL BLACK WOMEN'S HEALTH PROJECT, 1237 Ralph David Abernathy Blvd. SW, Atlanta, GA 30310; (800) ASK-BWHP. NBWHP maintains a national network of self-help groups as well as international groups in Kenya, Belize, Barbados, Nigeria, Canada, and Brazil. Call to find a group near you or to learn how to start a chapter in your area.

THE NATIONAL SELF-HELP CLEARINGHOUSE, 25 W. 43rd St., room 620, New York, NY 10036; (212) 354-8525. Call for a referral to a regional clearinghouse of self-help support groups in your area.

23

The Healing Power
of Spirituality

We are a spiritual people. The unseen, omnipresent force that is a part of all of us and all of us are a part of provides us strength and comfort. For some people the spirit is God or Allah, for others it is sistermother, and for still others it is simply Spirit. Having strong spiritual ties can help us stay healthy. Just as we must keep our minds and bodies nourished, we must feed our spiritual sides through prayer, meditation, and ritual.

Spirituality has been a part of African tradition since long before the birth of Christianity. According to *Black Women in Antiquity,* edited by Ivan Van Sertima, Neith, a goddess worshipped by North Africans, can be traced back to 4000 B.C. Ancient Egyptians worshipped Hathor, the moon goddess, among other Black female deities. She was both the donor of life and the protector of the dead. She was also regarded as the goddess of sensuality and was strongly linked with dance, song, and music.

Our Africans ancestors who were taken against their will to the New World brought their ancient religions with them and adapted them to the dictates of American Christianity. Some of them clung to the old

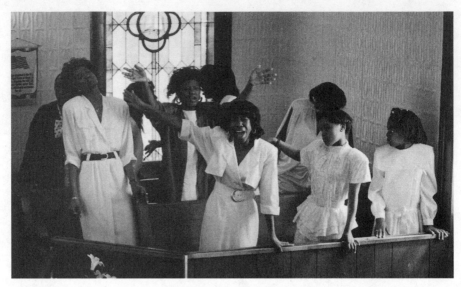

The J. Patterson Choir of the Progressive Baptist Church in New York City expresses spiritual joy through music.
(Photo: Marilyn Nance)

ways, taking the African religions underground. Deprived of our talking drums, spirituals became our new secret code.

Steal away, steal away, steal away to Jesus,
Steal away, steal away home,
I ain't got long to stay here.

The master might have thought slaves were singing of freedom in the great hereafter, but we were dealing with more pragmatic matters: Freedom in the here and now—with the help of Jesus, of course.

Our slave foremothers used spirituality as a tool against oppression. The church gave us the forum for using that strength to fight back. Dr. Martin Luther King, Jr., the Reverend Jesse Jackson, and many other men and women have turned the pulpit into a political platform to demand justice. And we don't have to look any further than the example of Malcolm X to see the power of spirituality to transform.

As sisters, we've been the backbone of Black spirituality. Strong women such as Mary McLeod Bethune, Fannie Lou Hamer, and Septima Clark relied on the power of the spirit to force a change in the landscape of African-American lives.

How Spirituality Fits into Your Life

Spirituality is a rock to hang on to when the world is rushing out of control. It is the unseen force that gives you the courage to push when you'd much rather pull. It shows the way when it seems there is no way. It makes sense out of nonsense and encourages you to have faith—help is just around the corner.

It's the balm that soothes and heals your inner wounds. With spirituality, you rest easy knowing that whatever ails you, enrages you, troubles you, or gets on your last nerve, this too shall pass. It's the map to inner peace on a road that never ends. And it ain't just about being deep.

Spirituality makes you leave the pity party. It lightens you up. All of a sudden, you find that you are laughing at yourself. Laughing with yourself. And with others. Even when it hurts. Simply put, feeling the spirit brings you joy.

And as countless sisters who have gone before you and who are living it every day will testify, spirit is the salve needed to heal and transform. Here's how three Black women find sustenance through spirituality:

Like most parents, New Jersey children's book publisher Cheryl Willis Hudson fretted as she watched her teenage daughter come of age. Life seemed to move a lot faster than when she was a teenager growing up in Virginia during the civil rights era. Back then her greatest struggle was trying to get a library card at the local (segregated) library. Today, it seemed, the challenges facing her daughter, Katura, and other young people were much greater. For one thing, there was so much pressure to be sexually active at an earlier age. And then there was the ever-increasing violence in the community.

Cheryl wanted to make sure that Katura had the tools she needed to make a graceful entry into womanhood. The more she talked to other African-American mothers of teenage girls, she saw that she was not alone in her fears. "It's a quantum leap from childhood to the things you're expected to know as teenagers and grown people," says Cheryl. "All of us had been influenced by sixties activism. We wanted to pass some of that enthusiasm and excitement on to our daughters. We asked ourselves 'What are we going to do to help these children? They're going to be women. How do we help them to grow up to be decent human beings?'"

The seven mothers decided to create a rite-of-passage ceremony for their daughters similar to the ones performed in some African societies. To prepare themselves and the girls, they organized monthly seminars in topics ranging from self-esteem to careers to African crafts. Sometimes the girls met separately; at other times mothers and daughters learned together. The young people were a little reluctant at first. "They looked at it like it was some 'African thing' their parents were forcing them to

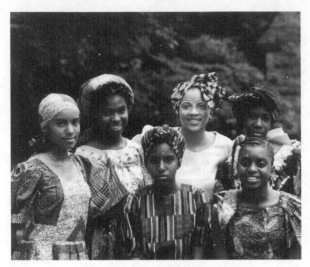

Cheryl Willis Hudson's daughter, Katura, and her friends on the day of their coming-of-age ritual ceremony. *(Photo: Dee Watts-Jones)*

do," Cheryl recalls. "It was like, 'Why do you have to be so Black?' But we wanted to pass on some information, fill in some spots for things we thought we were missing in our own relationships with our daughters. And ours was a struggle to always connect it to an African-American perspective."

The night before their final ceremony, the girls spent the night together. Since they were making a formal break from girlhood, the idea was to put them in confinement so that they could bond as sisters. Cheryl didn't see fourteen-year-old Katura at all until the next day. At the ceremony, both mothers and daughters wore African dress; the girls wore their braided hair tightly wrapped in African headdresses. Later, to symbolize their passage into womanhood, they slowly unraveled their wraps. There was drumming and dancing. To represent the African custom of orally passing down one's heritage, a griot (storyteller) offered libations to honor the ancestors, and a minister recited traditional prayers. As the proud mothers introduced their daughters, each girl went through a "rebirth," traveling through a birth-canal line formed by both mothers and daughters. They emerged at the end, born-again women.

"We all shouted and sang and ate a whole bunch of food," says Cheryl. "I think I came a little closer to understanding myself and looking at my daughter in another light. It forced me to see her as an individual. Parents tend to always see their offspring as children. But this was a wonderful opportunity to see her grow. The tables were kind of turned. It gave me an opportunity to form a spiritual bond with other women my age. It was really a unifying experience."

Anita Beard is a nun. Growing up Catholic, even at the tender age of seven, Anita knew she would be a nun. Her parents hoped she'd outgrow the idea. In high school, she did the normal teenage things: She dated, went to the prom, hung out with her friends. But as soon as she graduated from high school, she left town and joined a Pennsylvania convent, confident that she was ready to take on the vows of chastity, poverty, and obedience. Anita loved convent life. She cherished the daily ritual of

Before I embraced the spiritual life, I battled with confusion and depression. I went back and forth in a real tug of war: I knew I wanted spirituality in my life, but I didn't know what kind. I experimented with a lot of different religions. I went to Jewish synagogues. I danced in the street with the Hare Krishnas. I even joined an Egyptian temple in St. Louis.

In 1973 I went through a transformation. I was pregnant at the time, and when I went into labor, it was for twenty-three long, hard hours. Within twelve hours the baby died. In a period of less than two days, I knew what it was to really, really struggle to bring life forth. To look upon it with all its magnificence and then see the power of death take that away. It shook me profoundly. I did not want to be here on this planet. I became suicidal. I felt like, I don't have to do this existence; I can take myself out.

I took a handful of pills. But instead of dying, I had an out-of-body experience. I saw myself leaving my body and sitting up on the ceiling. I was having a debate with myself. And then I was shown images of things that would occur in my life. The message was: It's time to change the program. Cut the crap and grow up. I knew I had to live the best kind of life I could in this lifetime.

As I embarked on my spiritual recovery, I embraced Yoruba, an ancient African religion that believes in ancestor reverence and nature worship. The tradition came over here with the slave trade. It survived, despite the oppressors' attempt to make us over in their Christian image.

In Yoruba, we believe that humankind experiences God on two levels: The visible—creation and proof of the existence of a Creator—and the transcendent or invisible force. So we worship and respect Nature, the physical and visible.

We also revere our ancestors, those whose earthly conduct was good for the community. We have access to those who have gone before us. They are here to help us—if we let them. Each day when I get up, I salute the ancestors. I give thanks for my mind and body. I speak to the altars I've set up in my house, and I ask for my share of ache for the day. Ache is the power that runs all things, the power to positively affect changes.

I believe in a real spirituality that is about how you live and not how you don't live. With a lot of traditional Western religions, we're taught that being on this earth is a curse. You know, hurry up and go to heaven for your reward. That bill of goods got old real fast. Really living your life is what is holy.

"Really living your life is what is holy."

—LUISAH TEISH,
YORUBA PRIESTESS AND
AUTHOR OF *JAMBALAYA:
THE NATURAL WOMAN'S
BOOK OF PERSONAL
CHARMS AND PRACTICAL
RITUALS*

prayer and devotion. It was the obedient part she had trouble with—and the isolation.

"I've always asked questions. I've not been one to take anything at face value. I was raised and encouraged to question, and that was frowned upon in the convent. I was invited to leave. I kind of felt my whole world had crashed. That was all I had wanted all my life. It's one thing to say you want to leave, it's not for you. It's another thing altogether to have the religious community reject you, when deep down in your heart, you really felt you were being called."

Back in Chicago, a disappointed Anita found work as a secretary with the local telephone company. She took advantage of the company's tuition-aid programs, earned a bachelor's and a master's degree, and worked her way up the management ranks. Outwardly her life was successful, but inside she knew something was amiss.

In 1980, wanting to be of service to the Catholic church, Anita joined a lay ministry program and became actively involved with her parish. Still, it wasn't enough. She longed for fulfillment and peace. That yearning had never really left her.

Through the "actions of the spirit," Anita discovered what she'd been looking for: a convent without walls, one that would allow her to live with and take care of her ailing mother while holding down her corporate job. In 1985, she finally took her vows. "Being a vowed religious woman is a choice that I celebrate every day. It's the only choice for me. There's no perfect solution, but I believe in the universality of the church. There's a greater sense of guidance that comes from God."

Today Anita attends daily mass and sets aside time each morning to meditate and center herself. She still hangs out with her friends, wears fashionable clothes, and earns a decent living. But each month, to keep within reason her vow of poverty, her expenses must be approved by her superiors. Her friends and family salute her choice. And as for the others—colleagues and strangers—unless they bother to ask or need someone to pray with, no one knows she's a nun. "It's not a badge I wear. And it's not meant to be worn as a badge. I don't look to be treated any differently, nor do I want that. I'm here as a quiet witness in the midst of contradictions, greed, and the desire to get ahead. People are really searching for something solid. I'm striving to give witness, to let people know that there's something more than what they're getting paid to do."

*   *   *

In four different cities in four corners of the country, more than one thousand African-American women have joined BarbaraO in a ritualistic healing circle. Along with Yoruba and Akan priestesses, the women performed rituals and breathing exercises designed to heal themselves and the planet. While the healing circles have stopped, BarbaraO is marketing a health and healing video designed to show Black folks how to incorporate wellness rituals into their daily routines.

Healing is something BarbaraO, who played Yellow Mary in Julie Dash's award-winning film *Daughters of the Dust,* takes seriously. In her fifties and with a calm, clear demeanor and the smooth skin of a twenty-year-old, she is a living testament to what a healthy, spiritual life can provide. "African-Americans are stuck in a self-destructive mode," says BarbaraO. "And humankind is heading toward catastrophe. But we can tap into the healing forces through positive visualization, deep breathing, nutrition, rituals, yoga, and color and sound therapy. But to change ourselves—and our world—we have to change how we look at things. Healing is really an expansion of consciousness. Healing is what our soul is about. We are ten lifetimes behind in our spiritual growth. We have to do this work. We don't have a choice.

"Women have to realize that we're the wombs of the planet. We have to take responsibility for that. If we heal ourselves, then our relationships and our community and the planet gets healed. But you have to take the responsibility to start at home."

Beginning at home means taking the time out to establish your own wellness ritual. Each morning, BarbaraO prays and meditates, giving thanks for her blessings before performing a series of yoga positions called the "sun salute." After bathing and eating a breakfast of lemon water and fresh fruit, she is ready to face the day. She tries to end her day as peacefully as she began it: with a shower or bath, a series of stretches, and positive affirmations. She pours libations to the ancestor spirit guides. And once again, she gives thanks.

After years of searching and trying on different philosophies, BarbaraO says she has finally found what she believes is the answer: "The harder we work to be healthy, physically and spiritually, the more we clean our vessel—body and soul—the more we can be a vessel for the Almighty. But getting to that point takes time. Sometimes you've got to let go and let God have it. Give it up. There was a time when I had so

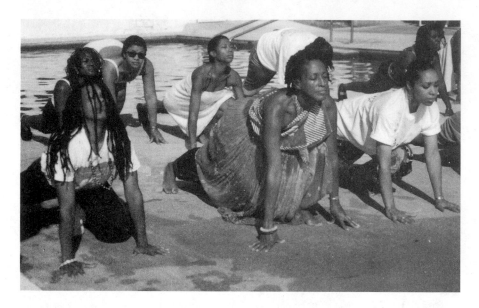

BarbaraO, front center, leading a group in the "sun salute" yoga exercise. *(Photo: Sheila Turner, SisterShip)*

much work to do on a project, I didn't know what to do. I just dropped to my knees and said, 'God, you've got it. I won't make a move that you won't take.' We have to be like a child and have faith in possibilities. We have to have faith that some kind of order is inside."

How to Tap into Your Spiritual Self

While many may profess to know the "true path," there is no set way to be spiritual. The fact is, while we are on the earth none of us can really know for sure what the truth is. Tapping into the life source—whether you call it spirit, energy, Creator, Allah, or God—is an intensely personal search that means different things to different people. You may have given up on religion years ago, but that doesn't mean you can't enjoy a rich spiritual life—there are more ways to pray than just in a pew.

There are things that you do every day to get in touch with your spirituality, whether it's walking along a beach, meditating, going to church, or performing rituals. Iyanla Vanzant, author of *Acts of Faith: Meditations for People of Color,* offers these tips:

Be still. Listen to yourself. Instead of asking others for advice, seek your own counsel. Meditation can help you learn to quiet your mind.

Begin each day focusing totally on yourself. In the morning, spend at least fifteen minutes alone. Think about what you want to accomplish that day. Talk to the mirror. Pray. Meditate.

End your day exactly as you started, focusing totally on yourself.

Examine your day. Take yourself into account. Ask yourself: How could I make it better? Did I keep my promises to myself today? Celebrate your strengths, and commit yourself to strengthening your weaknesses.

Keep the commitments you make to yourself. If you say you're going to do something, do it. If you're not going to do something, evaluate why and don't beat yourself up about it. Be honest with yourself. When you do this, you learn to trust yourself.

Forgive yourself and others. You may not like what someone did, but you can forgive. "Forgiveness is a major step toward spiritual growth," writes Vanzant, "but it must come from the heart." By forgiving others—and yourself—you move out of anger, shame, guilt, and fear and are free to experience love, joy, happiness, success, and peace. You don't have to physically confront someone to forgive them. Try writing a forgiveness letter. And when you're done, burn it, tear it up, or throw it away.

When you begin your spiritual path, unclutter your brain at least once a day by writing out your thoughts, feelings, dreams. Later, you can cut down your writing to just once a week. But do it—and be consistent. By writing out your thoughts, you free your mind. And later you'll have a written record tracking your own spiritual progress.

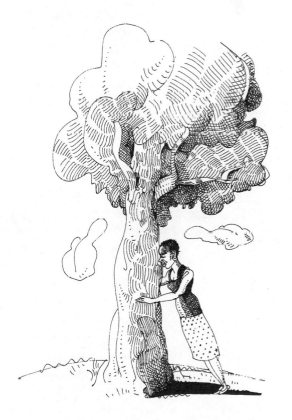

In times of trouble, get yourself to water—whether it is the river, ocean, or bathtub. Cry and pour your heart out to God.

Do a new thing. Whatever you used to do, don't do it that way anymore. Cut your hair. Or grow it. Change your makeup. Walk to the office. Take a class. Make a new friend. Move. Push yourself to grow out of your rut.

Talk to the elements instead of other people. Ask for help. Try asking a tree, "I need to be strong like you," or tell a rock, "I need my foundation strengthened." If you feel in need of spiritual assistance, go within yourself.

Learn to distinguish between the inner voice of your human self, your ego, and your spirit. The human voice will tell you about your lack and limitations. The ego is the para-

Communing with nature is one way to get in touch with spirituality. *(Drawing: Yvonne Buchanan)*

"God has never, ever, let oppressed people down."

—REVEREND RENEE MCCOY, pastor, FULL TRUTH UNITY FELLOWSHIP OF CHRIST CHURCH, DETROIT

God has always been central to my life. I grew up Catholic. And I grew up a lesbian. But when I left the Catholic church more than fifteen years ago, it wasn't because of gay rights. It was because of race. I just couldn't deal with the way the church excluded people of color. I felt like I had no place. Later, the church's unwillingness to embrace lesbians and gays kept me from going back.

But the Black church isn't guilt-free on this either. Far from it. I go to mainline churches, and I hear Black ministers denouncing homosexuality. They almost always say, "God didn't make Adam and Steve." Mainline churches, including the Black church, are so invested in a God who has very little creativity. I see Black gays and lesbians feeling depressed because of the rejection from the traditional churches. They don't feel God is active and present in their lives.

But I believe that God is capable of many manifestations of love. I serve a God who, as the kids say, "is living large in the world." I feel sorry for people whose God isn't larger than themselves. I want God to heal the world. And if God is the only thing that heals, I've got to believe that God loves the whole world.

I was ordained as a minister at the Universal Fellowship of Metropolitan Community Churches, a denomination of over three hundred churches around the world that focus on gay and lesbian issues. I left three years ago to start my own church right here in Detroit. I just felt it was time for me to work from a Black lesbian and gay focus. We needed a church that comes straight out of the Black tradition. With AIDS, our community is looking at our mortality dead in the face—more than others are. It was time, and there was a need.

I tell my congregation how great they are every week. Every chance I get to tell them that they are good and beautiful, I do. I tell them how God works in their lives and that God has never, ever, let oppressed people down. I really believe you've got to look at your life and understand that no matter what negative messages you're getting from the rest of the world, God is there, steadily working.

The greatest power in the world is love. And God is that love, and love is for everybody. You can't stop it, and no power on the earth is going to stop it. The Gospel calls the church to be about one thing: the business of liberating the world. And that's exactly what I'm trying to do, each and every day.

noid voice telling you what others think or are saying about you. Spirit is the quiet voice that pushes you beyond your limits, to trust and have faith.

Honor your ancestors. Recognize their traditions. By honoring those who have gone before us, we keep their light alive. Afrocentricity isn't about mimicking the things Africans did years ago but about honoring the principles they gave us, such as valuing the family, hard work, and community. Doing so gives us a sense of continuity.

Learn to let go of fear, worry, and anxiety.

Remember that there's nothing wrong with you. Expect the best. Always.

How Meditation Heals

Meditation is not a religion. It is a science that originated five thousand years ago and has been used by many other cultures, including some in Africa. With meditation, you learn to calm the flurry of your thoughts to find stillness and inner peace. On a practical level, meditation gives you deep, conscious relaxation, reduces stress and tension, and helps you to free yourself of negative thoughts and behavior. You will tap into your spirituality and learn that you alone have the power to effect change in your life.

To meditate, set aside twenty minutes each day. You must be consistent. Pick a certain time each day, and stick with it. Devya, president of Devya & Associates, a New York City meditation center, offers these tips:

Find a place in your home, a room or a corner that is quiet and free from traffic. A retreat. If you like, you can put things in it, such as religious symbols, African art, pictures of ancestors, and flowers, that signal that you are coming to this place to commune with your higher self.

Sit in a cross-legged position on a firm cushion or in a comfortable, upright chair with a shawl draped around your shoulders, and wear loose, comfortable clothing.

Close your eyes. Tell yourself that you are taking this time just for you. This is a notice to your subconscious that you don't want any nonsense. It will yield to your wishes, and eventually you will develop a habit that you will look forward to.

Focus on your breathing with the intent of calming yourself. Notice how your abdomen expands when you inhale and then contracts as you exhale. The more you focus on your breathing, the calmer you will become.

Begin to exhale, imagining the breath flowing down to your ankles. As you inhale, imagine your breath flowing to the crown of your head. Continue, imagining the breath stopping at the knees, then to the spot on your spinal column where your navel is located. Take the breath to the spot between your breasts, then to the hollow of your throat, then to the "bridge" where the nostrils let air out over the top of the lip. Inhale and exhale at the bridge about ten times.

Now switch the focus of your breath to along the spinal column, imagining the breath sweeping up to the crown of your head. Inhale and exhale along that point, slowly and deliberately at first, and then with total abandon, about sixteen or seventeen times.

Next relax your breath, bringing it back to the bridge. You may feel light-headed, as if you are in a trance. At this point, begin to just be in the silence and that space you have created. If any thoughts pass into your mind—and they will—allow them to pass through undisturbed. Ignore them, as if the thoughts are a ticker tape. Let your thoughts have no meaning for you. As you become more practiced, you will be able to stay in that state for longer and longer periods of time.

When you are finished, rub your hands together lightly, then put the palms of your hands over your eyes. Open your eyes, looking only at your palms, then follow your hands with your eyes as you bring them to your lap. This will ease the transition back into the real world.

Remember, you are training your mind to be still. It will be difficult at first. It won't happen overnight. Your mind and body will want to fidget. But be gentle with your mind. Don't fight with it or scold it. It is tremendously powerful, much bigger than you. Don't forget: You are looking for a partnership with your subconscious.

For More Information

BOOKS

Acts of Faith: Daily Meditations for People of Color, Iyanla Vanzant, Simon & Schuster, 1993.

Black Pearls: Daily Meditations, Affirmations, and Inspirations for African-Americans, Eric V. Copage, Quill, 1993.

Black Religion and Black Radicalism: An Interpretation of the Religious History of Afro-American People, Gayraud S. Wilmore, Orbis Books (Maryknoll, N.Y.), 1983.

Black Women in Antiquity, Ivan Van Sertima, ed., Transaction Publishers (New Brunswick, N.J.), 1984.

Carnival of the Spirit: Seasonal Celebrations and Rites of Passage, Luis Ah Teish, HarperSanFrancisco. 1994.

Daily Motivations for African-American Success, Dennis Kimbro, Fawcett Columbine, 1993.

In the Spirit: The Inspirational Writings of Susan L. Taylor, Susan L. Taylor, Amistad Press, 1993.

I Asked for Intimacy: The Stories of Blessings, Betrayals, and Birthings, Renita Weems, LuraMedia (San Diego, Calif.), 1993.

Jambalaya: The Natural Woman's Book of Personal Charms and Practical Rituals, Luisah Teish, HarperCollins San Francisco, 1988.

Just a Sister Away: A Womanist Vision of Women's Relationships in the Bible, Renita Weems, LuraMedia (San Diego, Calif.), 1988.

No Hiding Place: Empowerment and Recovery for Our Troubled Communities, Cecil Williams and Rebecca Laird, HarperCollins San Francisco, 1993.

How to Have a Flood Without Drowning, Barbara King, DeVorss & Co. (Marina Del Rey, Calif.), 1990.

Oya: In Praise of an African Goddess, Judith Gleason, HarperCollins San Francisco, 1992.

Righteous Discontent: The Women's Movement in the Black Baptist Church, 1880–1920, Evelyn Brooks Higginbotham, Harvard University Press, 1993.

Ritual: Power, Healing and Community, Malidoma Some, Swan Raven & Co. (Newberg, Ore.), 1992.

Sisters of the Yam: Black Women and Self-Recovery, bell hooks, South End Press (Boston), 1993.

Soul Quest: A Healing Journey for Women of the African Diaspora, Denese Shervington, M.D., and Billie Jean Pace, M.D., Physicians Health Management (New Orleans), 1994.

Tapping the Power Within: A Path to Self-Empowerment for Black Women, Iyanla Vanzant, Writers and Readers Publishers (Emeryville, Calif.), 1992.

Transform Your Life, *Barbara L. King, DeVorss & Co. (Marina del Rey, Calif.), 1989.*

The Unsung Heart of Black America: A Middle-Class Church at Midcentury, *Dona L. Irvin, University of Missouri Press, 1993.*

Upon This Rock: The Miracles of the Black Church, by Samuel G. Freedman, HarperCollins, 1994.

Walk Tall: Affirmations for People of Color, Carleen Brice, Recovery Publications, 1994.

Afrocentric Guide to Spiritual Union, Ra Un Nefer Amen, Khamit Corp. (Brooklyn), 1993.

Way of the Orisa, P. J. Neimark, HarperCollins San Francisco, 1993.

Wouldn't Take Nothing for My Journey Now, Maya Angelou, Random House, 1993.

PART V

LOVING

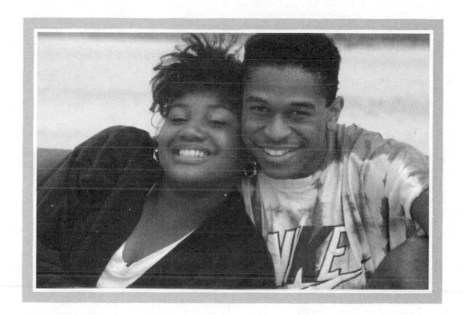

24

Loving Ourselves

Picture an African sister, straight-backed, head held high, swathed in colorful cloth, walking proudly with beauty, dignity, and strength: That's what self-esteem looks like. In all parts of the diaspora, Black women have hurdled numerous obstacles and still managed to be phenomenally productive along the way. Our female ancestors, grandmothers, mothers, aunts, cousins, sisters, and sister friends provide role models and are "sheroes" for all whose lives they touch. Other well-known Black women personify high self-esteem and positive self-image: sisters such as civil rights and women's rights activist and scholar Angela Davis, our first Black congresswoman Shirley Chisholm, pro-choice activist Faye Wattleton, Olympian athlete Wilma Rudolph, welfare and tenant-rights activist Bertha Knox Gilkey, former congresswoman Barbara Jordan, children's rights advocate Marian Wright Edelman, congresswoman Eleanor Holmes Norton, athletic superstar Jackie Joyner-Kersee, *Essence* editor Susan Taylor, television personality Oprah Winfrey, writers Toni Morrison and Alice Walker, and the list could go on and on. These are women who can inspire us all.

Given what we've been through in this country, it's a wonder we have

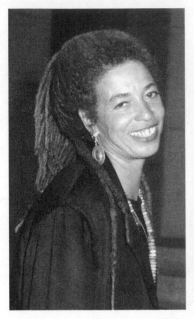
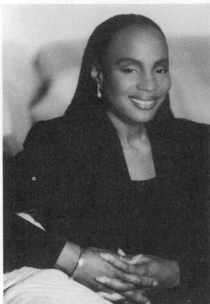
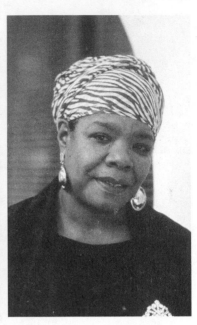

Left to right, activist and scholar Angela Y. Davis, *Essence* magazine editor-in-chief Susan L. Taylor, and poet Maya Angelou epitomize dignity, pride, and strength. *(Photos: Globe Photos, Inc. [Angela Davis and Maya Angelou]; Dwight Carter, courtesy* Essence *magazine [Susan Taylor]).*

been able to survive and, for many of us, thrive—much less possess self-esteem. Slavery, racism, sexism, family problems, making ends meet, raising children in a dangerous world, fighting illness, supporting our lovers—these and other historic and current battles would be enough to flatten women made of lesser stuff. And these kinds of problems have crippled even the best of us. But somehow, most of us make it; we wrestle the demons and come out on top. While some of us carry the weight of our burdens like lead balloons, others of us move buoyantly through life with "pep in our step and glide in our stride," in spite of missteps along the way. The difference, in all likelihood, is a strong, stable, and positive sense of self.

Poet Maya Angelou, who herself radiates self-esteem, said it best in her poem "Still I Rise":

> *You may write me down in history*
> *With your bitter, twisted lies,*
> *You may trod me in the very dirt*
> *But still, like dust, I'll rise.*

Does my sassiness upset you?
Why are you beset with gloom?
'Cause I walk like I've got oil wells
Pumping in my living room.
Just like moons and like suns,
With the certainty of tides,
Just like hopes springing high,
Still I'll rise.
Did you want to see me broken?
Bowed head and lowered eyes?
Shoulders falling down like teardrops,
Weakened by my soulful cries.
Does my haughtiness offend you?
Don't you take it awful hard
'Cause I laugh like I've got gold mines
Diggin' in my own back yard.
You may shoot me with your words,
You may cut me with your eyes,
You may kill me with your hatefulness,
But still, like air, I'll rise.
Does my sexiness upset you?
Does it come as a surprise
That I dance like I've got diamonds
At the meeting of my thighs?
Out of the huts of history's shame
I rise
Up from a past that's rooted in pain
I rise
I'm a black ocean, leaping and wide,
Welling and swelling I bear in the tide.
Leaving behind nights of terror and fear
I rise
Into a daybreak that's wondrously clear
I rise
Bringing the gifts that my ancestors gave,
I am the dream and the hope of the slave.
I rise
I rise
I rise.

—from *And Still I Rise*, Random House, 1978

What Is Self-Esteem?

To borrow the words of a song, self-esteem is "something inside so strong." If you look and listen closely, you can tell when a sister has high self-esteem. Maybe that sister is you. She doesn't necessarily have to be beautiful or well-dressed, but a certain happiness and confidence shine through. She's comfortable in her skin and secure within herself, not threatened by others. She isn't jealous of other women—their relationships, their jobs, their money, their clothes, their beauty, their size—because she's satisfied with what she's got. She likes her work whether she makes a lot of money or doesn't get paid at all. She has loving relationships because she can listen and share, nurture and be nurtured. Her life may not be perfect, but she doesn't stay down for long because she is assured that her own skills, ingenuity, friends, and family will help her overcome any obstacle. She doesn't rely on money or a man or clothes or any outside stimulus to make her happy; she truly loves herself, and the reflection of that love is her wealth and her beauty.

Self-image (also labeled self-concept or self-perception) is one of the most fundamental aspects of our identity, the way in which we define ourselves and our place in our communities and the world. The two domains of self-image most critical to healthy psychological functioning are *self-esteem* and *self-efficacy*. Self-esteem or self-worth refers to our valuation of ourselves in relationship to others. Part of this valuation is personal, and part is tied to feelings about Black people as a whole. Self-efficacy refers to our perceived competency, or what we believe we can accomplish.

Racism and sexism have a marked effect on the self-esteem and self-efficacy of our people. As researchers Gloria Powell and Marguerite Beale Spencer found, many Blacks have high self-esteem but low self-efficacy. These people understand that racial discrimination, rather than individual failings, explains many of the problems in our community, and that fact doesn't affect their self-*esteem*: "I know I'm a good person, and I understand that my people aren't stupid and lazy; we've been systematically oppressed." But that very understanding may get in the way of self-*efficacy:* "I know I'm a good, smart, industrious person, but as a Black woman (or man) I'll never get anywhere in this society because of systematic oppression."

For others of us, it's the opposite: high self-efficacy but low self-esteem. These brothers and sisters identify strongly with mainstream culture and are often highly accomplished and successful. Yet because they have little connectedness with their African origins or Black identity, their self-esteem is low. They don't believe that discrimination is a prob-

As a child, I didn't know that having dark skin was a big deal. I mean, everybody in my family was very dark. Both my parents are from Nigeria and unmistakably African.

When school started, I didn't have any problems—at first. I had lots of friends, and they all adored me. Believe it or not, they were mostly white. To white kids, Black skin was Black, no matter how dark or light, and it was a novelty. Things did change by the time I reached seventh grade and two (lighter-complected) "sistas" transferred to my school. Reluctantly, I had to give up the "only" title and watch as my white friends became fascinated with the new girls. But nothing could prepare me for the color craziness that was to follow.

For college, I was Howard-bound, to the land of Black pride, togetherness, and personal support. Still I was a little nervous and apprehensive, and it turned out to be for good reason: There seemed to be a silent caste system there. Need I say what determined your place in it? What a shock to see Black students at an all-Black college checking out each other's complexions.

I remember one day I was walking with some friends, and some brothers yelled out the normal mating call: "Yo, cuties, what's up?" Though we all ignored them, I became their chosen target. "Fuck you, then, you black ugly bitch." Shocked, crushed, and humiliated, I managed to show little or no emotion. But that was the beginning of the end. I stayed for one semester and applauded when Spike Lee's School Daze came out and told the truth. It portrayed my experience to the hilt.

My Black friends back home were no better. A light-skinned girlfriend once said to me, "Let me tell you something, honey. A fly light-skin girl like me never has to worry about anything, because men will always be attracted to me because I'm a red-bone, and you know how men feel about red-bones." What can I say?

Eventually, I transferred to a predominately white university where instead of intraracial color prejudice, I experienced blatant, out-and-out racism. I remember sitting down in class and noticed my name written on the desk, along with that of an old boyfriend who had skin as dark as mine. Underneath our names, someone had drawn stereotypical caricatures and written "Niggers go home, back to Africa."

That was the last straw. From that day on I decided I wasn't going to cower or withdraw every time a comment or reference was made about my Black skin. Every day I tell myself, "Yes, I am a Black woman. Yes, I am a dark-skinned woman. And yes, I am beautiful."

I thank God for letting me find my beauty and worth in this world. It makes me feel good to say, "I am Black, I am dark, I am African and proud of it."

"I am Black, I am dark, I am African and proud of it."

—Ebun Phillips-Bowen,
SOCIAL WORKER,
Roosevelt, New York

lem, so when it occurs, they automatically blame themselves. These are the kind of people who seem to have it all together professionally, but their personal lives are a mess, fraught with confusion, identity crises, substance abuse, and bad relationships.

Rather than focusing on oppression and negative images, the key is to think and to teach children to think positively and proactively. It's important to understand that oppression has kept our people down and given us fewer opportunities than have been given whites. At the same time, as a people we have overcome tremendous barriers. Throughout history, people of African descent survived trials and tribulations that would've killed off folks with less determination, resilience, strength, and creativity. Understanding that to the core results in high self-esteem ("Society's image of Blacks is wrong—I'm a good, competent person") and high self-efficacy ("Despite oppression, I can do it").

Our Image in the Media and Its Consequences

The insidious nature of negative role modeling is particularly critical considering that the entertainment industry (music, television, and movies) plays an integral role in our lives and can shape the minds of our children.

Black women are represented in mainstream media by myriad images, from denigrating (e.g., the crack-addicted, promiscuous, pregnant "welfare mother") to exalting in Eurocentric terms (e.g., the gorgeous, articulate, upper-middle-class "superwoman" who can run an organization, take care of a family, "read" a sassy cab driver, and still have the energy to do volunteer work in the community). Neither of these images is accurate: The first one insults and incorrectly stereotypes us, and the second makes us feel inadequate, because we can never live up to the impossibly high Clair Huxtable standard. Unfortunately our brothers often perpetuate these damaging images of Black women by calling us names like "bitch," "ho," and "skeezer" in comedy skits and rap songs.

This stereotyping by white men and women, Black men, and even, more sadly, one another taxes us and further depletes our energy reserves. Even those of us who are brusque, mouthy, meticulously attired, seemingly emotionally healthy, perhaps a little intimidating (exhibiting high self-efficacy in terms of professional productivity and social responsibility) may harbor very low self-esteem. We may be lonely, afraid, and tied to abusive mates.

Specifically, poor self-image may manifest itself psychologically in the following ways:

Affective disorders such as depression (with symptoms including sleep disturbance with early morning awakening, appetite disturbance with weight loss or gain, crying spells, low energy, constipation, loss of interest in normally pleasurable activities)

Underachievement

Substance misuse and abuse, sexual risk taking

Participation in nonsupportive/abusive relationships

Eating disorders such as anorexia nervosa and bulimia

Violence (child abuse, homicide, suicide)

Unemployment or underemployment

Sexually transmitted disease spread

Self-Esteem and Black Children

One of the most heartbreaking studies on self-esteem took place several decades ago. In 1950 Mamie P. and Kenneth B. Clark demonstrated that young Black children preferred white dolls to Black dolls, projecting negative societal stereotypes onto the latter and imbuing the former with glowing, socially endorsed qualities. In a repeat study in the late 1980s, researchers were surprised to find that not much had changed: Black children still chose white dolls.

A number of factors have been cited as barriers for our children and adolescents in their struggle for a stable identity. A distorted history of people of African descent hurts all of us. Though that is changing as multicultural textbooks and curricula move into the mainstream, many of our children are still deprived of the rich historical contributions of our ancestors.

The breakdown of our families and communities has taken a toll on the self-esteem of our youngsters. Research has shown that African-American students in racially isolated Southern schools have higher self-esteem than their local white peers and urban Blacks. Gloria Powell attributed this finding to the Southern Black students' sense of the power and achievements of the adult members of their strong and cohesive African-American community. Still, in many communities, the African ideal that "it takes a whole community to raise a child" seems to be dying away. Though our extended family networks remain vital to our culture, the tradition of community members who enriched the Black child's life and "stood in" for parents who were overwhelmed is less common, undermined by desegregation.

With role models, stable families, and quality schools all lacking, television and its negative images of Blacks and women plays an overly

"I have finally begun to cherish me."

—VALERIE WILSON WESLEY, WRITER, NEWARK, NEW JERSEY

I had my first fat fit when I was fifteen. I stood in front of the mirror and hated every part of me with a passion that shook me to my soul. My feelings about myself—my sense of self—were tied to the way I looked, and I looked fat, and fat was unacceptable. There were other things that shook my sense of self-esteem, like being the only Black youngster in a white school—but being overweight was the worst.

Until recently, I used to have the fat fits at least once or twice a month. I could count on having them at the start of every season when I had to change my wardrobe and something didn't fit quite right. Or I'd have a fit whenever I felt bloated or ate too much.

Now I understand how very distorted my self-perception was. When I look at my seventeen-year-old daughter, who has a body much like I had when I was young, I see how very beautiful she is. She is shapely with full breasts and full hips. She looks womanly, much rounder and fuller than the models you see in Seventeen and Elle magazines. So far she likes her body and herself—and that is one of the things I can pat myself on the back for. She doesn't go on the punishing diets that I once endured. She doesn't stand in front of the mirror and curse the way she looks and feel bad about herself. She doesn't have the same love/hate affair that I once had with food. When I look at her, the depth of my misconception about my body size and self-image astounds me.

One of my earliest memories of my mother and her sense of my growing female body were her comments about the size of my stomach and her pleading that if I "could just hold it in I would have a nice little figure." But she was as hard on herself as she was on me. In countless ways, her own self-confidence was undermined. She didn't like herself as a whole, she liked certain parts of herself—her legs, her hair—but not the whole package. She passed those feelings on to me about my body.

Other conflicting messages about food and body size marked my childhood. Eat and hate yourself for doing it. Lose control and hate yourself when you do. Don't be fat. Fat is slovenly and ugly and lower-class. But food is love. Food is acceptable. Food is sophistication. Food is knowledge. Food is much more than simple sustenance.

It has taken me twenty-five years of shame about my body to finally put these things in perspective. Because my sense of food and of my body size were so distorted, it took me years to see and accept myself as a physical being. Exercise has been essential to me. I began to learn that feeling good about myself came from feeling the potential of my body—the strength and capabilities. When I jog or lift weights or stretch and feel the strength and mobility *of my muscles and limbs, I love myself. I love to move, to run, to feel strong.*

Along with that awareness of myself as a physical presence came my complete awareness of myself as a person. I will never again let anyone tell me that I should feel ashamed of my body because of the way it looks. It is mine. I have finally begun to cherish me, all of me. What others may see as too large, I finally claim as my own. I am strong. I can run two and a half miles without getting tired. I finally belong to me, and my self-esteem has never been higher.

influential role in the lives of our young people. In a 1989 Wayne State University survey of ten-to-eighteen-year-olds, peers and television/radio influenced children and young adults more than did home—which similarly outranked school and church. This contrasts with 1950, when home was most influential, followed by school, church, peers, and TV and even 1980, when home was followed by peers, TV, and finally school.

Despite all of the ways society and its images can break down our children's self-esteem, a strong Black community can help boost it. In our community we have our own standards of beauty, so that Black women and girls aren't judged by the white ideal. Black folks are likely to believe that broad noses, brown eyes, kinky hair, and Black skin *are* beautiful—even though the larger society tells us they are not. The saying "nobody want a bone but a dog" shows our respect for large, lush bodies. The appreciation that comes from within our community helps bolster our self-esteem. All of us must continue that tradition by teaching all children that Black is *very* beautiful.

Learning to Love Yourself

Too bad we can't snap our fingers and—*poof*—be full of self-esteem and self-efficacy. It's not that easy, but it's also not impossible to maintain the love we have for ourselves, reinforce it, and help it to grow. Here are some suggestions:

Confront issues from your past. Facing up to painful experiences from the past can help raise self esteem. Anger and bitterness turned inward lead to low self-esteem, so it's best to work on forgiving and letting go. Try to do it with a therapist whom you trust and are comfortable talking to. Or you can make the journey with the help of books, friends, family, a self-help support group, and spiritual leaders.

Be true to yourself in your choice of jobs and romantic partners. Many "sell out" for material gain or acquiesce to familial and societal pressures at the cost of personal happiness and satisfaction. Think of this poster quoting an unknown writer: "Do not follow where the path leads. Rather go where there is no path and leave a trail."

Be alone. Spend time with the person you should love most—yourself. Go on walks, write in a journal, take leisurely hot baths, meditate, listen to music, or just sit quietly and allow yourself to think in solitude.

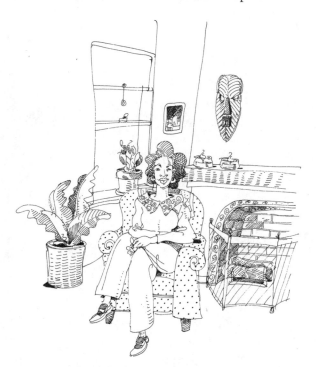

Taking care of yourself by spending time alone can be rejuvenating. *(Drawing: Yvonne Buchanan)*

Invest in yourself. Partnered or single, parent or childless, work to create an environment of people and space that reflect and support you. Instead of filling every minute of your time with work and other responsibilities, get involved in activities that you truly enjoy. And surround yourself with objects that you love, such as African cloth, candles, art, photographs of your ancestors, and mementos.

Take action and get involved. Self-empowerment begins with resisting fatalism and backing up your beliefs with actions. Don't be "all talk and no walk"; be a doer instead. Get involved with organizations or programs that represent your sociopolitical stance, attend church, or start a community group of your own. There is so much work to be done in the world, and doing your small part will give you a sense of empowerment and mastery. Remember the slogan "If you aren't part of the solution, you're part of the problem." Plus, giving to others is really a gift to yourself.

Clarify your aspirations, and set some goals and objectives. Expect to modify or replace them as you grow, but you need to feel that your life has some purpose and direction beyond basic survival. As Langston Hughes wrote: "Hold fast to your dreams, for when dreams die, life is a broken-winged bird that cannot fly."

Embrace Afrocentrism and "womanism" (Alice Walker's Black feminist construct) personally and politically. Whether we realize it or not, racism and sexism are alive and well and take a daily toll on our self-images as we're assaulted by negative societal attitudes. So it's important for each of us to celebrate our blackness and femaleness, to respect and uplift other people of African descent, especially other sisters. We shouldn't use derogatory terms such as "nigger" and "bitch," nor should we be hyper-critical of our own people. We should recognize and understand that women and people of color are oppressed in our society, but not let that obvious fact keep us from moving forward and loving ourselves.

Surround yourself with positive role models. We don't outgrow our need for role models and mentors, particularly informal ones. Pursue romances, friendships, acquaintanceships, and coworker relationships with people whose decisions and life choices you admire, and who inspire, appreciate, and support the best in you. Sheroes and heroes pop-ulate our daily lives; we need only to open our eyes to find them. And avoid "misery loves company" scenarios on an ongoing basis. There is emerging neurochemical evidence to suggest that "bad moods" are con-tagious, particularly for women as a result of our being (perhaps over-) socialized to nurture others and foster relationships.

Credit your intuitive assessments. Women and people of African descent have often been ridiculed and penalized for their intuitive, gut-level responses. Tune in to your inner voice, and consider it an additional source of input.

Be proactive, not reactive. Think of the cliche "An ounce of prevention is worth a pound of cure." Don't wait for problems to become entrenched and magnified before addressing them. Early intervention is much more likely to be effective, and taking action is easier when you're not feeling overwhelmed.

Acknowledge and validate your own feelings. Don't be afraid to allow yourself to feel bad if you are unhappy. The key is identifying your feel-ings, verbalizing them, and finding healthy, constructive, and socially appropriate ways of expressing them and dealing with them, especially the negative ones. Denying or burying them only leads to depression or other self-destructive outlets.

Examine your relationships. We sometimes need to let go of people who are or become negative influences in our lives. A part of finding and maintaining personal happiness is identifying our priorities in relation-ships and not compromising on those relationship requirements that we consider major. The immediate pain of loss is more than compensated in the long run by the self-esteem and integrity derived from insisting on fair, respectful, and loving treatment by a mate. Maintaining high stan-dards also exhibits the kind of security that attracts others who might be more suitable.

Address your spiritual needs. Spiritual grounding is critical to optimal functioning. It helps us deal with adversity, especially grieving, as well as prosperity—which can be both stressful and fleeting if not kept in perspective. As human beings, we need to feel that our lives have meaning and purpose, that they fit into a "grand scheme." For many Blacks, this need is fulfilled within a Christian religious setting. But there are many other philosophies and religious expressions that resonate for others of us. The key is in finding yours.

Above all, keep in mind that although as Black women we've been put to the test in every way, we have survived. When you feel down, keep thinking of this poem by Mari Evans:

> *I*
> *am a black woman*
> *tall as a cypress*
> *strong*
> *beyond all definition still*
> *defying place*
> *and time*
> *and circumstance . . .*
> —from *I Am a Black Woman,* William Morrow and Co., 1970

Raising Healthy, Free, Secure Daughters

A highly publicized 1991 report called "Shortchanging Girls, Shortchanging America" noted that at the age of nine, a majority of girls were confident and assertive with positive feelings about themselves, but by the time they reached high school, less than one-third felt that way. Interestingly, Black girls in the study started out with higher self-esteem and said they were much more self-confident in high school compared with white and Latina girls.

"In healthy Black families there is a very high premium placed on individual and personal self-worth," explains Janie Victoria Ward, an African-American advisor to the study. "[Black] girls are given very strong messages about independence and assertiveness from their mothers, and in the culture there's a lot of support for feistiness and being your own woman."

What's more, asserts Dr. Ward of Simmons College in Boston, "All women are bombarded with messages about being thin, tall and blond, but whites may be more troubled than Blacks by their failure to match those images."

We must fight to create and maintain self-esteem in Black girls and young women. While there is no all-inclusive childrearing "formula" guaranteeing high self-esteem in our developing girls, the following suggestions are based on current research findings and some pretty compelling anecdotal evidence.

Take a hard look at yourself. Make sure you're happy and secure, or you won't be able to teach your daughter to love herself.

Support, with your time and other available resources, the development of competencies suited to your child's aptitudes and interests, even if they fall in traditionally "masculine" domains, such as artistic endeavors, academic prowess, athletic pursuits, mechanical/electronic tinkering.

Praise and reward your child more for her competencies than for her looks or decorum (such as her ladylike manners).

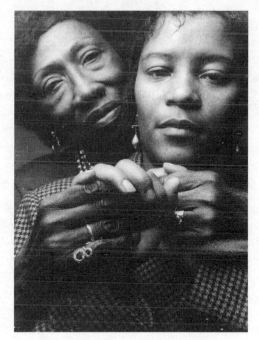

Strong mothers cultivate strong daughters.
(Photo: Albert Trotman/Allford Trotman Associates)

Frame references to Africa, physical features reflecting African descent such as dark skin or full lips and African-American cultural values in positive terms: Don't "dog" other Black folks or our culture because that will produce or reinforce internalized racism and self-hatred.

Teach children to appreciate the rainbow of skin colors and hair textures. Take your daughter to see the movie *Daughters of the Dust* so she can see that beautiful Black women come in all colors.

Choose your battles with care. Especially as girls reach puberty, self-expression, peer approval, and detachment from parents assume premiere importance—don't destroy rapport and open lines of communication with trivial arguments about leg-shaving, clothing tastes, or hairstyles.

Encourage lofty dreams, but emphasize the hard work and persistence necessary to make those dreams a reality. Whenever possible, provide concrete "how-to" information relevant to those goals.

Be mindful of self-fulfilling prophecies—a child told that she is "no count" and "no good" and "just like her no-good father" is more likely to grow up to be just that.

Surround your child with positive African-American role models and, if possible, mentors of both sexes; those with shared interests or involved in career pursuits to which she aspires are particularly helpful in provid-

Defending Ourselves

Nowhere has the real-life "double jeopardy" of gender and race for Black women been as vividly dramatized on the small screen as in the Anita Hill–Clarence Thomas debate during his confirmation hearings for the Supreme Court.

Following the tradition of our foremothers who have always pulled together to respond to assaults on our character, a group of more than one thousand African-American women refused to allow the attack of Professor Hill to turn into another attack on our self-esteem. These sisters took out a three-quarter-page advertisement in the November 17, 1991, edition of the Sunday New York Times *and other publications with this message:*

African American Women In Defense of Ourselves

As women of African descent, we are deeply troubled by the recent nomination, confirmation and seating of Clarence Thomas as an Associate Justice of the U.S. Supreme Court. We know that the presence of Clarence Thomas on the Court will be continually used to divert attention from historic struggles for social justice through suggestions that the presence of a Black man on the Supreme Court constitutes an assurance that the rights of African Americans will be protected. Clarence Thomas' public record is ample evidence this will not be true. Further, the consolidation of a conservative majority on the Supreme Court seriously endangers the rights of all women, poor and working class people and the elderly. The seating of Clarence Thomas is an affront not only to African American women and men, but to all people concerned with social justice.

We are particularly outraged by the racist and sexist treatment of Professor Anita Hill, an African American woman who was maligned and castigated for daring to speak publicly of her own experience of sexual abuse. The malicious defamation of Professor Hill insulted all women of African descent and sent a dangerous message to any woman who might contemplate a sexual harassment complaint.

We speak here because we recognize that the media are now portraying the Black community as prepared to tolerate both the dismantling of affirmative action and the evil of sexual harassment in order to have any Black man on the Supreme Court. We want to make clear that the media have ignored or distorted many African American voices. We will not be silenced.

Many have erroneously portrayed the allegations against Clarence Thomas as an issue of either gender or race. As women of African descent, we understand sexual harassment as both. We further understand that Clarence Thomas outrageously manipulated the legacy of lynching in order to shelter himself from Anita Hill's allegations. To deflect attention away from the reality of sexual abuse in African American women's lives, he trivialized and misrepresented this painful part of African American people's history. This country, which has a long legacy of racism and sexism, has never taken the sexual abuse of Black women seriously. Throughout U.S. history Black women have been sexually stereotyped as immoral, insatiable, perverse; the initiators in all sexual contacts—abusive or otherwise. The common assumption in legal proceedings as well as in the larger society has been that Black women cannot be raped or otherwise sexually abused. As Anita Hill's experience demonstrates, Black women who speak of these matters are not likely to be believed.

In 1991, we cannot tolerate this type of dismissal of any one Black woman's experience or this attack upon our collective character without protest, outrage, and resistance.

As women of African descent, we express our vehement opposition to the policies represented by the placement of Clarence Thomas on the Supreme Court. The Bush administration, having obstructed the passage of civil rights legislation, impeded the extension of unemployment compensation, cut student aid and dismantled social welfare programs, has continually demonstrated that it is not operating in our best interests. Nor is this appointee. We pledge ourselves to continue to speak out in defense of one another, in defense of the African American community and against those who are hostile to social justice no matter what color they are. No one will speak for us but ourselves.

For information about purchasing a poster-size copy of this statement, write to Kitchen Table: Women of Color Press, P.O. Box 908, Latham, NY 12110, (518)434-2057.

---

ing guidance in hurdling barriers, acquiring necessary skills, managing obstacles, and negotiating the system. Keep in mind, however, that your child's primary role model is you. Discuss your own personal and occupational struggles, successes, and failures, especially those communicating proactive ideas toward racial/ethnic or gender barriers ("you have to be twice as good to succeed," not "no way a Black woman can get ahead in this society").

Provide for your child's spiritual development and guidance, whether formal or informal.

For More Information

BOOKS: Black Women's Lives

Just about any book that discusses our history, our ancestors, and the lives of brave sisters will help boost your self-esteem and that of your friends, family, and children. Go to a library or Black bookstore and browse until you find something inspiring! You can also check out:

Black Women in America: An Historical Encyclopedia (2 vols.), Darlene Clark Hine, editor, Carlson Publishing (Brooklyn), 1993.

Children of the Dream: The Psychology of Black Success, Audrey Edwards and Dr. Craig K. Polite, Doubleday, 1992.

I Dream a World: Portraits of Black Women Who Changed America, photos by Brian Lanker; Stewart, Tabori & Chang, 1989.

Notable Black American Women, Jessie Carney Smith, editor, Gale Research (Detroit), 1992.

When and Where I Enter: The Impact of Black Women on Race and Sex in America, Paula Giddings, William Morrow & Co., 1984.

BOOKS: Self-Esteem

For Black Women Only: A Complete Guide to a Successful Life-Style Change: Health, Wealth, Love, and Happiness, Ingrid D. Hicks, African-American Images (Chicago), 1991.

In the Company of My Sisters: Black Women and Self-Esteem, Julia A. Boyd, NAL/Dutton, 1993.

Recovery of Your Self-Esteem: A Guide for Women, Carolynn Hillman, Fireside, 1992.

Revolution from Within: A Book of Self-Esteem, Gloria Steinem, Little, Brown & Co., 1992.

Sisters of the Yam: Black Women and Self-Recovery, bell hooks, South End Press (Boston), 1993.

Women and Self-Esteem: Understanding and Improving the Way We Think and Feel About Ourselves, Linda Tschirhart Sanford and Mary Ellen Donovan, Viking Penguin, 1985.

25

Loving Our Men

Gather a group of Black women together, and ask them about their husbands, lovers, grandfathers, fathers, uncles, brothers, and sons. As they speak, listen to their tones rather than their tales. You'll hear a mixture of warmth, exasperation, patience, weariness, annoyance, pleasure, and pain. But shining through all the talk will be the sound of love. As they themselves might say colloquially, "Black women *love* them some Black men!"

Like women everywhere, they have the option of choosing men from other races or not choosing men at all. But Black women know that Black men are more than just the original model for "tall, dark, and handsome." They embody all the wonderful attributes Black women gravitate to naturally. Through thick and thin, ups and downs, and through the ages, Black women have admired, wanted, needed, and loved Black men.

But strife and tension have crept in and created a wedge between Black women and men. Sometimes it seems as if we are at war. African-American feminist Michele Wallace pointed this out in her landmark 1979 book *Black Macho and the Myth of the Superwoman*: "I am saying among other things, that for perhaps the last 50 years there has been a growing distrust, even hatred, between Black men and Black women. It has been nursed along not only by racism on the part of whites, but also by an almost deliberate ignorance on the part of Blacks about the sexual politics of their experience in this country. It is from this perspective that the Black man and woman faced the challenge of the Black Revolution—a revolution subsequently dissipated and distorted by their inability to see each other clearly through the fog of sexual myths and fallacies. This has cost us a great deal. It has cost us unity, for one thing."

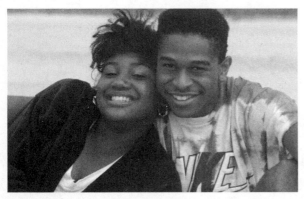

Finding a loving mate can be a wonderful learning experience. (*Photo: Diane Allford/Allford Trotman Associates*)

Though Wallace was harshly criticized for her book, it opened the eyes of many Black women.

If there is a battle, it raged on in 1990 with Shahrazad Ali's controversial, self-published book *The Blackman's Guide to Understanding the Blackwoman*. To this Black female author, Black women are for the most part dirty and sex-crazed, have smaller brains than Black men, and all too often only open their mouths to spew obscenities that force men to slap them. Ali's ridiculous book fed the anger that some Black men harbor against Black women and that Black women hold against themselves and opened up a painful wound that exists between the sexes.

The battle continued in 1991 from coast to coast on television as Professor Anita Hill testified that Supreme Court nominee Clarence Thomas had sexually harassed her. Though Thomas was confirmed, for the first time Americans saw educated African-Americans—a man and a woman—pitted against each other, and Hill went on to become a feminist heroine. The battle raged on in 1992 as a young Black woman, Desiree Washington, accused boxer Mike Tyson of rape, and he was sent off to prison. Young Black men proudly sport T-shirts emblazoned with Tyson's photo and the phrase "I'll Be Back."

Our relationships with men—both public and private, loving and embattled—cannot be viewed in a vacuum. Our African past, enslavement in America, and the harsh economic, political, and social conditions that persist up to today have all contributed to the ways in which Black women and men relate to each other.

Marriage and the Family in Black History

Traditionally and in contemporary African societies marriage is a merger of families. While a couple may meet and develop a friendship that could lead to marriage, there are long-standing formalities that they and their families have to go through before marriage can be arranged. Things are changing in Africa, especially among urban populations, but in the past a couple that married became part of an already-existing extended family network on the man's side. Survival of that network, guided by the principles of respect, restraint, responsibility, and reciprocity were emphasized over and above the modern-day nuclear family.

The Effects of Slavery

The age-old traditions of courtship, marriage, and family were virtually destroyed by the system of slavery. In America, African men and women were treated as property, an unpaid labor force held in bondage to build and maintain the agricultural lifeblood of the South. Marriage between slaves was not legal since both the man and the woman had slave masters and no rights as individuals. In addition to working in the field, male slaves were used as studs to impregnate Black women, who were made to bear as many children as possible. The offspring would, in turn, either work the land or be sold for profit. Some couples, even those from different plantations, were allowed to choose their own mates, but they always lived under the threat that either of them or their children could be sold. In lieu of legal marriages, the couple would have a ceremony called "jumping the broom," in which the man and woman jumped over a broomstick handle held a foot or so off the ground by two other slaves to cement their union.

In spite of this inhuman system that wrenched families apart, Black men and women did have courtships, and there were feelings of kinship and family among Blacks, particularly those on the same plantation. Slaves who escaped and went north or west would often search for those who had successfully gone before them. Emancipation in 1865 and the period of Reconstruction that followed was a time of reunion for countless couples and extended families that had been unwillingly split up over the years.

After Slavery

Freedom didn't live up to the high expectations held dear by the former slaves, largely because of deep-seated hatred and bigotry. White America, particularly defeated Southerners, put into place a system of discrimina-

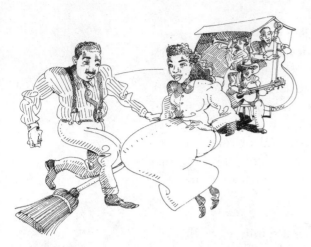

Marriage between slaves was illegal, so couples devised their own ceremony called "jumping the broom."
(Drawing: Yvonne Buchanan)

tion in jobs, education, and housing (known as Jim Crow laws) that effectively kept Black men and women in subservient positions while protecting and elevating whites.

During Reconstruction and into the early decades of the twentieth century, Black men and women were, for the most part, relegated to the low-paying, backbreaking fields of agriculture and service. Women found work doing the same domestic chores they had performed under slavery. A number of Black men counted themselves lucky to be able to work for the railway as sleeping-car porters, a step up from being sharecroppers, farmhands, and menial laborers. The doors to better-paying jobs in manufacturing and skilled trades such as construction, plumbing, and carpentry were shut to Black men.

Under such adversity, Black families did the best they could. Strong family bonds and the Black church were instrumental in imparting self-esteem to African-Americans. Women regarded their men as heads of household, and men worked long hours in their hometowns and on the road to earn money to care for their families. There was a shared sense of struggle between Black men and women in the larger community as everyone tried to move beyond the legacy of slavery. There was optimism that life would improve with hard work and education.

Black families and communities in the 1920s really believed better days were ahead. A number of men served in the armed forces during the two world wars. But the American victories in these wars turned sour when honorably discharged Black veterans found themselves still at the bottom of the ladder in every sector of society. Between the wars, the Great Depression swept across America, and although whites were almost as poor as Blacks, they maintained their centuries-old attitude of superiority and an economic upper hand.

The Depression was so devastating that the U.S. government was forced to institute Aid to Families with Dependent Children (AFDC), or welfare, as it was and still is called. To prove that children in poor families were truly dependent on welfare, there had to be no able-bodied man in the household. The welfare rules did not take into consideration Jim Crow's effectiveness, the fact that even when Black men were with their families they very often could not get jobs to fully support them. To meet the requirements for welfare benefits, Black men had to be absent or pretend to be absent from their families—an emasculating, humiliating predicament. Even now this pitiful condition is still a reality in much of this country.

The charade that so many Black families had to live by (and that many still live by) took its toll on relations between men and women. Men, especially poor men, felt powerless, unable to fulfill the roles of provider and protector that society expected of them, and women felt unable to help them. Both felt trapped in a cycle of poverty where, ironically, they were better off apart than together. And both were bitter at a system that worked to undermine Black family life.

The pressure on Black couples and families to merely survive continued through the second half of the forties and into the fifties. The 1960s saw the beginning of the civil rights movement and an attempt by Blacks and fair-minded whites to finally do away with institutionalized racism. Desegregation was the byword, and Black men and women worked side by side to bring about change. Expectations were high that at last the long-hoped-for new day was dawning. Blacks enrolled in college in record numbers, and graduates found new opportunities open to them, due in part to federal legislation and to a willingness to allow a select number of Blacks into the previously all-white enclaves of business and government.

Women's Liberation

Right on the heels of the civil rights movement was women's liberation or the feminist movement, which adapted many of the tactics of the former to enact or alter laws for the benefit of women—over half of the population. Black women and white feminists have always had an uneasy relationship. The issues feminists raised all too often placed Black women in the position of having to choose gender concerns over race concerns. Feminists pointed at men (white men and their laws, traditions, and wishes) as the root of their anger. The most outspoken women were accused of man-bashing and bra-burning. Black women, on the other hand, were sensitized to the emasculation our men have suffered at the hands of the same white men who victimized white women. It was difficult for Black women to blame Black men for all their problems when both had suffered side by side for so long. Activist Fannie Lou Hamer often found herself at odds with white feminists. "I got a Black husband, 6 feet 3, 240 pounds, with a 14 shoe, that I don't *want* to be liberated from," she once said. "We are here to work side by side with this Black man in trying to bring liberation for all people."

Though some would consider it a contradiction in terms, Black feminists did emerge, and some, like Wallace, were brave enough to accuse Black males of sexism and even point to the degradation of women within the Black Power Movement. Wallace and other feminist writers like Ntozake Shange *(for colored girls who have considered suicide/when the rainbow is enuf)* and Alice Walker (*The Color Purple* and other novels) have been shot down by African-American male literati as being anti–Black male.

By the early 1970s, the Pandora's box that held the muffled, strained cries of Black gender strife—over preferential hiring, who was head of household, and a thousand other large, small, and extremely sensitive issues—was opened, and a resolution to the conflict has yet to be found. In fact, things intensified in the 1980s and presently as poor Blacks got poorer and the middle class tried to keep its head above water. Instead of pulling together as we have done in the past, too often Black men and women blame each other for the struggles and oppression we have to deal with every day. We bring home our anger at the world and get mad at each other.

What We Must Do

In order for Black men and women to have healthy, loving partnerships it is first critical for all women to understand that no woman *needs* a man to complete her. Many women are happy and healthy without male relationships, content to take a break and focus on themselves.

Not until you love and respect yourself can you have a healthy relationship with a man. And many, many brothers and sisters have happy, satisfied long-term unions. Supportive relationships generally have these components:

Wholeness. Both the man and the woman are whole people, not looking for completion through the relationship. And, of course, since no two people are exactly alike, each attempts to understand, appreciate, and accept their differences.

Communication. Both the man and the woman try to communicate wants and needs clearly—and to listen to the needs and wants of the other. The purpose of their interactions is to understand and be understood.

Letting go of judgments. Each tries not to negatively judge the other—or him or herself. Both the man and the woman attempt to take responsibility for their own behavior and not heap blame on the other.

I've never been married, but I'd like to be. Most guys think I look like a walking commitment. I'm nice and I'm good, and I have a five-year-old son. A lot of men won't date women with children because it's responsibility.

I was involved with my son's father for eight and a half years.

We called ourselves best friends. When I told him I was pregnant, he told me he was getting married to someone else. He never told me he was even thinking about it until then. About the child, he said, "Get rid of it." I made three attempts to go to an abortion clinic. But I couldn't do it. After that he wouldn't talk to me. He's in Richmond with his wife and baby.

At this point I don't really date, and I was celibate for three years after my son was born. I once lived with a guy for four years, and I think we would have gotten married eventually. But the guy worked really slowly, and at the rate he was going I would have been about forty, so I left. Another guy I probably would have married got caught up in a metaphysical thing; he went crazy looking for God.

Despite what's happened to me, it doesn't affect the way I feel about Black men. They have it hard in this society, but I know there's some good brothers out there. Because we outnumber them and they have so many choices, they figure when they're ready they can pick one. Maybe it's that the one-on-one is too much when Black men are faced with so many women. They can just go out and have fun.

Sometimes I get lonely, and I wish I could be like some women and cross the color barrier, but I just can't do it. I think my son would be confused. I worry about my son. He's never seen his father. He doesn't get sad or depressed about it, yet I know he needs that father-son thing.

I'm going to wait for a man I can have a partnership with—not just companionship, but a male role model for my son who can live with us. A fifty-fifty partnership, a thing that's real. But in the meantime, I just go out and do my own thing. I try to stay active. When I come home from work I go for a run. It takes out a lot of frustration and makes me feel better. On weekends I take my son to see a show or something, and I go to jazz clubs with friends. I attend readings at a library or bookstore and read books—especially books by Black women. Mostly I just try to relax.

> *"I'm going to wait for a man I can have a partnership with—not just companionship."*
>
> —Jennifer Daughtry, principal staff clerk for a manufacturing company, Atlanta

Forgiveness. All healthy relationships contain some degree of conflict. But a couple that wants to work things out doesn't hold long grudges and works to forgive and accept the other.

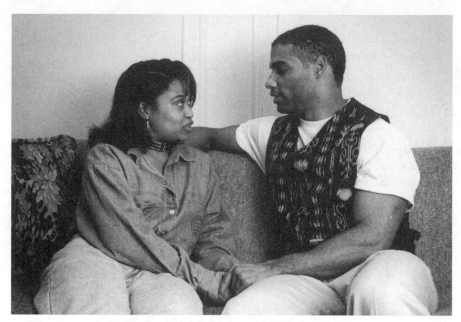

Men and women must communicate to keep relationships strong. *(Photo: T. L. Litt/Impact Visuals)*

Sometimes couples need outside help in order to work out their differences and conflicts. It may be difficult to consider going to a psychotherapist or marriage/family counselor. However, it is critical and calls for setting aside our historic reluctance to seek help. The weakening of traditional extended ties makes it difficult to turn to our parents, grandparents, aunts, and uncles to help resolve marital and family disputes. Black men in particular resist psychotherapy. But today there are trained Black therapists who are in tune with the background of Black men and can work with them and their families to resolve difficulties.

Some Black men may never go for counseling or sit around and talk with other men about their lives. But Black couples *can* work on their relationship together. It will take time, openness, and hard work because each brings the baggage of past disappointment and pain, but the lines of communication can be opened. Here are some guidelines suggested by Linda James Meyers, an assistant professor of clinical psychology in the departments of psychology and Black studies at Ohio State University.

A first step is something couples actually need to do separately. Each of you should take an honest look at yourself and learn to love and accept that self.

Sit down together and determine what kind of relationship you have and what kind you'd like to have. Do you have the same goals and aspirations? It's important for each of you to know what you want and

My husband, Leroy, and I have been married for over twenty-five years. We met at an election day eve party on November 8, 1968, and got married the following June. From that first day we knew we'd be together, but it's not a picture book. You have to work.

One reason our marriage has worked is because we were married six years before we had our children. That way we got a chance to grow up, get to know each other, and work together as a team. But once we had the children, we had financial troubles. My husband was in school, and he had to go to work part-time. My first daughter weighed only two pounds, and I had to stay at home with her and, later, with the other children. I used to baby-sit in order to make money to buy food. My mother kept the kids, and we'd paint people's houses for money so he could keep gas in his car.

Those times were so bad that our marriage could have gone either way. He could have left me, or I could have gone back to my mother. Leroy and I had hard days, but because of the love between us it made us stronger.

I also had a lot of trouble with his family. They are light-skinned people, and I wasn't good enough because my hair wasn't hanging down my back. I had problems with his father. The man tried to rape me, but my husband didn't believe me. That put a whole lot of stress on the marriage. Finally I told him it was either them or me, and he chose me.

For Black couples, racism also puts stress on the marriage and family. My husband's a social-work administrator for the state. He's taken them up on discrimination charges three times, and it's cost us a lot for lawyers. But whatever he did, it was my job to support him. Sometimes I feel drained, but if I get just a little back, it's good. As long as I'm getting something out of it, I'll be there.

But I guess I'm lucky. Leroy listens, he treats me as an equal, and he's a good father. Sexually, sometimes I just want to be hugged, so I tell him and he listens. I always say that if something happened to Leroy, if God took him away, I don't think I'd ever marry again. He's my best friend, and I'm his. I can see myself being a little old lady and us holding hands.

> "Leroy and I had hard days, but because of the love between us it made us stronger."
>
> —JEANETTE SMITH, BANK OFFICER, BROOKLYN

expect from the relationship and the future. You don't necessarily have to agree, but it clarifies just where each of you stands: Do you want a home? Where? Do you want children? How many? You can even discuss such things at pets and plants. When hopes, dreams, and desires are talked about honestly, no one has to make assumptions about what the other wants or needs.

Make sure you take the time to have a loving, sexual relationship. This physical part of marriage can be very satisfying if each of you lets the other know what feels good.

Bring a sense of fun to the relationship. Laugh together.

Work at developing nonverbal understanding. Sometimes it's hard for one partner or the other to talk about certain things, but there can be silent, heartfelt understanding between a couple.

Work toward developing your spiritual selves; encourage each other to look inward and reach for a higher self.

Make a commitment to each other. If a couple determines that they are truly committed to their relationship, they can work through whatever obstacles they may encounter.

You may be in a relationship where your partner is unwilling to seek solutions with or without outside help. Here are some things that might help you:

Go for counseling by yourself; it'll show how serious you are about getting help.

Don't feel guilty. You're entitled to your feelings.

Don't hold a grudge or indulge in spiteful, vindictive acts toward your partner. Let go of what's past, and look forward to a more positive future.

Get support from other women. Friends, sisters, mothers, aunts, and grandmothers have seen and heard much of what you're going through. They can offer a sympathetic ear and good, homey advice. If something hasn't happened to them, it happened to someone they know, and they'll be generous in sharing their wisdom and old-fashioned straight talk.

Take some time off; go away for a day or two or a week. A change of scene and a temporary break can uplift your spirits and give you a new outlook.

In the thick of an argument that's hot and heavy, take a "strife break": call time out, leave the room, change the subject. Then return to the subject once the two of you have "cooled out."

Seek spiritual guidance. This could be in the form of a book, audiotape, sermon, or words from a teacher, preacher, or other spiritual person. Listen and be soothed.

In the midst of the strife, we must look ahead to the future. One of the best and most important things we can do is to teach our young sons and daughters to love, trust, and respect the opposite sex.

We should also discuss Black men and Black male-female relationships as a community. Consider attending and encouraging the men in your life to attend the Annual Black Man Think Tank, which is held in

January at the University of Cincinnati. For more information contact the University of Cincinnati, Division of Student Affairs and Services, Ethnic Programs and Services, 330 Tangeman University Center, M.L. 0092, Cincinnati, OH 45221-0092; (513) 556-6008.

Interracial Relationships

Until as recently as the late 1960s, interracial marriages were banned in sixteen states. But now Black-white relationships—what filmmaker Spike Lee calls "jungle fever"—are growing in the U.S. According to the Census Bureau, Black-white marriages tripled during the seventies and eighties, and these unions are on the rise.

In most cases, interracial pairings involve a Black man with a white woman—which has long been a sore point for many sisters. In fact, interracial liaisons between Black male activists and white female civil rights workers during the sixties created much tension in the movement.

Though Black men are four times more likely than Black women to marry outside of the race, the number of Black female-white male couples is also increasing. These pairings are seen on the streets in big cities, in movies (such as *The Bodyguard,* with Whitney Houston and Kevin Costner) and on television. Many reasons explain the increase. For one, the societal taboo against interracial dating is falling away, especially in urban areas. Plus, thanks to the civil rights and women's movements, Black women have entered colleges and the corporate workplace in larger numbers and end up coming into contact with white men more. And during this time of a so-called "Black male shortage" some sisters have turned to white men for love and companionship.

Many interracial couples report that "love in black and white," especially in our racially polarized society, can be difficult. Dealing with parents—both Black and white—who aren't comfortable with Black-white relationships can be challenging, as can raising biracial children who are straddling two cultures.

For more information on interracial relationships, contact the Association of Multi-Ethnic Americans, P.O. Box 191726, San Francisco, CA 94119-1726; (510) 523-AMEA, which acts as a clearinghouse for information on inter- and multiracial relationships of all kinds and sponsors a confederation of more than ninety interracial support groups across

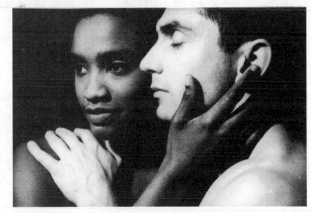

Black female/white male pairings are on the rise.
(Debbie Egan-Chin)

the country. Check out the magazines *New People,* a publication that deals with the concerns of interracial couples, families, singles, and racially mixed individuals (P.O. Box 47490, Oak Park, MI 48237; [313] 541-6943) and *Interrace,* which covers the concerns of interracial activities (*Interrace Magazine,* P.O. Box 12048, Atlanta, GA 30355; [404] 364-9690).

Books to read: *Mixed Blood: Intermarriage and Ethnic Identity in 20th Century America* by Paul R. Spickard, *Love in Black and White* by Mark Mathabane and Gail Mathabane, and *Racially Mixed People in America* edited by Maria Root, which contains an extensive bibliography of interracial books and publications and was written mostly by multiethnic authors.

His Health

In 1990 a study that appeared in *The New England Journal of Medicine* painted a bleak portrait of our men's health. It revealed that Black men in Harlem are less likely to reach age sixty-five than men in the impoverished Third World country of Bangladesh. Harlem's high rate of poverty contributes significantly to the problem, but the illnesses that plague Black men cannot be blamed solely on economic factors. Poor nutrition, smoking, heavy alcohol intake, lack of exercise, and stress round out the picture for Black men of all classes.

What's more, many men are loath to visit doctors. While we women must go to clinics, physicians' offices, and hospitals for Pap smears, mammograms, prenatal care, and childbirth, many Black men *never* set foot into health-care facilities—until it's too late and something has gone wrong. Many Black men don't trust the medical system. Others are afraid or believe that seeing a doctor is a sign of weakness.

This reluctance to get checkups and tests leads to the high rates of illness and early death among our men. Men are ignoring or seeking treatment late for heart disease and high blood pressure; cancer of the lung, esophagus, and stomach; stroke; diabetes; liver disease, and other serious health problems. Prostate cancer is also a major killer among Black men. It is 50 to 70 percent higher in African-American men than in white, and it kills our men two to three times more often.

We can help keep the men in our lives—mates, friends, relatives—healthy by encouraging them to make the lifestyle changes many of us have made. That means:

- Exercising at least three times per week for twenty minutes or more per session

- Cutting down on fat, salt, sugar, and cholesterol in the diet, while eating more fruit, vegetables, and whole-grain, high-fiber foods
- Taking steps to control stress by talking about problems and meditating or practicing yoga
- Drinking more water and less alcohol
- Quitting smoking and avoiding drugs
- Learning to listen to the body and understand its signals
- Getting yearly health exams that include blood-pressure tests

Our men must get the facts about prostate cancer. The prostate is a walnut-size gland located below the bladder that manufactures the seminal fluid that transports the sperm. After age fifty, men become more susceptible to prostate cancer as well as another disorder called benign prostate enlargement or BPH. (BPH isn't usually life-threatening, but it does cause discomfort.)

The American Cancer Society (ACS) recommends that men forty and older get a rectal exam every year to test for the disease. Men over fifty should also consult their doctors about getting a prostate-specific antigen test, which measures levels of prostate protein in the blood; an increase may be a sign of prostate cancer.

The warning signs of prostate cancer are:

- Pain or burning while urinating
- The need to urinate frequently, especially at night
- Weak or interrupted flow
- Inability to urinate or difficulty starting or stopping urine flow
- Blood in the urine
- Continuing pain in the lower back, pelvis, or upper thigh

For more information contact the Prostate Health Council, c/o American Foundation for Urologic Disease, Inc., 300 W. Pratt St., Baltimore, MD 21201; (800) 242-2383; the American Cancer Society at (800) ACS-2345; or the National Cancer Institute at (800) 4-CANCER.

For More Information

BOOKS

Black Macho & the Myth of the Superwoman, Michele Wallace, Routledge, Chapman and Hall, 1990.

Black Men: Obsolete, Single, Dangerous? The Afrikan American Family in Transition: Essays in Discovery, Solution and Hope, Haki R. Madhubuti, Third World Press (Chicago), 1990.

Black and Single: Meeting and Choosing a Partner Who's Right for You, Larry Davis, Noble Press (Chicago), 1993.

"Black Men and Women: Partnership in the 1990s," in *Breaking Bread: Insurgent Black Intellectual Life,* bell hooks and Cornel West, South End Press (Boston), 1991.

Court of Appeal: The Black Community Speaks Out on the Racial and Sexual Politics of Thomas Vs. Hill, Robert Chrisman and Robert Allen, eds., Ballantine, 1992.

Crisis in Black Sexual Politics, Julia Hare and Nathan Hare, Black Think Tank (San Francisco), 1989.

Friends, Lovers and Soul Mates: A Guide to Better Relationships Between Black Men and Women, Darlene Powell Hopson and Derek S. Hopson, Simon & Schuster, 1994.

He Says, She Says: Closing the Communication Gap Between the Sexes, Lillian Glass, G. P. Putnam's Sons, 1992.

"Holistic Lovemaking," in *Heal Thyself,* Queen Afua, A & B Books Publishers (Brooklyn), 1992.

Jumping the Broom: The African-American Wedding Planner, Harriette Cole, Henry Holt, 1993. Contains history of Black marriage.

Love Lessons: A Guide to Transforming Relationships, Brenda Wade with Brenda Lane Richardson, Amistad Press, 1993.

Mad at Miles: A Black Woman's Guide to Truth, Pearl Cleage, Cleage Group Publication (Southfield, Mich.), 1990.

"The Many Places of Black Men, A Report of the Commission on African American Males," The Office of the Manhattan Borough President, N.Y., June 1992.

Nurturing Black Males, Ron Mincy, ed., The Urban Institute Press (Washington, D.C.), 1994.

Race-ing Justice, Engendering Power, Toni Morrison, Pantheon Books, 1992.

Strategies for Resolving Conflict in Black Male and Female Relationships, La Francis Rodgers-Rose and James T. Rodgers, Traces Institute Publications (Newark, N.J.), 1985.

Uncivil War, Elsie B. Washington, Noble Press (Chicago), 1994.

You Just Don't Understand: Men and Women in Conversation, Deborah Tannen, Ballantine, 1991.

26

Women Loving Women

"We are everywhere": This popular slogan emblazoned on buttons and T-shirts serves as a banner of truth. Lesbians—women who have their most intimate relationships with other women—can be found in every conceivable area of society, and each woman has a different way of living her life. But all lesbians have something in common: an element of pain over society's refusal to recognize their relationships. Black lesbians and gays have to battle double oppression: Racism from whites and homophobia from straight Blacks. And Black lesbians also face sex discrimination. And oppression and rejection are most painful when they come from friends and family members. This kind of strain can take its toll: A 1994 UCLA study found that African-American lesbians have rates of depressive distress as high as those of HIV-infected men.

Nonetheless, there has been a strong presence of lesbians in African-American history, although this presence generally has been hidden. Moms Mabley, dubbed the Funniest Woman in the World, was a lesbian, as was her contemporary, pianist and blues singer Gladys Bentley, who donned a tuxedo and top hat when she performed in the 1920s and 1930s. Acclaimed

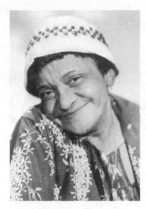

The late, great comic Moms Mabley was a lesbian. *(Photo: Schomberg Center, New York Public Library)*

playwright Lorraine Hansberry, author of *A Raisin in the Sun,* discovered her love for women during the late 1950s but kept it a secret, in part because of the predictably negative response of the Black nationalist movement of which she was a passionate supporter. The legendary blues singer Bessie Smith lived passionately, loving both men and women.

We celebrate other Black lesbians, living and dead, including poet Angelina Weld Grimké, poet and activist Pat Parker, singer and activist Mabel Hampton, filmmaker Michelle Parkerson, writer June Jordan, and poet and essayist Audre Lorde. You can call up the names of many other brave lesbians—your ancestors, family members, and sister-friends—for strength and guidance and to pay homage to.

Why Some People Are Gay

No one knows exactly how many people are gay. The most frequently cited and widely accepted estimate is 10 percent, which would mean that one in every ten people is a lesbian or gay man. In recent years, however, this number has been disputed.

Some people—gay and straight, experts and laypeople—believe that homosexuality is learned behavior, while others believe that it is biological, a hormonal or genetic consequence. The bottom line is that no one really knows why some people are attracted to others of the same sex. Many people believe that there's a broad range of sexuality but that most people choose to express only their heterosexual selves because of the constraints of society. Writer Alice Walker, for example, chooses to call herself pansexual.

Lesbians themselves feel that their sexuality is as natural as taking in breath. "I can't *not* be gay," says Lydia, a San Francisco lesbian who realized she was gay about ten years ago. "Once I admitted—to myself—that I was attracted to other women, I was finally able to be myself. Before that I was so busy hiding and pretending and denying that I didn't even know myself. Now my lesbianism is part of my identity, just like my Black skin, my long arms, and nappy hair."

Because most straight people don't understand lesbians and gays, myth after myth has been invented about them. The most common are:

Whites force homosexuality on Blacks. No one—Black or white—can force another person to have feelings she doesn't really have.

Being gay is a choice. The majority of people wouldn't choose to be gay or lesbian because it often brings rejection, ridicule, scorn, and violence. People can't make longing and desire disappear, but they can choose whether or not to express it or repress it.

Women who are raped or sexually abused become lesbians as a refuge from men and male sexuality. Many lesbians have not been raped or sexually abused, and many straight women have.

Lesbians hate men. Many lesbians have male friends both gay and straight.

Lesbians and gay men shouldn't raise children. No studies show that being raised by gay people does any harm to children. And being raised by a gay parent doesn't mean a child will be gay. Think about it: Most lesbians and gay men were raised by heterosexual parents. Many lesbians and gay men are raising children.

Lesbians prey on young girls. Statistics confirm that the overwhelming majority of sexual abuse and rape involves a straight man abusing a woman or girl.

Lesbians and gay men are anti-God. Many lesbians and gay men are deeply spiritual, and lesbians and gay men have long been an integral part of the community of Black Christians.

How Do You Know If You're Gay?

Just as there is no uniform answer about why some women are lesbian and others are heterosexual, there is no one way to discover sexual identity. Some adolescents go through a period of homosexual experimentation, but end up being straight. Other women marry and have children, but later discover their lesbianism.

Michelle Adams, a civil rights attorney who lives in New York City, remembers feeling different as early as age five. "I didn't want to be a boy, but I was hard pressed to figure who I did want to be."

Often even our feelings toward women during childhood are so repressed or confusing that only in retrospect do we recognize what they meant. Linda Grubbs, an administrative assistant from New Jersey, dated men well after high school and didn't feel different until much later. But looking back, she says, she is able to recall much earlier inklings of an interest in women. "I had dreams about my sister's third-grade teacher. They were sexual dreams about kissing her, running my fingers through her hair. I definitely didn't know what it was about at the time."

Yvonne Mercer, a Bronx guidance counselor in her fifties, discovered her lesbianism later in life. She spent nine years in a convent, then was married for two and a half years to a man before admitting her attraction to other women. She has now been involved with a female partner for nearly ten years.

Rhonda Williams, a professor of African-American studies at the

"Everything I ever wanted in a person, I've gotten from Nancy."

—NAME WITHHELD,
HOSPITAL SUPERVISOR,
NEW YORK CITY

Nancy and I have been together for thirteen years, and just like any other relationship, it's not easy. It hasn't been honey and cake for all this time. We have our ups and downs like anybody else.

It was very bumpy in the beginning. She didn't know whether this was the life for her or not, and her husband was saying he was going to come back. I took her over to talk to a minister, and when I came to pick her up, she walked out smiling. Whatever he told her, she's been able to deal with it from then on.

She has four children, and I've developed a good relationship with them. We never told them outright that we were lovers, but over the years, as much time as I've spent here, they know we are more than just friends. When two of them were at home, I would be like a second mother to them. Nancy used to work at night, and I would come here, make sure they ate, and be there when they went to sleep. In the beginning I tried to get her to tell them because it wasn't fair to them. She feels they know about the relationship by the way they treat the two of us together. We're just one family, we get together, and I'm not an outsider. We do Thanksgiving here and then go to my mother's for Christmas. My brothers and sisters accept Nancy like a sister, she's the godmother to my youngest brother's son.

I think our relationship has worked so well because we talk. We work at it, and that means you don't let every little nitpicking thing get in your way of the love that you have for each other. Whatever is on our minds must be cleared. It's hard; sometimes we don't want to talk about it, but if it must be discussed, we go ahead and discuss it. The biggest thing that can tear a relationship down is lack of communication. I think that if those lines of communication stay open, the relationship will continue to flourish. I don't consider myself married, but I've made sure whatever I have will go to her if something should happen to me. We don't have a lot of money or anything, but we have a will, and we just bought a cemetery plot. We just keep looking at the future, thinking about early retirement and looking at houses down in Georgia.

Everything I ever wanted in a person, I've gotten from Nancy. She's a very giving person and a very loving person, and she's not afraid to show me she loves me. That makes my love flow just as freely.

University of Maryland at College Park, was also married before she met a woman she was attracted to. "I enjoyed sex but found out I could enjoy it more with women."

Self-identification as a lesbian can occur long after a woman enters relationships with women. Even though Michelle Adams had a sexual relationship with another adolescent girl while in high school, it wasn't until she went to college and began reaching out to the lesbian community on her college campus that she began to identify herself as a lesbian.

Coming Out

Keeping a veil of secrecy around who we love and how we love, and especially hiding what may be the most compelling and important part of our lives from our close friends and family, can be depressing, tiring, isolating, and confusing. Relationships with loved ones are strained and conversations become restricted because such an important aspect of our lives is censored.

But coming out can be just as difficult. For some women, it's a wonderful process—awakening, freeing, and gratifying. But it can also be a nightmare of rejection and ridicule, of job loss, the loss of one's children, and even violence. Ayofemi Folayan, a wordsmith, performance artist, and "actorvist" who lives in Los Angeles, knows this intimately. When her

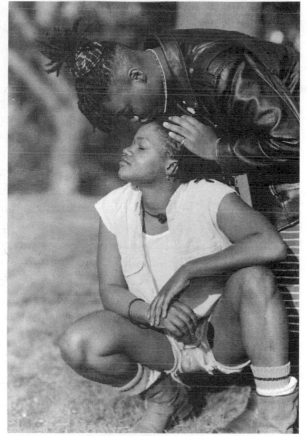

Being comfortable with sexuality can help foster loving relationships. *(Photo: Lisa Ross)*

parents discovered her lesbianism, they had her committed to a mental institution for six months.

Though most lesbians avoid that kind of horrible fate, many still feel anxiety about coming out. For other lesbians, however, coming out has brought them closer to their friends and family members. Says Lydia of San Francisco: "Since I've come out to my mother, we are much closer. She was angry and upset at first, but once she accepted the reality that I was not going to marry a nice Black man and have a big, fancy wedding to which all her friends could come, she was able to let go of her fantasy of me and get to know the real me. Now we relate to each other on an honest level."

For some women, coming out is political, for others it is personal, but ultimately the decision to come out is a choice each woman must make for herself, in her own time. Some people come out to one close friend but don't share the information with family members. Others tell their families but not the people they work with.

Parents and Friends of Lesbians and Gays (PFLAG), a national support network, suggests asking yourself the following questions before coming out:

Are you sure about your sexual orientation? Confusion on your part will increase your parents' confusion and decrease their confidence in your judgment.

Are you comfortable with your gay sexuality? If you're wrestling with guilt and periods of depression, you'll be better off waiting to tell your parents until you are more accepting of yourself.

Do you have support? In the event your parents' reaction devastates you, there should be someone or a group that you can confidently turn to for emotional support and strength.

Are you knowledgeable about homosexuality? Your parents will probably respond based on a lifetime of misinformation from a homophobic society. If you're informed, you'll be able to assist them by sharing reliable information and research.

What's the emotional climate at home? Choose a time to tell them when they aren't dealing with such matters as death of a close friend, pending surgery, or loss of a job.

Can you be patient? Your parents will require time to deal with this information if they haven't considered it prior to your sharing. Give them from six months to two years.

What's your motive for coming out now? Never come out in anger or during an argument. Do it because you love them and want to become closer.

Do you have available resources? Get a book your parents can read, or contact your local PFLAG chapter.

Are you financially dependent on your parents? If you suspect they are capable of forcing you out of the house or withdrawing college finances, you may choose to wait until they do not have this weapon to hold over you.

What is your general relationship with your parents? If you've gotten along well with them, chances are they'll be able to deal with the issue in a positive way.

What is their moral societal view? If they tend to see social issues in clear terms of good/bad or holy/sinful, you may anticipate serious problems.

Now I am comfortable with myself and with my identity, but if I hadn't come out, I probably would have attempted suicide and succeeded. It was too much pressure to be someone and something I was not.

I don't think about why I'm gay. I'm not sure if I believe in the genetic line, but I've known since I was five. Something had to be inborn, it was not placed in me by somebody. There was always a warmth I felt toward females that I didn't feel toward males.

I dated quite a few boys, but I never slept with any of them. They always looked kind of feminine. I had my last boyfriend my junior year in high school. I remember closing my eyes and wishing he was a woman. It was then I made a very conscious decision to stop dating boys.

Having gay feelings was just one of many things going on in my childhood. I was upper-middle-class and Black, so I was ostracized in many ways. White kids were calling me a nigger, and Black kids were telling me I was white. The fact that I had feelings toward women was just one more thing that made me different from everybody else.

When I was seventeen, everything got to be too much, and I tried to commit suicide by slitting my wrists. I felt I was living a lie, and I didn't have any brothers or sisters to confide in. My parents were all that I had. I felt there was no way I could come out to them and death would be more desirable. I was in the bathroom, and I had just begun to cut my wrist, and my father knocked on the door. My parents threw me into therapy. I had to work through so much, including being incested by a cousin.

After about three months, I was comfortable enough to come out to my parents. I told them I was a bisexual, even though I knew damn well I wasn't; I thought it would soften the blow. My mother went into hysterics, and my father came in to see why she was yelling, so I had to tell him. My father said, "You're not bisexual, you're not confused. You're gay or you wouldn't have brought it up," and he was right.

Coming out definitely didn't make my relationship with my mother any better. My mother ended up blaming herself, and then she blamed my father. She would say things like "Don't bring home any woman who looks like a man. I know what you people do. None of those people are welcome in my house." My father was as supportive as he could be with my mother grandstanding.

I moved out and went to college, and things were better. I found a lesbian community and had my first relationship with a woman as a freshman. I've had to struggle with a lot of ignorant people, but I survived, by looking out for myself and relying on my inner strength. Despite the problems, it was

---

"*This is who I am.*"

—NAME WITHHELD, STUDENT, OXEN HILL, MARYLAND

very important for me to come out. I don't want people to assume I fit into a certain mold because I'm female or because I'm Black. I don't want anyone to assume I'm straight. This is who I am.

———————

Is this your decision? Don't be pressured into coming out if you're not sure *you'll* be better off by doing so—no matter what their response.

For more information contact the Federation of PFLAG, Inc., 1012 14th St. NW, suite 700, Washington, DC 20005; (202) 638-4200, and ask for the pamphlet "Coming Out to Your Parents." Also read "Coming Out," by Linda and Clara Villarosa (*Essence,* May 1991), in which mother and daughter (the editor of this book) offer both sides of the coming-out experience.

Coping with Challenges That Affect Lesbians

Discrimination
Civil rights protection for lesbians and gays remains elusive. Sodomy laws, which still exist in nearly 50 percent of the states, outlaw homosexual activity between consenting adults. These laws are used to discriminate against lesbians and gays in employment and housing, public services, custody, government jobs, and religious institutions. For Black lesbians and gay men, racial discrimination compounds the problem.

Increasingly, lesbians and gay men are fighting back against oppression. Civil rights laws protect us from discrimination based on sexual orientation, and some cities have specific laws that ban bias against gays and lesbians. Some progressive companies (and some city governments) recognize lesbian and gay households and extend insurance and other benefits generally limited to married couples to the "domestic partners" of gay or lesbian employees.

Some straight Black people get angry when they hear that lesbians and gay men are demanding civil rights protection. However, discrimination is discrimination whether it's against Black folks or gay men and lesbians; it's always wrong.

To find out more about fighting against bias, especially if you feel you've been discriminated against on the basis of sexual orientation, contact the Lambda Legal Defense and Education Fund, 666 Broadway, 12th floor, New York, NY 10012-2317; (212) 995-8585; or 6030

Wilshire Blvd. #200, Los Angeles, CA 90036-3617; (213) 937-2728; or the National Gay and Lesbian Task Force, 1734 14th St. NW, Washington, DC 20009; (202) 332-6483.

Violence

As Black folks, we know that when people are angry or hurt, they sometimes take out their pain on other groups of people. Gay men and lesbians are too often the victims of violent crime committed by people— Black and white—who don't understand them, are angry at them, or who randomly and irrationally hate them.

Every year thousands of lesbians and gay men are "bashed," violently attacked because of their sexual orientation. In fact, in 1992 a woman from Salem, Oregon, was murdered by skinheads because she was a Black lesbian. The National Gay and Lesbian Task Force estimates that in 1992 anti-lesbian/gay crime increased 4 percent, with 1,822 incidents reported in five cities. Sadly, however, most crimes go unreported.

If you are afraid or have been the victim of antigay violence, contact the Gay and Lesbian Anti-Violence Project, 647 Hudson St., New York, NY 10014; (212) 807-0197. If you need legal advice or representation, contact Lambda Legal Defense and Education Fund, 666 Broadway, 12th floor, New York, NY 10012-2317; (212) 995-8585; or 6030 Wilshire Boulevard #200, Los Angeles, CA 90036-3617; 213-937-2728.

Battering

Like straight men and women, lesbians sometimes reach the boiling point and lash out at those people closest to them. Social worker Valli Kanuha maintains that battered Black lesbians are reluctant to seek help because "the triple jeopardy they face as women living in a sexist society, lesbians living in a homophobic society, and as people of color living in a racist society forms a complex web of silence and vulnerability with very little protection. In this often isolated existence, lesbians of color in violent relationships are further hidden because of the shame and fear associated with domestic abuse." For more information, read the chapter "Compounding the Triple Jeopardy: Battering in Lesbians of Color Relationships" in *Diversity and Complexity in Feminist Therapy*, edited by Kerry Lobel, or *Naming the Violence: Speaking Out About Lesbian Battering* by Kerry Lobel and the National Coalition Against Domestic Violence Lesbian Task Force.

If you are in an abusive relationship, call WOMAN, Inc. (a lesbian domestic-violence program) at 333 Valencia St., suite 251, San Francisco,

CA 94103; (415) 864-4722/4555; the National Coalition Against Domestic Violence National Office at P.O. Box 18749, Denver, CO 80218-0749; (303) 839-1852; or the Gay and Lesbian Anti-Violence Project at (212) 807-0197.

Alcoholism and Drug Addiction

Experts believe that a disproportionate number of lesbians and gay men are alcoholics. The higher rates may be a response to the emotional pain of being gay caused by societal rejection. It is exacerbated by the tendency for social life to be structured around bars and nightclubs, environments that encourage alcohol consumption. A study of 1,566 lesbians conducted between 1985 and 1987 revealed that 30 percent were in recovery, and a 1983 survey of lesbians in Los Angeles found that 33 percent were addicted to drugs or alcohol.

If you are drinking too much or using illegal drugs, explore the reasons. Are you uncomfortable with or feeling guilty about your sexuality and using drugs and alcohol to feel better? If so, get to the root of the problem by seeking help in the form of therapy or group counseling. Most gay community centers can hook you up with a support group, and AA groups in some areas are predominately gay or *specifically* geared toward lesbians and gays. Call (212) 870-3400 or contact your local chapter for more information.

If you need help getting off drugs or giving up alcohol or would like more information, contact one of the following groups that specialize in substance abuse in the gay community: the National Association of Lesbian and Gay Alcoholism Professionals, 1147 S. Alvarado St., Los Angeles, CA 90006; (213) 381-8524; or the Pride Institute, 14400 Martin Dr., Eden Prairie, MN 55344; (612) 934-7554 or (800) 54-PRIDE.

Multiple Problems of Lesbian and Gay Youth

Every day lesbian and gay youth are bombarded with antigay images and messages from the society at large and within the microcosms of the school and neighborhood. The compounded problems of isolation, lack of family support, and the prevalence of substance abuse and depression make lesbian and gay youth more likely to drop out of school and three times more likely to attempt suicide.

According to the Hetrick Martin Institute, a not-for-profit agency that offers a variety of social and educational services to gay youths, 26 percent of gay youths are either expelled or forced to leave their homes because of continual conflict over their homosexuality. Researcher Joyce Hunter, a cofounder of Hetrick Martin, conducted a study of African-American and Latino lesbian and gay youth in New York City in 1990 and found that 41 percent reported being victims of violence from family, peers, and strangers. In a separate study in 1992, Hunter found 83 percent of young lesbians had used alcohol, 56 percent had used drugs, and 11 percent had used crack.

The following organizations can provide referrals and/or assistance to young folks struggling with their gay identity: Sexual Minority Youth Assistance League (SMYAL), 333 1/3 Pennsylvania Ave. SE, Washington, DC 20003; (202) 546-5940/5911; the Hetrick Martin Institute, 2 Astor Pl., 3rd floor, New York, NY 10003; (212) 674-2400; or Indianapolis Youth Group, P.O. Box 20716, Indianapolis, IN 46220; (317) 541-8726.

Lesbian Parenting

For many people the words *lesbian* and *mother* don't go together—but that's because most people are ignorant about the fact that millions of children are being raised by gay women. The American Bar Association estimates that six million to fourteen million children are being raised in at least four million gay or lesbian households. Lesbian mothering is particularly common among Black women because a large number of lesbians have children from marriage or a previous relationship with a man.

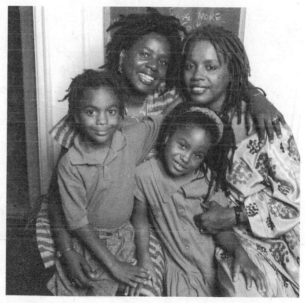

Studies show that children raised by lesbian parents are as emotionally healthy as those raised by heterosexuals. *(Photo: Lisa Ross)*

Numerous studies show that children who grow up in lesbian and gay homes face no disadvantage compared with those who are reared by heterosexuals. In a review of studies published in a 1993 issue of the journal *Child Development,* children raised by gay parents are no more likely to have psychological problems than those raised by straight parents. Children of gay parents are likely to suffer teasing and ridicule from narrow-minded children. But to remedy that, we must fight homophobia rather than discourage lesbians from becoming parents.

Three dozen studies reviewed by a psychologist at the University of

Virginia showed no evidence that being raised by a lesbian mother affects gender identification. In other words, lesbians are no more likely to raise gay children than are heterosexuals.

Lesbians find inventive ways to raise children, relying on networks of family and friends for support and assistance. Most lesbians recognize the importance of a male presence in their children's lives, so some women coparent with gay males or have male family members and friends play an important role.

Likewise, coming out to children is a deeply personal decision; only individual mothers must decide if and when the time is right. This decision may largely be based on the way a woman feels about her lesbianism. Some women come out to their kids while they are very young and increase the sophistication of discussions as the child matures. Others choose to wait until their children are old enough to be aware of sexuality.

Open discussion and frankness cannot shield a child from negative societal messages about her or his mother's sexual identity. A child may also begin to experience ridicule from schoolmates beginning in adolescence. Fortunately most children are primarily concerned about their relationship with their mothers and are very protective of that bond. Assure children that your sexual identity does not affect your relationship with them, and be open to answering more specific questions older children may ask.

For information about the legal aspects and methods of lesbian parenting read *The Lesbian and Gay Parenting Handbook: Creating and Raising Our Families* by April Martin. You may also contact the Lesbians of Color Project, c/o National Center for Lesbian Rights, 870 Market St., suite 570, San Francisco, CA 94102; (415) 329-NCLR, for free legal advice on parental and other issues and parenting workshops. The Gay and Lesbian Parents Coalition International, P.O. Box 50360, Washington, DC 20091; (202) 583-8029, is a support group based in Washington, D.C., with forty chapters in the United States and Canada. Also call for information about books for children of lesbians and gays and coming out to your children and others.

If Your Child Is Gay

As a parent, your first response to learning that your child is gay may be all about you; you may feel shocked, angry, hurt, or guilty about some personal inadequacy or a mistake you may have made in raising her. You are entitled to all of your feelings, but as soon as possible you need to stop and respond to the needs of your child.

Chances are you became aware of changes in your child's behavior and the way she related to you and the rest of the family. She may have been distant and secretive, but remember that she was actually lonely and desperately afraid. She was afraid of your reaction, that you would reject her, that she would lose her mother as a consequence of discovering herself. The only thing she needs to hear is that you still love her and that you will always love her. Remember that lesbian and gay youth are three times more likely to attempt suicide than other young people, and lesbian and gay suicides comprise 30 percent of youth suicides committed annually. Your support is essential.

Reserve judgment and negative comment until you contact a therapist or a support group that can help you better understand your child's sexuality. PFLAG notes that many parents go through these stages when confronted with a child's homosexuality:

1. Shock. On learning that a child is gay, parents may experience a paralysis that makes them unable to react and leads to
2. Denial. After getting over the shock of learning their child is gay, parents may attempt to pretend that they never learned about their child's sexual identity. This denial may take the form of an obsessive interest in the child's dating life or even arranging dates with the opposite sex.
3. Guilt. Because of the negative images that typify the lesbian and gay identity, parents may mistakenly believe they made parenting mistakes that caused their children to become gay.
4. Expression of feelings. Once some time has passed, there will be a need to express the reactions to homosexuality that can be hardest for the child to hear since they are likely to echo the negative opinions of society.
5. Personal decision making. At this point parents may decide to sever ties with the child indefinitely or that while they do not understand or accept their child's homosexuality, they do want to continue to have a relationship with their child.
6. True acceptance. Many parents never reach this stage. True acceptance means they no longer view homosexuality as an unfortunate reality; that they are able to discuss their child's personal life with as much comfort as they would with a heterosexual child; and that they can treat their child's lovers as they would a child's spouses.

To get the support you need contact PFLAG, which provides support groups and information to parents of lesbians and gays and helps them understand each other. The group can refer you to meetings in your area, offer suggested readings, answer questions and send pamphlets geared toward parents and youths such as "Why Is My Child Gay?" and "Can We Understand?" You can also look in the library for the May 1991 *Essence* article "Coming Out," which provides a frank look at how a mother dealt with her daughter's lesbianism.

Health Issues Facing Lesbians

Generally speaking, lesbians share the same health concerns that straight and bisexual women have. But there are some issues that affect lesbians differently. Two in particular are breast cancer and AIDS. For a more in-depth look at lesbian health issues, read *Alive & Well: A Lesbian Health Guide* by Cuca Hepburn and Bonnie Gutierrez or *Lesbian Health: What Are the Issues?* edited by Phyllis Noerager Stern.

Lesbians and Breast Cancer

Suzanne Haynes, an epidemiologist at the National Cancer Institute in Washington, D.C., says that though national statistics show that breast cancer will hit one in eight women in the United States, for lesbians the numbers could be as high as one in three.

Haynes is quick to note that her suspicions are based on an assortment of data that has yet to be fully tested. Nonetheless, she points to four basic factors that increase the risk of getting breast cancer and that may be more common among lesbians. The best documented of these is the link to childbirth, which shows that women who never get pregnant have a 60 percent greater risk of breast cancer than women who do. Although lesbians are perfectly capable of giving birth, a study of two thousand lesbians conducted by the National Lesbian and Gay Health Care Foundation found that 84 percent had no children.

Other studies suggest that obesity and alcohol consumption, which for a number of complicated reasons seem to affect greater numbers of lesbians than women in general, also increase the risk of breast cancer. (And Black women, gay or straight, are more likely to be overweight than white women.) Finally, several studies indicate that lesbians are less likely to get routine medical checkups that can detect breast cancers before they become fatal.

To learn more about breast self-examination, see chapter 18, "Checkups and Tests We Can't Live Without"; for more on breast cancer see chapter 7, "We Are at Risk." The following organizations also provide information and support for lesbians living with cancer or who want to know more:

Lesbian Services of Whitman-Walker Clinic, 1407 S St. NW, Washington, DC 20009; (202) 797-3585.

Mary-Helen Mauntner Project for Lesbians with Cancer, P.O. Box 90437, Washington, DC 20090; (202) 332-5536.

Women's Cancer Resource Center, 3023 Shattuck Ave., Berkeley, CA 94705; (510) 548-WCRC.

Lesbians and AIDS

Though AIDS is ravaging the Black community, taking a particularly high toll on gay men and heterosexual women, lesbians have often been called "God's chosen people": As of 1992, only two cases of AIDS transmission between women have been documented by the Centers for Disease Control (CDC).

Lesbian health experts, however, warn against ignoring safe sex practices in the face of the devastating AIDS virus. Studies seem to indicate that woman-to-woman transmission is difficult, but it's certainly not impossible. And since the CDC has only recently begun to fully investigate AIDS in women and has never done specific studies on women who sleep with women, there's really no way of knowing how many lesbians have AIDS.

If you're not involved in a monogamous relationship and/or don't know your lover's sexual history, there are many good reasons for practicing safer sex. One is that many lesbians do have sex with men, either regularly or occasionally, and can contract HIV more easily from men. Lesbians can also contract HIV if they are IV drug users and share needles. In either case it's important to remember that a woman can be infected with HIV and not know it, either because she hasn't yet developed symptoms or because she hasn't been properly diagnosed. This woman can then pass the virus on to her female sexual partners.

Safer sex can also prevent the spread of other sexually transmitted infections (STI's) that lesbians can and do share, some of which can lead to very serious health problems. For tips on how to practice safer sex, including the use of dental dams and plastic wrap, see chapter 27, "Sexuality and Having Sex Safely."

There are many health clinics and organizations around the country that are sensitive to the special needs of lesbians with HIV and AIDS. Contact the Lesbian AIDS Project, Gay Men's Health Crisis, 129 W.

20th St., 4th floor, New York, NY 10011; (212) 337-3532, for information and referrals.

If you or someone you know needs more information on AIDS, call the Centers for Disease Control National HIV and AIDS Information Hotline: (800) 342-AIDS (open twenty-four hours a day).

Meeting Other Lesbians

One of the most difficult aspects of being a lesbian is feeling isolated. Meeting other Black lesbians in particular can be quite difficult. For various social and personal reasons, many of our sisters may not be openly lesbian. The white lesbian community is seemingly larger and more organized, but many of us may prefer to find our own community. Still we manage to find one another through that sixth sense called "gaydar." But just in case, here are some good avenues for meeting other lesbian sisters:

Political/activist organizations. Volunteer for groups such as the Black Gay and Lesbian Leadership Forum in Los Angeles or the People of Color Steering Committee in New York. AIDS advocacy, health advocacy, lesbian and gay rights, feminism, and political-interest groups are also a great way to meet like-minded sisters.

Community sports centers have information about where to pick up a basketball, soccer, or football game if you aren't already a member of a league or team.

Nightclubs, bars, and social organizations. Most major cities have a few lesbian bars that Blacks may frequent. Also check gay weeklies for parties that may be given by Black women, or check bulletin boards at your community center. Organizations such as Sisters of Something Special, STRUT, and African Ancestral Lesbians United for Societal Change provide activities in the New York area.

Support groups. Find a support group such as the Black Lesbian Support Group in Washington, D.C., where you can meet women in a safe, open environment. Check gay publications or at your local gay community center for notices of meetings.

Writing, dance, singing, or other creative groups. You can meet lesbian sisters in groups such as the Lavender Light Chorus in New York or the Ache Project (a group of lesbians who produce the journal *Ache: A Journal for Women of African Descent*) in the Bay Area.

Lesbian and gay community centers. Various organizations meet in these centers, which host a variety of events such as lesbian movie nights, crafts fairs, lectures, and parties.

Personal ads. Black gay publications such as *BLK* list personals and advertise dating services as do nearly all gay newspapers.

For contact information, see the listings below.

Bisexuality

Until recently, bisexuals were lumped together with lesbians and gays or assumed to be straight. Many gays think bisexuals are using bisexuality as a shield that allows them to obtain heterosexual privilege and frees them from the stigma of homosexuality. But while many lesbians and gays go through a stage of identifying themselves as bisexual, and some may have infrequent heterosexual relationships, it is possible to be attracted to both sexes. Bisexuals assert that just as gays and lesbians feel strongly attracted to members of the same sex and heterosexuals prefer the opposite sex, they have strong feelings for both sexes; that expressing themselves sexually with both women and men allows them to have a richer sexual experience.

The pull of social and political demands from both sides makes it difficult for many bisexuals to step up and claim their identity. Fortunately, many bisexual women have formed support groups and political organizations and exercise their right to sexual freedom. For more information about bisexuality, read "Bisexuality Coming Out of the Closet" (*Essence,* October 1992); *Bi Any Other Name: Bisexual People Speak Out* edited by Loraine Hutchins and Lani Kaahumanu; *Bisexuality: A Reader & Sourcebook* edited by Thomas Geller; and *Closer to Home: Bisexuality and Feminism* by Elizabeth Reba Weise.

The New York Area Bisexual Network, 208 W. 13th St., New York, NY 10011; (212) 459-4784, holds discussion groups, socials, safer-sex workshops for women and has a support group especially for women of color. (You can call the New York–area number for a referral in your area.) Also, BiNet USA, P.O. Box 7327, Langley Park, MD 20787; (202) 986-7186, and the Bisexual Resources Center, 95 Berkeley St., Boston, MA 02116; (617) 338-9595, offer resources and referrals.

For More Information

ORGANIZATIONS

AFRICAN ANCESTRAL LESBIANS UNITED FOR SOCIAL CHANGE (formerly Salsa Soul Sisters), c/o The Center, 208 W. 13th St., New York,

NY 10011; (212) 620-7310. Serves lesbians and is committed to the spiritual, cultural, educational, economic, and social empowerment of African ancestral women.

ASTRAEA NATIONAL LESBIAN ACTION FUND, 666 Broadway, suite 520, New York, NY 10012; (212) 529-8021. A feminist, grass-roots multicultural, multiracial lesbian foundation that gives grants to lesbian causes, foundations, and organizations.

THE BLACK GAY AND LESBIAN LEADERSHIP FORUM, 1219 S. LaBrea Ave., Los Angeles, CA, 90019; (213) 964-7820. Holds the National Black Gay and Lesbian Leadership Conference annually.

THE BLACK LESBIAN SUPPORT GROUP, c/o Whitman Walker Clinic, 1407 S Street NW, Washington, DC 20009; (202) 797-3593. Offers various services, in addition to peer support, including a book club and a spring retreat.

FEDERATION OF PFLAG, INC., 1012 14th St. NW, suite 700, Washington, DC 20005; (202) 638-4200. PFLAG has 340 local chapters across the U.S.

LESBIAN HERSTORY ARCHIVES, c/o Lesbian Herstory Educational Foundation, Inc., P.O. Box 1258, New York, NY 10116; (718) 768-DYKE. Gathers and preserves records of lesbian lives and activities.

NATIONAL COALITION FOR BLACK LESBIANS AND GAYS, Box 19248, Washington, DC 20036. This national political and educational organization is geared toward helping Black lesbians and gays address homophobia, racism, identity, and other issues that affect them.

NATIONAL GAY AND LESBIAN TASK FORCE, 1734 14th St., Washington, DC 20009; (202) 332-6483. A national grass-roots political organization.

THE SHANGO PROJECT, National Archives for Black Lesbians and Gay Men, P.O. Box 2341, Bloomington, IN 47402-2341; (812) 334-8860. Gathers and preserves materials that document aspects of the African-American lesbian and gay experience.

UNITED LESBIANS OF AFRICAN HERITAGE, 1626 N. Wilcox Ave., #190, Los Angeles, CA 90028; (213) 960-5051. A nonprofit organization dedicated to the visibility, unity, and empowerment of Black lesbians.

Most states and/ or major cities have national lesbian and gay community centers that provide services from coming-out support groups to suicide prevention to lesbian movie nights. Most centers also have organizations for people of color, and Black members hold annual events such as Kwanzaa and Black History Month celebrations. Call information for local addresses and phone numbers.

BOOKS

Lesbian Couples, D. Merliee Clunis and G. Dorsey Green, Seal Press, 1993.

Odd Girls and Twilight Lovers: A History of Lesbian Life in Twentieth-Century America, Lillian Faderman, Viking/Penguin, 1992.

Hidden from History: Reclaiming the Gay and Lesbian Past, Martin Bauml Duberman, Martha Vicinus, and George Chauncey, Jr., eds., NAL Books, 1989. (Read the chapter called "A Spectacle of Color: The Lesbian and Gay Sub-Culture of Jazz Age Harlem.")

Black Women's Health Book: Speaking for Ourselves, Evelyn C. White, ed., Seal Press, 1990. (Read "Taking the Home Out of Homophobia" by Jewelle Gomez and Barbara Smith.)

All the Women Are White, All the Blacks Are Men, But Some of Us Are Brave: Black Women's Stories, Gloria T. Hull, Patricia Bell Scott, and Barbara Smith, eds., The Feminist Press, 1982.

The Rights of Lesbians and Gay Men: The Basic ACLU Guide to a Gay Person's Rights, Nan D. Hunter et al., Southern Illinois Press, 1992.

Sister Outsider: Essays and Speeches, Audre Lorde, Crossing Press, 1984. (Includes essay about raising a son.)

Zami: A New Spelling of My Name, Audre Lorde, Crossing Press, 1983.

MAGAZINES

Ache: A Journal for Lesbians of African Descent, P.O. Box 6071, Albany, CA 94706; (510) 849-2819.

BLK, The National Black Lesbian and Gay Newsmagazine, Box 83912, Los Angeles, CA, 90083-0912.

Black Lace, Box 83912, Los Angeles, CA 90083-0912. Black lesbian erotica.

COLORLife!, P.O. Box 1518, Ansonia Station, New York, NY 10023.

27

Sexuality and Having Sex Safely

Sexuality is a complex and natural form of human expression. No one really understands it perfectly, and each woman's sexual needs and attractions are as unique as her signature. What we like and who we like to do it with is influenced by an array of factors including genetic makeup, childhood environment, cultural values, and exposure to new ideas. Sexuality can be a deeply personal, intimate experience of pleasure and discovery.

Black Women's Sexuality

For African-American women, our sexuality is further complicated by racist, sexist stereotypes that affect our feelings about being sexual. During slavery, control of our sexuality was taken away from us. Our ancestors were bred like cattle to produce an unlimited supply of free labor. White slave owners also raped Black women freely, then justified their inhuman behavior by labeling Black women as sexually insatiable, always "wanting it." To survive, our ancestors responded by playing into the stereotype or desexualizing themselves as mammies or repressed religious women.

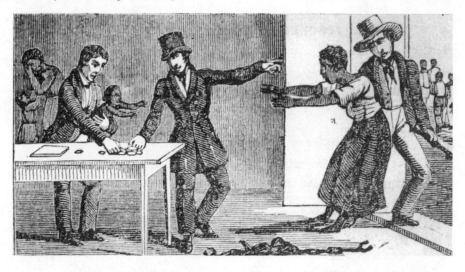

During slavery, Black women were raped and bred like cattle. *(Photo: The Bettman Archive)*

Gail E. Wyatt, Ph.D., a UCLA professor of psychiatry and an expert on Black women's sexuality, has spoken and written eloquently of the vestiges of those stereotypes that remain with us today. She believes that negative images of Black women's sexuality impact us in the bedroom. In her study "The Sexual Experience of Afro-American Women," Dr. Wyatt reveals that many of us battle with the stereotype of the "loose" or sexually knowledgeable woman. "Many Black women will not initiate sex or communicate what they find pleasing during sex because they feel it will reflect badly on them, as if they've 'been around,'" Dr. Wyatt says. Other women in her study were traumatized by sexual abuse or rape, which greatly affected their sexual functioning, or they simply felt guilty, afraid, or inhibited.

According to June Dobbs Butts, Ph.D., a sex therapist and assistant professor of psychiatry and behavioral sciences at Meharry Medical College in Nashville, the impact that sexual stereotypes and narrow media images have had on us is far-reaching. "In this materialistic and commercial society, appearance and external approval have become more important to us than how we actually feel inside," she says. "Many women don't know to trust their own internal instincts when it comes to their sexuality. Often we look to our partners for approval, and in the process we ignore our own needs." The unfortunate result is that many women's sexual experiences are less than satisfying because they do not feel comfortable voicing their needs.

Recently that has begun to change as African-American women are speaking for themselves about what it means to be sexual. Contemporary authors have contributed to a redefinition of our sexuality through work such as that collected in *Wild Women Don't Wear No Blues: Black Women Writers on Love, Men and Sex,* edited by Marita Golden. The diverse images these writers present have helped us reclaim our sexual identity and examine how negative stereotypes have affected our behavior.

Pleasuring Yourself

Dr. Wyatt's research reveals that women who have gratifying sex lives commonly attributed their satisfaction to several factors:

They were able to verbally and nonverbally communicate their needs.
They prefer to actively initiate sex and try new things.
They had sex often and were highly orgasmic.
They had overall positive feelings about having sex.

To have good sex, you must first explore your body—touch yourself—and become familiar with what gives you pleasure. Although Dr. Watts's research shows that Black women are much less likely than white women to masturbate, it is not wrong or sinful but an important part of overall sexual health. According to the book *For Yourself: The Fulfillment of Female Sexuality* by Lonnie Barbach, studies show that women who masturbate reach orgasm 95 percent of the time and often have stronger orgasms than during sex with a partner, have increased sexual desire and more positive feelings about sex, and are more orgasmic with their partners.

The best way to begin your exploration is to become familiar with your body. Make time for yourself. Find a quiet and relaxing environment; maybe take a bath or turn the lights off in the bedroom and light some candles. Free yourself from distractions; allow yourself to become absorbed in this experience.

You may want to get a small hand mirror so you can see as you touch and investigate. Start by observing your breasts. Notice the dark ring around your nipples called the areola. During various stages in sexual excitement these will swell. Try touching your breasts in different areas, including the nipples. Experiment with different types of touches: stroking, massaging, rolling your nipple between your thumb and finger. Don't worry if you think your breasts are too big or too small; breast size has no effect on your level of sensitivity or ability to become aroused.

As you touch your breasts, you may begin to feel some sensation in your genital area. Position the mirror between your legs so that you can clearly see your vaginal area. Start at the top of the genital region where your pubic hair begins, just below your abdomen. Touch your pubic hair and be aware of its texture and color.

Next touch the lips of your vagina; they'll feel soft, fleshy, and sensitive. With your fingers, pull open your outer lips. Inside is another set of lips, called the inner lips. Every woman's vaginal lips have a unique shape, and yours may have several folds, or they may be dark in color. Open your inner lips and you'll see a protective fold of skin, called the clitoral hood. If you pull this back, you will expose a small, round organ about the size of a pea. This is your clitoris, which for most women is the most important organ for sexual pleasure. Unlike any other human organ, the sole purpose of a woman's clitoris is to provide sexual pleasure.

Explore different types of touch to your clitoris. Each of us has different preferences, and it may take some time to discover what works for you. If you feel too self-conscious about touching yourself, try running water from a bath or shower over your clitoral area. You may enjoy less direct stimulation, like placing the palm of your hand or a pillow between your legs and rubbing. Or you may want to rub your finger across it and try out different speeds and intensities (hard and slow, soft and fast, two fingers). Most women are not able to reach orgasm unless they have some type of clitoral contact. So if you have never played with your clitoris or have never climaxed, you will find this is the most effective way to increase your sexual enjoyment.

As your hand moves just past your clitoris, you'll notice a small opening, your urethra, through which urine passes. For most women the urethra plays an insignificant role in sexual pleasure.

If you continue downward, below your urethra, you will see a larger opening, which is your vagina. The degree of sexual pleasure derived from having the vagina stimulated varies from woman to woman. Many of us gain a great deal of enjoyment when touched around the opening of the vaginal canal. This area is very sensitive because there are several nerve endings here. The upper two-thirds of the vagina is less sensitive to touch but is responsive to pressure and stretching. At the uppermost area inside your vagina is your cervix, the lower part and neck of your uterus. Some women have discovered that deep thrusting during penetration pushes against their cervix and can add to their excitement. Other women, however, find it uncomfortable and jarring.

*"I am learning
to let my body
speak, to listen
to its naked
power."*

—BELL HOOKS,
FEMINIST CULTURE CRITIC
AND AUTHOR OF *SISTERS
OF THE YAM* AND OTHER
BOOKS, NEW YORK CITY

Mama, I can hear my sisters say, voices dripping with scorn and hurt; "She stands naked in front of the mirror, just staring, as though she aint got no shame. Anybody could be looking up and see her through the window." Naked with shame on auction blocks Black female slaves watched the world that was our body change. Nakedness that could not be covered must be forgotten, shrouded in cloaks of modesty, Victorian puritanism, religion without flesh—signs that repeatedly say This Black female body is not on the block, not of the streets, not for sale, not without shame. *Ours is a history of shame, written on the body we cannot erase.*

Imagine growing up with five sisters in two large attic bedrooms painted a dusky rose, rooms with slanted roofs and huge windows from ceiling to floor. Six brown girls living in a private world no males could enter. You might imagine this world would be a place where we would forget all puritanical notions about the body learned outside and live in our flesh anew. That was not the way it was. When we climbed the stairs to the sanctuary, we moved all the more deeply into the heart of our repressions. We denied the presence of the body.

Nakedness was forbidden. Nakedness hurt the eye, like when Adam first looked at Eve. In these two rooms we wanted never to be caught looking. We refused to see one another's bodies. We worked hard to turn our eyes away, to dress in the dark, in half light, to change when no one was there, to always—always—wear gown or robe, to never not wear panties, keeping underwear on even during sleep. We denied our bodies, our right to see and feel ourselves, to witness our brown bodies move gracefully through girlhood and beyond. We made no celebration to herald budding breasts, moon flow or rounded hips. We lived to forget—to never remember our bodies naked without shame. We dreaded our dark female flesh.

The blackness of our bodies held no deep meanings, the range of shades and colors between us so common as to be unworthy of note. More than blackness we shared being female, felt the awesome power and presence of woman becoming. That presence troubled us. We invented gestures of disregard, habits of being that allowed us to forget our bodies. We created closets where we stripped ourselves of flesh. We pretended to be invisible—that we could never be seen, not by any human eye.

To be invisible hurts. To live in our bodies but always away from them was to live always alone in states of fierce and sorrowful abandonment. As a Black girl in a house of woman being I wanted to see myself. I longed to cherish mirrored reflections, to understand naked brown-girl flesh becoming itself. At 12 I read The Book of Negro Poetry. *I learn these words by heart:*

"She does not know her beauty. She thinks her brown body has no glory." A poem called "No Images." I understand this title. How can there be images if we insist on remaining invisible, lost to the flesh.

In search of glory, I find my body. I search it out, standing naked in front of mirrors, watching, giving my body sight—visibility. I look at my Black-girl body, see it clearly, learn its trace, learn to place myself outside history. Reinventing paradise, a garden of nakedness, a place where brown flesh can be known and loved.

I search my body out in the dark, hands mapping familiar terrain. My skin is smooth, velvety soft, soft as marshmallows roasted over fire—the color of warm honey. When my tongue licks my arm, I taste the sweetness there— warm honey. I fall asleep at night, naked from the waist down, hands between my legs, warm and wet, holding the memory of orgasm, mountain peaks I climb alone—solitary transcendant pleasure. I sleep deeply now, can lose myself in dreams, sure that my brown body is a haven, a home the spirit can return to.

My sisters pull the covers back, try and capture my secrets, brown hands between brown thighs, hands deep in pussy as sweet as warm honey. "Why you gotta use that word," my sisters say, "Aint you got no shame."

Their taunts seduce, fill me with the knowledge that to live as a brown woman in my flesh without shame is pure rebellion. I am learning to let my body speak, to listen to its naked power. I celebrate freedom in the flesh They seek to silence me. Aint you got no shame! *I touch lips with my tongue, biting flesh with my small white teeth, watch the fullness of their swell, blood coloring them earth-red, naked brown woman without shame, refusing to keep her body hidden—refusing history.*

Many women get enormous pleasure from the simultaneous arousal of their clitoris and vaginal area. You may like to insert your finger into your vagina while stimulating your clitoris or breasts.

If you can, try contracting the muscle that surrounds the vaginal opening. This is the pubococcygeal muscle (or PC muscle), and women who regularly exercise it find increased sexual enjoyment during intercourse. Talk to your gynecologist about exercises to help improve the tone of your PC muscle, especially if you've gone through childbirth.

Many women love having their G-spots stimulated. Named after a

German gynecologist, Ernst Grafenberg, the G-spot is an area a couple of inches inside behind the front wall of the vagina—between the back of the pubic bone and the cervix. To locate your G-spot, insert your finger along the uppermost wall of your vagina, go in about one or two inches, and feel for a spongy lump. Women who experience pleasure from their G-spot report that it takes some toying with different kinds of stimulation to discover what feels good. If you do enjoy the sensation and reach climax, an ejaculate fluid may spurt from your vagina. Don't get hung up if you aren't aroused by touching your G-spot. Every woman's body is different, so try to discover what feels right for you. Behind your vagina is the anus. Some women like to have theirs stimulated, while others are uncomfortable with the idea or the feeling.

You may be feeling self-conscious or hearing negative voices that say that your genitals are ugly or "nasty." Try to relax and think of your sexual organs as just another part of your body. Just as you appreciate your eyes for helping you to see beauty, you can also appreciate your genitals for providing you with another form of human pleasure.

What Is an Orgasm?

As you begin experimenting with different types of touch to your body, you'll begin to feel aroused. Experts describe women's sexual responses in these phases:

Excitement Phase. This may begin as a tingling or tightening feeling around the genital area because it is filling with blood. The clitoris becomes swollen and sensitive, and the vagina lubricates itself by creating wetness.

Plateau Phase. At this point the genitals become engorged with blood and the vagina is very wet. The breathing and heart rates increase, and the feeling of excitement is very strong.

Orgasmic Phase. During orgasm or climax (or "coming"), the muscles around the vagina and pelvic floor contract rapidly. Then a sense of release, a wave, or warm feeling washes over the body. Some orgasms are very powerful and seem to take over the whole body, while others are smaller and more genitally centered. A combination of the released tension and the emission of brain chemicals called endorphins give us that feeling of exhilaration during orgasm.

Some women feel self-conscious about how they look when they have orgasms. They're afraid that they may look ugly or funny. Rather than judge yourself, concentrate on the feelings of enjoyment and accept the natural expressions your face and body will go through.

Resolution Phase. At this point the heart and pulse rate slow to normal and your genitals return to their normal size. Some women are able to become aroused again immediately after their first orgasm and may even be able to have another or several orgasms. However, other women find they are too sensitive to be stimulated into orgasm again.

Men's Sexual Response

To have pleasurable sex with a man, it's important to understand his body and how he becomes aroused. Though men's bodies are different from ours, they go through the same phases of excitement.

Excitement Phase. A man's genital area fills with blood as his penis goes from a limp state to an erect position. His penis will grow in length and width, his testicles elevate, and his breathing and heart rate increase. As with the size of women's breasts, the size of a man's penis has no bearing on his sexual functioning.

Plateau Phase. His increased arousal makes his heart and breathing rates increase, his genitals continue to become engorged with blood, and his testicles elevate fully. His urethra, the opening at the tip of his penis, enlarges and may emit seminal fluid, a clear secretion that can contain sperm.

Orgasmic Phase. His body contractions prompt him to ejaculate as semen squirts out of his penis.

Resolution Phase. His heart rate returns to normal, his penis becomes soft, and his testicles descend. Some men require more time than others between orgasms, but unlike women, they do not have the ability to become immediately aroused into multiple orgasm.

Communicating with Your Partner

In her novel *Waiting to Exhale,* Terry McMillan brings a common problem to light through her character Savannah. She is a thirtysome-thing professional sister, bright and independent, but she feels inhibited in talking to her partners about what brings her pleasure: "I wish I could tell some [men] that they should start by checking the dictionary under *F* for 'foreplay', *G* for 'gentle', and *T* for 'tender' or 'take your time.'"

A healthy sex life shared with a partner begins with communication.

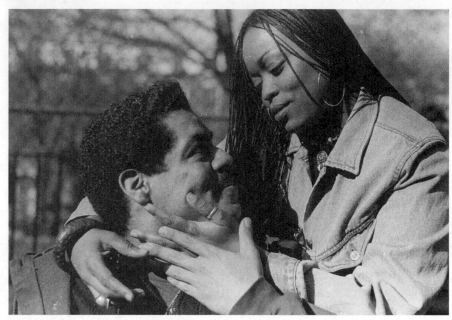

Healthy sex begins with communication. *(Photo: Lisa Ross)*

(In this age of AIDS and sexually transmitted infection, all women *must* discuss safer sex with their potential partners. For more information, see below.) As African-American women we are often socialized by well-meaning parents not to discuss sex for fear of being seen as loose or immoral. Unfortunately too many of us suffer in silence, growing more disappointed with each sexual experience.

Once you are sure that you want to move into a sexual relationship, it's important to share your preferences with your partner. Be willing to communicate what you want as well as to ask and learn. In her seductive poem "Teach Me" (from *Black Erotica*), Michelle Renee Pichon sensuously asks to be schooled in the classroom of her lover's body:

> *i want you to teach me*
> *the warmth of your breath*
> *the weight of your body*
> *i want to experience*
> *the trembles heat*
> *educate me with your*
> *mouth tongue shoulders arms fingers*

If you are having difficulty knowing where to begin, Dr. Wyatt has a few suggestions to help bridge the communication gap:

Think of what kind of sexual experience you want. Are you more interested in being held and caressed in a nurturing manner? Or are you hoping for more genital contact? Or do you like to incorporate both? Discuss it with your partner to see what ideas your lover may have.

Use pictures, videos, erotic books, or fantasies to describe situations that sound good to you. This will open a dialogue about preferences.

Guide your partner during foreplay and lovemaking with nonverbal clues such as moans, sighs, and body language. Or be direct and say, "I like that," "That feels good," or "Try touching me harder/softer." Reassuring your lover helps both of you feel comfortable and close.

If you have survived an abusive or traumatic sexual experience, share your apprehensions with your partner. Many survivors feel more comfortable if they can maintain a certain degree of control regarding the pace or direction of lovemaking.

Having Sex Safely with a Man

Once you've decided to have sex together, you and your partner must discuss ways to have *safer sex*. Sex educators call it "safer sex" because no form of sex other than celibacy (no sex) is completely without risk of passing along sexually transmitted infections (STI's), including the AIDS virus. Safer sex refers to any kind of sex during which bodily fluids are *not* exchanged, such as hugging, dry kissing, rubbing, stroking, massaging, reading or watching erotic material together, oral sex with a condom or other barrier, or intercourse (vaginal or anal) with a condom.

Some men don't want to wear condoms. They complain that it's unromantic, takes away their pleasure, or implies that they're diseased or untrustworthy. But as the saying goes, "No glove, no love." Make sure he understands that you won't have unprotected sex with him. Explain to him that you don't have sex without a condom. It's not a "trust thing," it's a "health thing." Tell him that you care about him, but you also care about yourself. If he still refuses, suggest that the two of you put off intercourse until you can work out your differences.

Though dealing with the condom should be his responsibility, you must take care of yourself to avoid the risk of contracting an STI. To use a condom correctly, follow these guidelines:

Have condoms available. Don't rely on the man to supply them. Choose latex condoms, and use them with a water-soluble lubricant containing nonoxynol-9 spermicide (which may help to kill the AIDS virus). Do not use oil-based lubricants (baby oil, petroleum jelly, mineral oil, cold cream, shortening) because they weaken the latex and can cause the condom to break.

Keep in mind that all condoms are not created equal and you'll need to experiment with different brands and types. Never use lambskin or natural condoms as they are porous and don't provide the same protection against STI's.

Condoms deteriorate with age, so check the expiration date. Store them in a cool, dry place, avoiding direct sunlight.

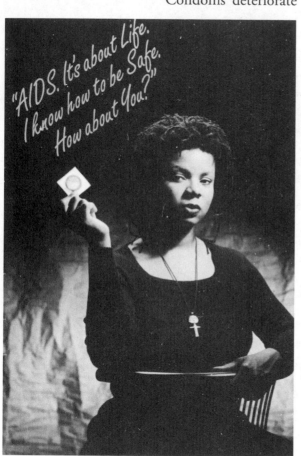

This poster reminds us to use condoms. *(Courtesy: The San Francisco Black Coalition of AIDS.)*

Condoms should become part of foreplay. As soon as you touch his penis, put on the condom.

Take the condom out of the package. If it's not lubricated, squirt spermicide into the tip and on the outside.

Unroll the condom directly onto his erect penis, making sure to leave a half-inch of space at the end of the condom to minimize the risk of breakage.

After he ejaculates, be careful that the condom doesn't come off inside you. Hold on to the rim as he withdraws so it doesn't slip off of his penis or spill, and then discard it. Never reuse a condom.

Though the risk of contracting AIDS during oral sex is less than it is through anal or vaginal intercourse, you should use a condom during oral sex. If he's performing oral sex on you, have him use a dental dam, a small latex square that is spread over the genital area to prevent contact with bodily fluids. You can find them at some shops, such as Condomania (located in Los Angeles, New York, San Francisco, Miami, and Las Vegas) or at dental-supply stores. You can also use a condom for protection: Cut the condom and use it as a barrier between his mouth and tongue and your genitals. You can also use plastic wrap.

Other excellent safe-sex accessories include latex gloves and finger cots (latex covering for the fingers). Gloves allow for worry-free penetration with hands and fingers for both partners. Any cuts, scratches, or sores on the hand (even those barely visible) should not come into contact with vaginal fluids. So check your local drugstore or surgical-supply store for the assortment of glove types: plain, powdered, or lubricated.

For additional information about safe-sex procedures, read *The Complete Guide to Safer Sex* published by the Institute for Advanced Study of Human Sexuality in San Francisco, or call the National HIV/AIDS Hotline run by the Center for Disease Control at (800) 342-AIDS (accessible twenty-four hours every day). Remember, a few moments of safer-sex preparation won't kill you, but *one* unsafe sexual experience can.

Safer Sex with Women

Though few cases of lesbians with AIDS have been reported, cases do exist. Health-care advocate Jacquie Bishop conducts safe-sex workshops for women of color throughout the New York area. She emphasizes that lesbians are as vulnerable to AIDS as heterosexual women because many have had or continue to have sex with men who engage in high-risk behavior. And some lesbians have used or do use intravenous drugs, and the virus that causes AIDS can be transmitted from woman to woman through vaginal fluids.

"Sadly, many lesbians understand the risk involved in having unsafe sex but don't always protect themselves," Bishop contends. "I offer tips to make safe sex sound appealing." Here are some of her recommendations:

Establish personal guidelines ahead of time. Either discuss that you are only willing to have safe sex or simply take the initiative during lovemaking to protect each other. Wear latex gloves or finger cots (a latex covering for the fingers) when touching her genitals or penetrating her with your hands.

When having oral sex, use a dental dam, a small latex square that is spread over the genital area to prevent contact with bodily fluids. You can find them at safe-sex shops such as Condomania (located in Los Angeles, New York, San Francisco, Miami, and Las Vegas) or at dental-supply stores. You can also use a condom for protection: Cut the condom and use it as a barrier between her mouth and tongue and your genitals. You can also use plastic wrap or cut a latex glove.

If you use a vibrator or dildo, put a condom over it. Wash "sex toys" after each use with a bleach solution.

Keep well-stocked supplies of latex gloves, condoms, dental dams, finger cots, and a water-based lube next to the bed, under a pillow, or under the mattress at all times. It allows you to be spontaneous and safe.

Be an active participant during sex. For example, if your lover is performing oral sex on you, help her hold the dental dam in place.

Think of creative activities that don't involve oral sex or penetration. Masturbation or erotic talk are sexy alternatives. Try reading erotica to each other. *Serious Pleasure* (edited by the Sheba Collective, San Francisco: Cleis Press, 1989), a collection of lesbian erotica, includes contributions by Black writers such as Jewelle Gomez.

For more information, contact the Lesbian AIDS Project at the Gay Men's Health Crisis: (212) 337-3531. Request a copy of "The Safer Sex Handbook for Lesbians." Also, see chapter 26, "Women Loving Women."

Sexual Dysfunctions

Anyone who is sexually active has encountered at least one troublesome situation. It may have been as minor as not being able to concentrate during lovemaking or simply not being in the mood. Unfortunately, a lot of us feel ashamed if we admit to having any problems with our sexual functioning. That shame can exacerbate problems, making us feel as if there's something wrong with us or our partner and adding tension to the relationship.

Knowing that you're not alone is often the first step in feeling comfortable enough to discuss the issues with your partner or, if need be, with a sex therapist. Terri A. Price, Ph.D., a psychologist and trained sex therapist, cites sexual stereotyping as the major reason that African-American women and their lovers don't seek help for their problems. "The primary and most compelling stigma we face is feeling we have to live up to the stereotype of being sexual superstars," states Dr. Price. "Not only do we have the pressure from the dominant culture, but we've also absorbed these myths in our own community."

Throughout her career counseling African-American couples with sexual dysfunctions, Dr. Price has noted several common problems. She urges couples to acknowledge the situation before it worsens and encourages either partner to seek help if the problems persist.

The leading cause of sexual conflict in a relationship is lack of communication. If you find it difficult to discuss any aspect of your sexuality, Dr. Price recommends beginning with one or two words. "Yes" and "no" are a good place to start and will help you gain confidence during sex. Communicating not only helps you feel in control of your body and pleasure but also allows for more intimacy between you and your partner. Many women believe that there is no greater aphrodisiac than openly talking to a lover.

Another prevalent issue among couples is dealing with past sexual traumas. If you or your partner has a history of sexual abuse, you may discover that communication is even more inhibited. Often the experience of sexual abuse is so painful that the survivor shuts down. Sometimes this translates into inhibited sexual desire, where he or she loses interest in sex or dissociates during lovemaking. Dissociation is a defense mechanism in which survivors learned to "disappear" or "go away" during the abusive act. Consequently all sexual acts become triggers for dissociation, making sex an unpleasant experience for both partners. Sex becomes less frequent, sometimes suspended for months or years, and tension within the relationship mounts.

It is essential, Dr. Price believes, for women or men suffering from the effects of sexual abuse to seek professional help from a trained sex therapist rather than blame themselves for a failed sexual relationship. Sexual abuse is a serious violation that demands patience and compassion from both the survivors and their partners.

Inorgasmia, or the inability to reach orgasm, is a frequent complaint among African-American women. In these cases women have difficulty getting aroused enough to have an orgasm because they are unable to communicate their needs to partners. Dr. Price has counseled women who are afraid to assert themselves because they fear being judged by their partners as promiscuous. Others have been raised with the belief that the man sets the sexual agenda and women are there to assist but not expect too much. And some women are just too intimidated to broach the subject for fear of disappointing, hurting, or losing their lovers. In all cases women often aren't familiar enough with their bodies or different types of sensations to even know what they would like. However, Dr. Price has seen encouraging evidence that women are gaining access to sexual information that has them questioning the quality of their sex lives. With increased education women acquire a vocabulary that they can use to experiment alone or communicate with their partners.

Some men have difficulty achieving or maintaining an erection, or they ejaculate too quickly. Most men and women don't realize that within the span of a man's sexual life, he's bound to have some difficulty getting an erection at least once. As obvious as this might seem, men feel an inordinate amount of pressure to always be ready. This kind of performance pressure, especially prevalent among Black men who also must combat sexual stereotypes, only heightens anxiety and can make it increasingly difficult to get an erection. Like a snowball effect, each sexual encounter brings on anxious feelings and thus the inability to get hard, which makes him more anxious, et cetera. Pretty soon a pattern sets in where the more he tries the more he fails.

According to Dr. Price, this problem can easily be addressed if the couple or individual seeks counseling early in the dysfunctional stages. Again the key is for both partners to begin communicating, including talking about their fear, anger, or resentment, or whatever might allow the couple to attain a level of intimacy. By not buying into the sexual myths, we can allow our partners to express any feelings they may have regarding their sexuality or issues that affect sexual functioning.

Couples who have been together for a long time often complain that they are bored with their sex lives. It's very easy for us to fall into mundane sexual patterns, especially if we've been together for years. Like watching old TV reruns, we always know what's going to happen next. Some couples are content knowing that they have foolproof techniques to satisfy each other. But others need to occasionally change or add to their sexual repertoire as the relationship evolves. What turned you on two years ago may do nothing for you today. Our bodies, lifestyles, stress levels, and economic circumstances change throughout our lives and can influence our sexual behavior. If these changes aren't discussed, they usually lead to conflicts that create tension or resentment.

Dr. Price notes that when couples don't nurture their sexual lives together, they often lose interest in sex. She suggests that couples work at being intimate together in a variety of ways, including taking time to be together, talking about their feelings for each other, and discussing issues that affect the relationship. Of course you and your partner should consult a sex therapist or couples counselor if the problems persist.

Growing older can also affect sexual health. For more on older women and sex, see chapter 8, "Our Bodies Growing Older."

How Medicines and Illnesses Can Affect Sexual Functioning

Many women aren't aware how dramatically a chronic illness or medication with strong side effects can affect their sex lives or the sexual functioning of their partners.

Below is a list of the many ways illnesses and medications can affect your sexual functioning. Discuss with your physician any sexual problems medication or illness may be causing. Never discontinue medication without talking to your doctor. Also, try discussing these issues with your lover or spouse; support and understanding can help ease the tension.

Antihypertensives, used to control high blood pressure, can cause drowsiness and decreased sexual desire; men taking antihypertensives may have trouble having an erection.

Many women with *diabetes* find their sexual interest falls off. Often as the disease progresses, patients experience nervous-system dysfunctions that make women less sensitive to touch and cause impotency in men.

Physical exhaustion and shortness of breath are common complaints among people with *heart disease.* Those who have survived a heart attack often express fears that the physical exertion of having sex may cause another attack. However, with the reassurance of their physicians, most people are able to return to normal sexual activity.

Sickle-cell disease can be a debilitating and painful illness. During an attack (which may last from a couple of days to several weeks), most people experience too much discomfort to have sex. Additionally, men with the disease have difficulty achieving erection or experience severe pain when they have one.

Women taking *hormones or birth control pills* may experience changes in their vaginal secretions. If sex becomes painful, try asking your lover to extend foreplay, or use a water-based lubricant such as K-Y Jelly.

People undergoing *chemotherapy* often suffer from extreme fatigue and anemia because the treatments deplete the body's normal defense mechanisms. Some women find that the discomfort they experience from the therapy decreases their sexual desire.

In many cases women who are taking *antibiotics* suffer from yeast infections that can make sex uncomfortable.

Medications such as *steroids, hypnotics, sedatives, antidepressants, anxiolytics (anti-anxiety drugs), narcotics,* and *muscle relaxants* may lessen sex drive.

Many over-the-counter medications can impair sexual functioning. And despite the initial lowering of inhibitions, illegal drugs and alcohol, especially with long-term use, can lead to sexual dysfunction.

For More Information

ORGANIZATIONS

AMERICAN ASSOCIATION OF SEX EDUCATORS, COUNSELORS AND THERAPISTS, 435 N. Michigan Ave., suite 1717, Chicago, IL 60611; (312) 644-0828. Call for a referral.

BLACKS EDUCATING BLACKS ABOUT SEX HEALTH ISSUES, 1233 Locust

St., Philadelphia, PA 19102; (215) 546-4140. For information about having sex safely and other sexual health issues.

IMPOTENCE INSTITUTE OF AMERICA, 2020 Pennsylvania Ave. NW, suite 292, Washington, DC 20006; (800) 669-1603 or (301) 577-0650. Offers information about the causes of and treatments for impotence, provides physician referrals, or furnishes a local contact for Impotents Anonymous, an AA-style support group for men.

SEX INFORMATION AND EDUCATION COUNCIL OF THE UNITED STATES, 130 W. 42nd St., suite 2500; New York, NY 10036-7901; (212) 819-9770. Provides information and publications on all aspects of human sexuality including HIV and AIDS.

BOOKS

The A to Z of Women's Sexuality: A Concise Encyclopedia, by Ada P. Kahn and Linda Hughey Holt, M.D., Hunter House, 1992.

Black Erotica, Miriam Decosta-Willis, Reginald Martin, and Roseann P. Bell, eds., Anchor Books, 1992.

Becoming Orgasmic: A Sexual Growth Program for Women, Julia R. Heiman and Joseph LoPiccolo, Prentice-Hall Press, 1988.

Eve's Secrets: A New Theory of Female Sexuality, Josephine L. Sevely, Random House, 1987.

The Family Book About Sexuality, Mary S. Calderone and Eric W. Johnson, HarperCollins, 1990.

Good Sex, Julia Hutton, Cleis Press, 1992.

The Hite Report: A Nationwide Study of Female Sexuality, Shere Hite, Dell Books, 1987.

Lesbian Passion: Loving Ourselves and Each Other, JoAnn Loulan, Spinsters/Aunt Lute Book Co., 1987.

Lesbian Sex, JoAnn Loulan, Spinsters/Aunt Lute Book Co., 1984.

My Secret Garden, Nancy Friday, Pocket Books, 1987.

Sex for One: The Joy of Selfloving, Betty Dodson, Crown Publishing, 1987.

Women on Top: How Real Life Has Changed Women's Sexual Fantasies, Nancy Friday, Simon & Schuster, 1991.

28

Loving Our Children

Legend has it that Frederick Douglass's mother, a woman enslaved on a plantation a dozen miles from where her infant son lived with his grandmother, would walk those dozen miles every day after her backbreaking work under a grueling Southern sun just to get a glimpse of him. After taking him in with her eyes, she'd turn around and head back to her plantation to face another day of work so arduous that we today cannot begin to fathom it. Our unique circumstances in these Americas has made the bond between Black mothers and their children just a little bit tighter and the work of raising children a lot harder.

Rearing a Black child to be healthy, educated, and emotionally secure in today's society is an awesome challenge. However, it can also be the single most satisfying thing you ever do.

The statistics can be depressing. Nearly one out of every two Black children in the United States is born into poverty, and our babies are more than twice as likely to die in infancy as their white counterparts. Black girls have a two-in-five chance of having a child before they reach their twentieth birthday and only a one-in-ten chance of being married.

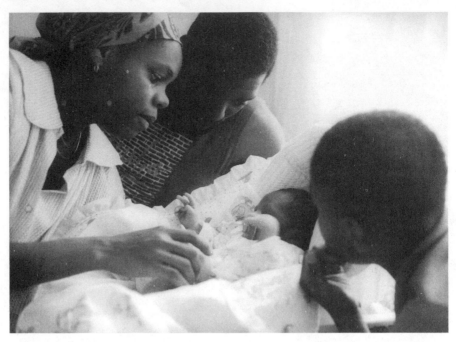

A new baby can bring a family closer together. (Photo: Diane Allford/Allford Trotman Associates)

One out of every three Black boys will be unemployed, and one out of twenty-four will be incarcerated while in their twenties.

These figures are alarming, and yet we know that there are success stories too—hundreds of them. Thousands. Millions. Single mothers are filling the shoes of two parents. They are holding down jobs and raising their children to be responsible, well-adjusted adults. Black boys are passing up gangs and drugs in favor of high school, college, and meaningful employment, and Black families are living together, working for and with one another, loving one another.

As a race, we have been lobbying our government, through civil rights and advocacy groups, to pass legislation to ensure that all of our children have the same opportunity to build fulfilling lives. A sister, Marian Wright Edelman, is the nation's foremost child advocate. Sadly, however, America is last or close to last among industrialized nations in spending on elementary and secondary education, reducing child poverty, and assuring children access to health care.

The bottom line is that much of what will determine whether the child you are raising becomes a success or a negative statistic depends on what you invest in terms of time, effort, and initiative as a parent. Experts agree that children who are well loved, well cared for, and well educated, both formally and in terms of developing good social skills,

I have five children aged from three to seventeen, who are depending on me for emotional and financial support. The fathers of these children played minor roles—they made them, then shucked off their responsibilities.

When I was pregnant with my first child, unbeknownst to me, her father had been a drug user and dealer. He had concealed this information from me for quite a while. When I found out that this man was involved in drugs, I thought, how could this man be any good for me, when he's no good to himself! We broke up and I was left pregnant, jobless, and scared to death of having to tell my parents about the baby. When I informed my father, he was not having it, so I decided to get on welfare.

Although welfare kept a roof over my head and put food on the table, I was not going to let the system make me complacent. I knew that being on welfare was just a temporary situation that I would have to tolerate in order to reach my goals. I swallowed my pride and kept my head held high.

I started applying to various local colleges, but when welfare got wind of this, they threatened to cut me off. Apparently the system only wants you to be self-sufficient enough to barely make ends meet. Eventually, though, I learned to manipulate the system to make it work for me, and I was accepted into a city college. I worked my ass off to make the grade.

College was a struggle. Mothering was a joy, but it had its struggles. Eventually, I got pregnant again, three more times, and each time it seemed that the chips were more and more stacked against me! My mornings were crazy. I would get up before the sun would rise to prepare five kids to take a couple to the baby-sitter and the rest to school. Then I would make a mad dash to classes all day, then deal with work study afterward. My evenings consisted of meal-making, kid-bathing, homework-supervising, baby-sitter-next-day preparations, then my schoolwork.

It took me nearly ten years to earn my nursing degree, but I did it. Graduation was the proudest day of my life! I made sure that all of my children were there to see me receive my diploma. I also told welfare to kiss my ass and got out of the system, as soon as my diploma was in hand! I am now working as an LPN, loving it, and expect to get flying colors on my RN exam. I feel like nothing can hold me back now.

"All of my children were there to see me receive my diploma."

—Wadyah Hassan, nurse, Jamaica, New York

---

tend to be the best equipped to make their way in this society. In this chapter we will examine just what's involved in seeing that our children get the love, care, and schooling they need to succeed.

Loving Your Child

Love may not conquer all, but when it comes to your child, its powers are wondrous. Talking with your children, hugging and cuddling them, and doing things together are among the best means of building self-esteem and passing along social skills.

Talking to Children

Asked whether or not they've talked with their children today, most parents' answer would be "Yes, of course." The operative word here, however, is "with." Many Black and especially single parents expend the bulk of their energy on life-sustaining matters such as earning a living and making ends meet. Conversations with the kids usually center on routine subjects like tasks that still need tending to, what's on television, and what's for dinner—and generally inspire little in the way of give-and-take. It's not that a parent doesn't care what's going on in her children's lives and heads; the problem is that she may not *communicate* her concern.

"Talking with" your children involves sharing your thoughts and then listening to theirs. For infants and toddlers such an exchange aids in the development of language skills. You may or may not be able to understand what your child is talking about, but she will pick up bits and pieces of what you are saying and recognize that you are interested in her response. In *The Black Child: A Parent's Guide*, child psychiatrist Phyllis Harrison-Ross and coauthor Barbara Wyden recommend that parents set aside fifteen minutes in the morning and fifteen minutes at night to talk with children about such subjects as school, friends, their interests, and what you did with your day. Such conversations—devoid of criticism and, unless requested, advice—provide your child with an opportunity to communicate directly or indirectly his thoughts. It also enables your youngster to feel included in your life.

You should also talk to your children about responsibility—their sense of responsibility to self, others, and the community. Build a foundation by teaching them to do things for others such as grandparents or younger siblings. Don't push it too much for fear of turning the child into a little adult, but make the discussion ongoing.

Talking About Race and Gender

During one of these "talking with" sessions your child's first questions or comments about race will arise. When it does come up, you should discuss the subject in a relaxed, natural manner. The issue of skin color or racial variations doesn't usually arise until age three. With younger children, you may want to use colors as a reference point by pointing to your arm or the child's to indicate brown or black. Preschoolers are more likely to be interested in their similarities or differences to others and will respond best to being told they are "Black" or "of African descent" like Mommy. As psychiatrists James P. Comer and Alvin F. Poussaint point out in their book *Raising Black Children,* "You are your child's source of pleasure and security and therefore somebody very positive. If you show enthusiasm about the fact that you are Black, your child will sense that being Black must be both positive and good."

When older children bring up race, it is important that they understand that your Blackness is a source of pride for you and the same should go for them. You may also want to point out that it can be a complex issue and that while people of one race may from time to time put another group of people down, all races have a history of achievements and individuals in which they can take pride.

Finally, you'd do well to keep in mind that children of all ages are keen observers and will quickly pick up on discrepancies between what a parent says and what a parent does. Make sure when you tell a child that Black is beautiful that your actions convey a similar message.

Teaching children about gender equality is equally important. You must make sure your sons understand that women are just as competent as men and that denigrating girls is not a sign of masculinity. Girls must learn that they are equal to boys and that they can do anything—math, science, sports, and so on. For more information on raising strong, healthy daughters, see chapter 24, "Loving Ourselves." For information on talking to your daughter about sex and sexuality, see chapter 9, "The Reproductive System and Menstruation."

Afrocentric Toys and Games

Black children no longer have to carry around little white dolls with long blond hair. Now many dolls look like us—even Barbie (made by Mattel) comes in Black skin. The Niya doll (Here Comes Niya, Fort Washington, MD; (301) 248-8587) can in English, Spanish, and Kiswahili.

Let your kids try board games with soul such as In Search of Identity (Identity Toys, Milwaukee) and African-American Discovery (Impact Publishing Company, Chicago). Even Bingo comes with Black history added (African American Bingo, Visions Research, Pittsford, NY).

In stores where products for us are sold, you can find other toys, games, and playing cards with Black faces.

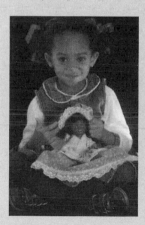

Many excellent Black dolls are available for our youngsters. *(Photo: Anthony Mills/Allford Trotman Associates)*

How About a Hug?

"It's ten o'clock," advises a TV public-service announcement; "Have you hugged your child today?" If you haven't, do it. Few people can resist the warmth and playful nature of a good squeeze, and children seem to bask in the physical display of a parent's affection.

With a newborn, Harrison-Ross and Wyden assert, most parents "instinctively handle their babies. . . . they play with them, pat them and stroke them so that they learn all of the good feelings of love." Through such contact, they also learn to like their skin because it gives them pleasure.

Hugs continue to be important as your child grows. They can be a source of comfort when your children are upset—helping them to relax and regain control while secure in your protection. Hugs can also help reaffirm in your children a sense of self with respect to their Blackness. When you compliment your child's hair, coloring, nose, or some other feature along with a gentle embrace, you reinforce the specialness of being Black.

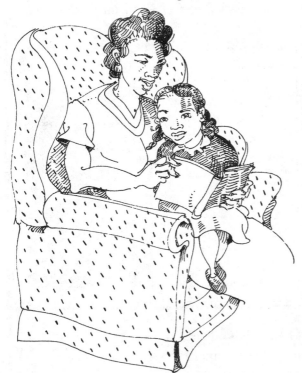

Reading together helps to create a bond between mother and child. (Drawing: Yvonne Buchanan)

Spending Time with Your Child

Like talking with your child, the quality of the time you spend together is key. Evaluate how much time you spend doing things with your child apart from chores and other routine tasks. Children and parents need to be able to spend time together that is just for play.

Reading is one activity that allows you to be close to your children and enhance their learning skills. Listening to a story, for instance, helps expand a young child's vocabulary and imagination. By reading a story again and again over time, children learn how to pronounce different words and understand what is taking place. Books are also a good way to teach values. If your children don't see many Black or female doctors or mechanics, they may be able to see them in books.

With young children it helps to set aside a certain time every day to read, such as before bed or after dinner, so that they learn that reading is an important parent-child activity to look forward to. Providing a structure such as books every night before bed also gives children a sense of safety and security. As your children grow, you may suggest that they read to you, thus allowing you to stay on top of pronunciation, reading, and comprehension. Adolescents may prefer something a little more independent: You may consider selecting a book that you both agree upon, reading it independently, and then setting a time to discuss it. Teens can also check out *YSB* (*Young Sisters and Brothers*, published in Rosslyn, Virginia) magazine for Black teens. The National Black Child Development Institute puts out the "African-American Family Reading List," which you can order for $2: 1023 15th St. NW, suite 600, Washington, DC 20005; (202) 387-1281. Or check out Black bookstores for other titles.

Hobbies and family outings are also important ways of spending time together and expanding your child's world. Visits to museums featuring Black exhibits, lectures on Africa, and/or contributions made to this country by people of African descent give your child a greater sense of appreciation for our people and our accomplishments. Even better: a trip to Africa.

Your Child's Health

Proper nutrition and health care are crucial to a child's physical and emotional well-being. Good food helps kids develop their bodies and their brains and helps ward off illness and disease. Routine checkups at your pediatrician's office or health clinic are the best way to keep children healthy.

Eating and Exercise

During the first half-year, a baby can get all the nutrition it needs from its mother. By the end of the first year, however, most of your child's nutrition will come from other sources. At that point, the principles for nutritious eating will be much the same as they are for adults. Your child should consume between 900 and 1,350 calories a day, with toddler-size servings of the recommended nutrients: proteins (fish, poultry, dairy products, and beans), carbohydrates (cereals, potatoes, and bread), fat (vegetable oil), calcium (fish, low-fat dairy products), and iron (green vegetables, enriched grains). A child should drink four to six cups of fluid (fruit juices, vegetable juices, soups, or water), with extra fluids necessary in the event of hot weather, fever, cold, diarrhea, vomiting, or respiratory infection. Doctors are also recommending that after age two parents limit the number of high-fat and salty foods.

As your children mature, you will want to make sure that they eat a variety of foods suggested by the U.S. Department of Agriculture. Ideally, a child's diet should consist of:

2 to 3 servings from the milk group (low-fat cheese, yogurt, milk, cottage cheese)

2 to 3 servings from the meat, egg, bean group (fish, poultry, eggs, beans, peanut butter, nuts)

3 to 5 servings from the vegetable group (potatoes, carrots, tomatoes, broccoli)

2 to 4 servings from the fruit group (oranges, apples, grapes, bananas, strawberries, blueberries, cantaloupe)

6 to 11 servings from the grain group (whole-grain bread, cereal, pasta, grits)

Although fats and oil should be part of a child's diet, limit the amount, especially of saturated fat found in meat and processed foods and cholesterol. Keep your child from developing an addiction to sugar by substituting dried and fresh fruit and juices for soda, desserts, and candy. Make sure salt intake is low (watch out for canned foods, which have high sodium content) and water intake is high.

Providing healthy, nutritious food for your child on a limited income is no easy feat, but there are several programs and organizations you can turn to for assistance. The Women, Infants and Children (WIC) program is for pregnant women, mothers who have just had babies, and infants and children under five who have health problems or are undernourished. Your local health department should be able to provide you with additional information. You may also be eligible for food stamps, which enable parents to buy food, beverages, and/or seeds to plant edible foods. Your local social-service department can tell you how to apply. In addition, many schools, child-care facilities, recreational centers, and after-school programs provide free or low-cost meals to children. For more information, call your local school district or state department of education.

It's also important that children get plenty of exercise. A 1992 *Prevention* magazine study found that in 1991 34 percent of kids were overweight, compared with 24 percent in 1984. The problem is more pronounced in our children: 41 percent of Black children are overweight. Our children watch more TV than white kids and get less exercise.

Children should exercise at least three times a week if not every day.

Turn off the television and get kids engaged in an activity they like. Exercise with your children: Take your son on a walk with you, or shoot baskets with your daughter. The activity will be good for both of you. Or sign your children up in recreational programs and encourage them to get involved in sports in school.

If your child has a health problem such as asthma, she or he should still participate in physical activity. Ask your pediatrician about the kind of fitness program best suited for such children and how long they should exercise.

Preventing Illness

There are nine childhood diseases that can cripple or kill. Making sure your child gets immunized on schedule will provide the best defense against these illnesses. Immunization means protection from hepatitis B, polio, measles, mumps, rubella (German measles), pertussis (whooping cough), diphtheria, tetanus (lockjaw), and haemophilus influenza type B. A 1991 CDC study shows that only 20 percent of Black children under two years of age received all the recommended vaccines, compared with twice the percentage of white children.

Children should have received a total of fourteen recommended immunizations by the age of two, plus booster shots. See the chart on p. 486 for the recommended immunization schedule.

Your pediatrician or family doctor should be able to provide all of your child's immunizations. To find out the names and locations of clinics providing free or low-cost immunizations, contact your local department of health or consult the telephone directory. It is important that you keep a record of your child's vaccinations, visits to the doctor, and health history. All children must have their immunizations to enroll in school.

In addition to the vaccinations, children should have a tuberculin skin test to check for tuberculosis when they are nine months, then at one- to three-year intervals thereafter. Your child should also have a blood test for sickle-cell disease. You should also check with your doctor or health clinic to find out whether your child needs additional booster shots or if other, new vaccines have been recommended. In some instances, a child may have a reaction to certain immunizations. Few of these reactions are serious; however, should one occur, notify your doctor or health clinic immediately.

Recommended Immunization Schedule

This chart, supplied by the American Academy of Pediatrics, tells you when to have your children immunized against common diseases.

	DTP	POLIO	MMR	HEPATITIS B*	HAEMOPHILUS	TETANUS-DIPHTHERIA
BIRTH				✔		
1–2 MONTHS				✔		
2 MONTHS	✔	✔			✔	
4 MONTHS	✔	✔			✔	
6 MONTHS	✔				◆	
6–18 MONTHS				✔		
12–15 MONTHS					◆	
15 MONTHS	●		✔			
15–18 MONTHS	●	✔				
4–6 YEARS		✔				
11–12 YEARS			★			
14–16 YEARS						✔

★ Except where public health authorities require otherwise.

◆ Depends on previous *Haemophilus Influenzae* type b vaccine given.

✱ Infants of mothers who tested seropositive for hepatitus B (HBsAg+) must receive hepatitis B immune globulin (HBIG) at or shortly after the first dose. These infants also will require a second hepatitis B vaccine dose at 1 month and a third hepatitus B vaccine injection at 6 months of age.

● For the fourth and fifth dose, the acellular (DTaP) pertussls vaccine may be substituted for the DTP vaccine.

Keeping Your Child Safe

The world can be a dangerous place for children, and Black youngsters are at particular risk for accidents of all kinds. But there are ways to keep your child clear of harm's way. Parents must also set limits on their children's behavior. Though it's hard to know how much discipline is the right amount, kids need structure and boundaries.

Everyday Health Risks

Seemingly benign objects and situations can often be hazardous to the health of your child. Left unsupervised, children can run into trouble with open doors, electrical wires, stairs, stoves and radiators, fire, furniture, poisonous household materials (disinfectant, window cleaners), and medications (including aspirin).

You can make your home childproof by having window guards installed (many states have laws that require landlords to install window guards in apartments that house small children), using gates, child locks, and safety caps, and by placing dangerous objects and materials well out of the reach of children. Contact the National Black Child Development Institute (address above and below) for more information about keeping children safe in the home.

As your children develop comprehension it is important that you advise them on a regular basis of potential dangers. A stern "no-no, that can hurt you" will suffice for babies and toddlers. With older children, you should explain that serious accidents can happen in an instant and that exercising caution around certain places, people, and things is their best insurance against harm.

Urban Black children are particularly susceptible to exposure to lead. Studies show that childhood exposure to lead can cause mental retardation, reduced IQ, reading and learning disabilities, impaired growth, short-term memory loss, sleep disorders, hearing loss, reduced attention span, and behavioral problems. For more information, see chapter 32, "Our Work, Our World."

Societal Dangers

In many Black communities, drugs, alcohol, and sexually transmitted infections pose serious health risks for our children. Your children's best protection against such temptations is for you to provide them with information as to the danger they present. Arm yourself with pamphlets and booklets, and share them with your children. Talk about how drugs, alcohol, and AIDS have affected your community and people you know. Help children develop ways of saying no to these threats so they will be able to look strong in front of their peers.

Observe your child carefully, keeping an eye out for changes in personality or lifestyle. Don't be afraid to ask questions; it's better to know.

Parents who believe their children may be in trouble should observe their kids' friends—who they are, what they are like. Don't be shy about enlisting school officials, clergy, other family members, and friends whom the kids respect and may confide in to try to get at the root of the trouble. Parents of children who are involved with drugs or alcohol should act swiftly and decisively to see that their kids receive medical

"My mom is the reason why I want to be a lawyer."

—KAWANA BENITA PETERSEN, HIGH SCHOOL STUDENT, NEW YORK CITY

I've never tried drugs, because my mother warned us about them since we were young. My father was a heroin addict. Maybe that's why I'm against drugs; I see what they could do to you.

I knew my father but not well. I loved him. He has been in jail for robbery, murder, and a bunch of stuff. He died last year of AIDS, and he was only forty-one years old. I am being raised by my mother, who is really mother/father. She and my grandmother did not want to tell me that my father had died of AIDS. I get depressed easily, and they were afraid that my school year would be ruined if I learned the truth about my father. I loved him, though, whether he had AIDS or not, even though he wasn't here for me. Yeah, I've missed having a father growing up, but maybe it's better because there was always one boss—my mother. Anyway, most of my friends are being raised by their mother only. My mom has a boyfriend, but she is the only person I really listen to. He does help my mother out financially, and I appreciate that.

I have a sister who is five years younger than me. Already she has been exposed to drugs—all kinds; she knows what's out here. She was almost raped by a young guy in my building. He is young and stupid; we're waiting to go to court. I don't know if they're going to do anything to him because he's only seventeen years old.

Sometimes I am afraid of dying at a young age, scared of being an innocent bystander at the wrong place and wrong time. I could go to a party, for instance, standing around, just minding my business, and a fight could break out—bullets and knives could go flying all over the place—I could get killed. Fear is also all over my high school—everyone is afraid. The fights are usually over something stupid like if you step on somebody's foot or something like that, you could lose your life.

The girls I know are afraid of losing their boyfriends, so they get pregnant thinking that the guys will stay with them. I think that is so stupid. I could never get pregnant now. I'm not ready for the responsibility of a child, and besides, these girls dump the babies on their own mothers to baby-sit. My mother already warned me that if I get pregnant, she will not be a baby-sitter! I still like to go out and party, and these girls still think that they can be free like me, even though they have a kid! I don't understand.

I admire my mom a lot. Although she's raised us on her own, she has always made sure that we came first, over anybody! I love my mom so much, and I respect her for trying her best with my sister and me. My mom is the reason why I want to be a lawyer. I want to make her proud of me, and I want to be successful. Maybe being a lawyer will make me not so scared of being out here.

attention and professional counseling. These are crisis situations when more than anything else children need their parents' guidance and support. Parents of sexually active children should speak to them frankly about birth control and safer sex.

Limits and Expectations

All children need structure, limits, and expectations set and lovingly enforced by parents; these provide a framework that keeps children steady and secure as they explore and grow. Together, the limits and expectations you set inform your children of the rules, regulations, and code of behavior you think is important for them to live by and the level of performance you believe them capable of achieving.

Experts indicate that children will begin to behave and perform in an unacceptable fashion when they sense that you believe they will do so, hence it is important that you convey to your children your confidence in their ability to live up to your expectations and within your limits. Parents who berate children as "good-for-nothing," for instance, are communicating to them that they are expected to fail. Positive reinforcement, in time, produces positive results—especially with our children, who may be receiving negative reinforcement from a racist society. It is also essential that you make your limits, expectations, and strategies for helping your child clear to teachers, caregivers, and anyone else who interacts with your child on a regular basis so that they work with rather than against you.

Black parents walk a fine line trying to deal with racism. While you don't want to convey to your children that discrimination does not exist, you also don't want racism to seem so all-encompassing that they will never be able to succeed and be happy. There is a tendency on the part of some Black parents to make their children believe that they have to be twice as good as their white counterparts to compete. Such admonishments, while well intended, invite stress, and children who believe that the limits and expectations they are faced with are too stringent may grow up to be neurotic overachievers or, conversely, drop out and give up entirely. Again, experts suggest emphasizing the positive. Tell your child that when she does her best, she can master almost anything.

The Importance of Discipline

To spank or not to spank is a debate that has been raging among experts. When it comes to black families, however, discipline takes on another dimension. In the past, harsh social conditions made many African-

American parents feel that they had to force children to obey so that they would not violate any of the racial rules that could bring harm to themselves or their families. As a result, many parents issued strict edicts that carried dire consequences for disobedience—with little explanation about why the punishment was so harsh. This kind of dogmatic discipline can promote docility, undermine self-esteem, and discourage curiosity and exploration.

The word *discipline* is derived from the Latin word for "teaching"; learning and thinking and enforcing discipline in this spirit can be extremely constructive. Your goal as a parent in meting out discipline should be to instill in your children a sense of right and wrong, to assist them in the development of self-control, to protect them from physical and/or emotional harm, and to teach respect for others.

While there are few situations when a whack may be necessary to let a child know that a parent means business (such as in a dangerous situation when a child may be too young to understand words), only talk can make punishment effective. Here are some suggestions:

- With babies, discipline is likely to have more to do with protecting them from things that are potentially harmful. Crying should never be seen as a punishable offense, and babies should not be hit. Patience is key here, for chances are that your child will repeat the offense over and over until your message begins to sink in. Distracting your child with a toy or placing the child in an alternative situation often helps to reinforce your wishes. As with all children, consistency and follow-through are essential.
- Make sure that your child understands that she or he is still loved even though you disapprove of the behavior. Children are never "bad boy" or "bad girl"; only the behavior is bad.
- When disciplining older children, explain why their behavior is unacceptable. If your children know that you believe they can do better, reasonable behavior will be something they will want to achieve. And talking with your child will also help you determine whether there are problems or circumstances that led to the behavior that also need to be examined.
- Refrain from nagging or trying to shame your child, as most experts agree that it is counterproductive.
- Learn to figure out when you need to do more than simply scold. In these situations, consider denying your child a privilege or insisting that she or he take a "time out." Sending a younger child to a chair

or another room to think about the bad behavior is often punishment enough. With older children, you will want to make sure the punishment is appropriate for the offense.

- Regardless of age, punishment is most effective if it follows on the heels of the undesirable action so that your child is fully aware of what the punishment is for.
- Know the difference between discipline and abuse. (For more on child abuse, see chapter 30, "Incest and Child Abuse.") If you do spank, never use an object. Temper spanking with hugs, rewards, and positive feedback.
- Let your own behavior set the standard for your children. You teach your child, by actions and words, the values and pattern of behavior she or he will carry through life. When you feel your anger or emotions getting out of control, take a walk or call a friend. Remove yourself from the situation. In recurring or more serious situations, consider seeking professional help. Parents Anonymous (800-421-0353) can provide crisis intervention and help for parents who feel overwhelmed and want to learn better ways of parenting.

Your Child and the Educational System

With all that your child has learned from birth to age four—walking, talking, recognizing people and places, colors and numbers—school should be a cinch. Sadly, though, for many Black children this is not the case. A 1990 study commissioned by the Washington-based Children's Defense Fund found that by age nine or ten Black students are twice as likely as white students to be two or more grades behind in school. By age sixteen or seventeen they are nearly three times as likely as whites to be two or more grades behind. Our students account for only 16 percent of the total school population, yet they make up 32 percent of school expulsions. Black children are half as likely to be placed in classes for gifted and talented students. Compared with whites, Black boys and girls are more than twice as likely to be spanked by teachers.

In short, the educational system in this country is failing many of our youngsters, and the only way that we as Black parents are going to reverse the situation is to invest our time, energy, money, and other resources in our children's education. Insuring that your child gets the most out of school means developing a constructive partnership with those teachers and school administrators who show a commitment to providing your child a good education. Don't be intimidated by teachers and other school staff; remember they should be working for you and your kids. You must find out whether the curriculum provides positive images of the African-American experience and speak up if it doesn't. It means taking an active role in improving and expanding those parts of the educational process that work and dismantling and finding alternative solutions for those parts of the system that have proven to be ineffective. Finally, and most important, it means communicating to your children in no uncertain terms that school is serious business and that learning is their job.

Educate yourself about Black children in the educational system. Some of the best books on the subject have been written by Jonathan Kozol, a white writer who spent time as a teacher in the public school system. Read his most recent book, *Savage Inequalities: Children in America's Schools.*

Separate but Effective?

The deterioration of the public school system in many of the nation's inner cities has led a number of African-American parents to consider a controversial solution: separate schools for young Black males.

Established on the premise that the present system is failing to educate Black children, especially boys, these academies separate Black males from Black females (and children of other races) and place them in smaller, nurturing classes taught primarily by Black men. Pilot programs and/or plans are now in the works in Detroit, Milwaukee, Baltimore, Portland (Oregon), and New York City.

At the Malcolm X Academy in Detroit, for example, children recite the Malcolm X Academy pledge every day, rather than the Pledge of Allegiance. It goes: "We at the Malcolm X Academy will strive for excellence in our quest to be the best. We'll rise above every challenge with our heads held high. We'll always keep the faith when others say die. March on till victory is ours: Amandla!" Instead of Halloween, students celebrate Heritage Day, dressing up like Black historical figures and giving speeches about them. Discipline is strict at the school, and children wear uniforms.

Critics of schools like this one denounce the system as a self-imposed form of segregation that, in an effort to save Black males, excludes Black girls, many of whom have also suffered educationally under the present system. It also shields Black males, leaving them unprepared for the real world, which includes men and women of all colors and is run by white males.

To learn more about Black male schools, read "Are Black Male Schools the Answer?" by Rosemary L. Bray in the October 1991 issue of *Emerge* magazine.

As an alternative to public schools and predominately white private schools, some parents choose independent Black schools. These are private schools that emphasize Afrocentricity. They can cost thousands of dollars a year.

For more information or to find a school nearby, contact the Institute for Independent Education, 1313 N. Capitol St. NE, Washington, DC 20002.

For More Information

ORGANIZATIONS

AMERICAN ACADEMY OF CHILD AND ADOLESCENT PSYCHIATRY, 3615 Wisconsin Ave. NW, Washington, DC 20016; (202) 966-7300. Provides information and referrals to parents and caregivers on psychiatric issues regarding children and adolescents.

AMERICAN ACADEMY OF PEDIATRICS, 141 Northwest Point Blvd., Elk Grove Village, IL 60007; (708) 228-5005. Advocates to insure access to health care for children and provides information to the public.

THE CHILDREN'S DEFENSE FUND, 25 E St. NW, Washington, D.C. 20001; (202) 628-8787. CDF's Black Community Crusade for Children is working to mobilize Blacks on behalf of our youth. To contact the Crusade specifically call (800) ASK-BCCC.

NATIONAL BLACK CHILD DEVELOPMENT INSTITUTE, 1023 15th St. NW, suite 600, Washington, DC 20005; (202) 387-1281. Services children and their families and focuses on child-care, health, education, and welfare issues.

NATIONAL CENTER FOR EDUCATION IN MATERNAL AND CHILD HEALTH, 200 N. 15th St., suite 701, Arlington, VA 22201-2617; (703) 524-7802. Provides information on child and adolescent health, nutrition, and illness and recommends services and programs.

NATIONAL MATERNAL AND CHILD HEALTH CLEARINGHOUSE, 8201 Greenboro Dr., suite 600, McLean, VA 22102; (703) 821-8955. Provides information and resource materials on child health.

PARENTS ANONYMOUS, (800) 421-0353. This hotline provides help for people who feel overwhelmed by parenting. Also offers local crisis intervention and services.

SINGLE MOTHERS BY CHOICE, P.O. Box 7788, FDR Station, New York, NY 10150; (212) 988-0993. A national organization that provides support and information for single women who are considering motherhood and for single mothers by choice.

SINGLE MOTHERS OF COLOR ON THE HORIZON, P.O. Box 06908, Detroit, MI 48206; (313) 894-7920. SMOC was formed to eliminate the negative images of households that are headed by single women. SMOC works within the community to develop workshops on parenting skills, strive for educational excellence, and promote family activities that affirm healthy bodies and minds.

WELFARE WARRIORS/WELFARE MOTHERS' VOICE, 4504 N. 47th St., Milwaukee, WI 53218; (414) 444-0220. This organization validates, supports, educates, and unites low-income mothers and teaches them to advocate for themselves. Welfare Warriors staffs a mothers' help line, (414) 873-MOMS, and publishes a quarterly newsletter, "Welfare Mothers' Voice."

BOOKS

Black Adolescents, Reginald L. Jones, ed., Cobb & Henry Publishers (Berkeley, Calif.), 1989.

The Black Child: A Parent's Guide, Phyllis Harrison-Ross, M.D., and Barbara Wyden, P. H. Wyden, 1973.

Black Children: Social, Educational and Parental Environments, Harriette Pipes McAdoo and John L. McAdoo, Sage Publications, 1985.

The New Child Health Encyclopedia, the Boston Children's Hospital Staff, edited by Frederick H. Lovejoy, Jr., M.D., and David Estridge, Delacorte Press, 1987.

Bringing the Black Boy to Manhood: The Passage, Nathan Hare and Julia Hare, the Black Think Tank, 1987.

Climbing Jacob's Ladder: The Enduring Legacy of African-American Families, Andrew Billingsley, Simon & Schuster, 1993.

Countering the Conspiracy to Destroy Black Boys, 2 volumes, Jawanza Kunjufu, African American Images (Chicago), 1986.

Developing Positive Self-Images & Discipline in Black Children, Jawanza Kunjufu, African American Images (Chicago), 1984.

Different and Wonderful: Raising Black Children in a Race-Conscious Society, Darlene Powell Hopson and Derek S. Hopson, Prentice-Hall Press, 1990.

Harvesting New Generations: The Positive Development of Black Youth, Useni Eugene Perkins, Third World Press, 1986.

Home Is a Dirty Street: The Social Oppression of Black Children, Useni Eugene Perkins, Third World Press, 1975.

Maggie's American Dream: The Life and Times of a Black Family, James P. Comer, M.D., New American Library, 1988.

The Moral Life of Children, Robert Coles, Houghton Mifflin, 1986.

Parenting by Heart, Ron Taffel with Melinda Blaua, Addison-Wesley, 1991.

Prejudice and Your Child, Kenneth B. Clark, Wesleyan University Press (Middletown, Conn.), 1988.

Raising Black Children, James P. Comer, M.D., and Alvin F. Poussaint, M.D., New American Library, 1992.

Savage Inequalities: Children in America's Schools, Jonathan Kozol, Crown Publishers, 1991.

To Be Popular or Smart: The Black Peer Group, Jawanza Kunjufu, African American Images (Chicago), 1988.

Young, Black, and Male in America: An Endangered Species, Jewelle Taylor Gibbs, ed., Auburn House Publishing (Dover, Mass.), 1988.

PART VI

KEEPING SAFE IN A
HOSTILE WORLD

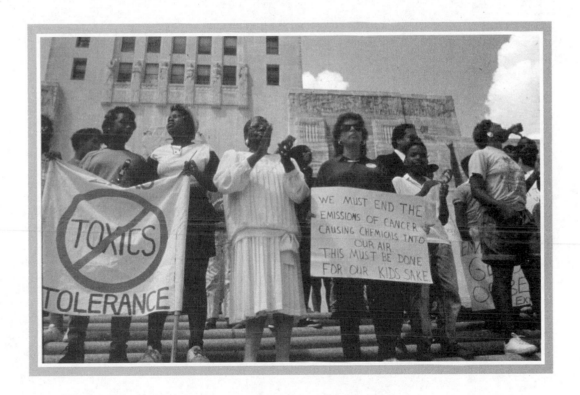

29

Violence
in Our Lives

Violence in our lives is now as regular as a Saturday night. Black women are mugged, beaten, raped, and murdered by men—both Black and white. They victimize us to silence us, to control us, to break our spirits and douse the fire in our souls. We are also the ones who wear black at the funerals of our loved ones who are killed in the overcrowded pressure cookers that are the communities we live in.

We bolt our doors and look over our shoulders as we walk down dark city streets.

But all too often, what we fear the least we should the fear the most. It's not always the drive-by shootings and gang warfare that are the most dangerous, though they certainly have taken their toll. And the Klan, though menacing, isn't an immediate threat to most of us.

The fact is, most of the time the face behind the gun, the knife, or the clenched fist is a familiar one. In 1990, more than half of all homicides nationwide were committed either by family members, friends, or acquaintances during a fight. And for us, the statistics are much more deadly: The rate of domestic homicides among African-Americans is eight times greater than that of whites. Among murdered Black women, two-thirds of the victims knew their killers; in more than four out of ten cases, the attacker was a family member.

The late Pat Parker summed up Black-on-Black violence simply in a poem from her collection *Movement in Black*:

> *Brother*
> *I don't want to hear*
> *about*
> *how my real enemy*
> *is the system*
> *I'm no genius*
> *but i do know*
> *that system*
> *You hit me with*
> *is called*
> *a fist*

Because so many deaths occur among acquaintances and often in the heat of the moment, buying a gun to arm yourself against anonymous strangers can backfire: It is forty-three times more likely that a firearm kept in the house will be used to kill a family member, friend, or acquaintance during an argument than that it will stop an intruder.

But we don't have to allow ourselves, our sisters, and our children to be brutalized. Neither do we have to accept the scenario of a lost generation, and we don't have to accept mayhem in our lives. We can't make poverty, joblessness, and the glamorized media images of violence vanish in an instant. But we can lobby our legislators to change laws, and we can talk openly with men about the sexual politics of rape and violence against women. We can try to make men understand that no means no, we can organize neighborhood block watches and teach our children through our own behavior how to handle anger without using physical force.

Violence is devastating and tragic. But it is not inevitable.

Rape

Every six minutes a woman is raped in America. Roughly one out of four American women will be raped in her lifetime; about one million rapes occur nationwide each year. Rape will continue to happen as long as women, especially Black women, continue to be devalued in our society. Day after day, movies, television, and music drives that message home: Black women are toys, a compilation of body parts ready to do the bidding of anyone who asks—or demands. As one popular song from the early nineties says, "She's playing hard to get. But she doesn't mean it. She really likes me."

As Black women, we are twice as likely to be raped as white women and less likely to report it. Many women never tell another soul that they've been raped. Rape is trivialized and ignored. So many women are afraid they won't be believed, and if they are, they'll be blamed for doing something to provoke the attack. Blaming the individual woman—the victim—often acts as a form of self-protection. Men may believe that "she asked for it," unwilling to face the reality that another man could do something so horrifying—especially a Black man to a Black woman. Women may also doubt the woman's story, because it may be too terrifying to admit that "If it happened to this woman *for no apparent reason*, then the same thing could happen to me."

But this blame-the-victim thinking obscures the reality of rape: Any time a woman is forced into a sexual act against her will, it is rape. Don't let anyone tell you that rape is about sex. It isn't about what a woman wore. It isn't about how she carried herself or whether she kissed her attacker. If she said no, and he ignored her, it was rape. Women shouldn't even engage in conversations about these peripheral issues. Rape is about power and control. It is an ugly act of violence.

Rape is one of the most sinister aspects of our history. On slave ships our ancestors were kept naked and vulnerable, ready prey for white slavers who used rape as a means to keep us in control. When we landed in the New World, our vulnerability continued on the plantations. We were easy targets for sexual exploitation by any male but especially by white men. We were viewed as property and loose women, ready for the taking.

The end of slavery didn't bring about an end to our victimization. Far from it. Long after emancipation, in the streets and on the job, white men continued to terrorize us. In fact, Deborah Gray White notes that "from emancipation through more than two-thirds of the 20th century, no Southern white male was convicted of raping or attempting to rape a Black woman. Yet the crime was so widespread that the staff of the National Commission on the Causes and Prevention of Violence admitted in 1969 that the few reported instances of the crime reflected not the crime's low incidence but the fact that 'white males have long had nearly institutionalized access to Negro women with relatively little fear of being reported'" (from *Conversations: Straight Talk with America's Sister President* by Johnnetta B. Cole).

"My internal scars haunt me."

—DEBRA JONES, SHEET-
METAL WORKER, NORFOLK,
VIRGINIA

I wear scars on the inside and the outside of my body every day of my life. I was violently attacked sixteen years ago during my teenage years by a man I didn't know. He nearly stabbed me to death after I thwarted his attempts to rape me. I remember that night in October as if it were yesterday.

I was on my way home from school when he approached me with a sob story about his dying mother. Finally, he persuaded me to go home with him under the pretense that my visit would console his mother. The stench of stale alcohol filled the air inside his apartment. I realized that his mother was pissy drunk as soon as he introduced us. After he briefly excused himself to the kitchen for a beer, I looked around the dingy apartment and started feeling uncomfortable. My fourteen-year-old instincts told me something wasn't right.

When he returned, he led me to the back of the apartment. Through the darkness of the room, I could make out a bare mattress lying on the floor. I asked him to please turn on the lights so that I could see, but he refused. I told him "no" when he asked me for sex. He kept pleading with me as he drank from his beer. I told him, "I have to go home now because it's getting late and I know my mother will come looking for me." After a while, he said, "Okay, I'll walk with you, but you're not going to get home safely."

My heart started pounding rapidly. I was so scared. My mind raced, searching for answers. I figured once we got outside I'd make a run for it. I tried to play it cool, but before I knew anything, we were standing in front of an abandoned building. I felt so alone and terrified.

He mumbled something unintelligible and without warning pulled out a 20-inch butcher knife. I stood, literally frozen at the sight of it. Suddenly, blood gushed from my throat like a water fountain. I ran holding my throat until I found an occupied section of the building. A woman had barely opened her door before I fell onto her living room floor, bleeding and semi-conscious.

He stabbed me in my throat and abdomen, missing my heart by a fraction of an inch. It took thousands of stitches and a year's stay in the hospital before I could return home. I made a positive identification of my assailant two days after the assault. He was arrested by the police, brought to trial, and released after serving only one year in a detox ward of a state facility. All because of sloppy police work.

I had an array of social workers and counselors involved in my healing process following the attack. Every time I looked around, my case was being referred to someone else. I told my story over and over again. I never trusted any of them. I felt they had labeled me crazy. Eventually I coped with my

anger through aggressive behavior. With so much pent-up rage, I had a diffi-
cult time dealing with people in general. I spent the rest of my teenage years
in and out of group and foster homes.

Today my internal scars haunt me. I learned just the other week that I
failed the psychological portion of the exam to become a police officer. I
exploded right there in the doctor's office because of his insistent line of ques-
tioning concerning the details of the attack. I'm trying, I'm really trying.
Now I just take it one day at a time.

But despite slavery's legacy of rape, the sad and ugly truth is that it is
not only the white man whom we need to fear. More often than not, it
is Black men who rape Black women. The rapist may be our father, husband, date, or stranger, but in eight of every ten rapes of Black women,
the rapist's face will be Black.

This is not something that our community finds easy to accept. We
might hold marches to protest the rash of Black-on-Black violence, but
it's not rape that many are thinking about when we pound city streets to
fight crime in our neighborhoods. Often the Black woman who steps
out of her place to point the finger at a brother is viewed as a traitor:
Witness the Mike Tyson rape case when Desiree Washington was vilified
for accusing the boxer of raping her in his hotel room. We cling to the
notion that we should be unified as a race no matter what—and no matter what is done to us.

Date or acquaintance rape makes us particularly squeamish. When a
victim, such as Washington or the sister who was gang-raped by a group
of St. John's University students, knows her attacker or attackers, we
want to dismiss it. "She knew what he wanted when she went to his
room," the reasoning goes. "What did she expect?" But rape is rape,
whether the rapist is your husband, the repairman, or your next-door
neighbor.

If you are raped, whether by a friend or stranger, there are certain
steps you should take immediately after you are attacked:

Make sure that you are safe, or get to a safe place.

Don't bathe or douche; don't wash your hair or hands. Don't gargle or
drink anything, and don't change your clothes. The urge to scrub away
the rape will be overwhelming, but you could be destroying evidence
that could be used to convict your attacker.

Leave the rape scene exactly as he left it. Don't disturb any physical evidence he may have touched.

Call the police or go to a hospital immediately, even if you do not think you're hurt. You may have internal injuries and not know it. Make sure that you are examined.

Seek counseling from a therapist, rape crisis center, crime-victims' assistance group, or church. Don't underestimate the impact of the rape. Being raped is devastating, and it will always be with you. It's important that you get help sorting through your feelings.

Whatever you do, don't ever, ever blame yourself. No one asks to be raped. Tell yourself that you did the best that you could under extremely trying and dangerous circumstances.

Report the crime. Your information just may insure that he never rapes again.

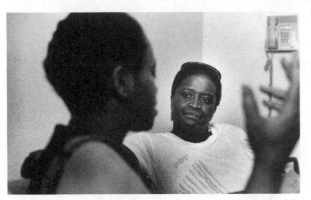

Counseling and support can help ease the feelings of devastation that follow a rape. *(Photo: John Goodwin; courtesy the General Board of Global Ministries, United Methodist Church)*

If someone you love has been raped, talk to the person. It may be painful, but don't sweep it under the rug. Encourage her to unburden herself and to seek counseling or a support group.

Battering

Battering is serious business, but all too often in our community it's a laughing matter. We spent years cracking up at Redd Foxx on *Sanford and Son* as he chased Aunt Esther around the room, threatening her with a fat lip. We snap our fingers to old blues songs where singers boast of using guns to dispose of unfaithful women. And we think nothing of dancing to rappers who brag about offing bitches and hos.

Many people gobbled up Miles Davis's autobiography, even though he unashamedly describes knocking Cicely Tyson, one of our most treasured actresses, around the room. Many others swallowed Shahrazad Ali's advice in her book *The Blackman's Guide to Understanding the Blackwoman,* in which she recommends the use of an open-handed slap to the mouth as a disciplinary tool to tame wayward women.

Battering is a hideous fact of life we don't want to own up to. It makes us squirm. Some of us reassure ourselves that it could never happen to us. "The first time a man hit me would be the last time he hit me, 'cause I'd have to kill him." Because we don't understand the complicated and often dependent relationship a woman may have with her batterer, we look down at a battered sister and wonder "Why doesn't she just leave?" or "She must like it." That leaves us with the wrong notion that only weak women get hit.

But the fact is, the battered woman is everywoman. She's straight, lesbian, married, single, African-American, Asian, white, or Latina. Violence against women is an equal-opportunity crime. You're not exempt if you're rich or middle-class. It doesn't matter if you're a take-no-prisoners type or if you're shy and introverted. Given the right—or the wrong—circumstances, it could happen to you.

Domestic abuse is a reality for more than 50 percent of all women who will be abused at some point in their lifetimes. (Child abuse and incest are also types of domestic violence; for more on these topics see chapter 30, "Incest and Child Abuse.") Battering is the single highest cause of injury to women in the United States. Every day, another four women are killed by their husbands and lovers.

Battering can be difficult to recognize and define. It doesn't necessarily mean that a woman's being beaten to a pulp. Battering tends to go in stages and can escalate. It may start with verbal abuse and then intensify into a push or shove and then a slap or kick. As the verbal insults and physical beatings get worse and worse, a woman may not have the strength to fend off her attacker.

And while it's easy for an outsider to say she would leave after the first blow, leaving a violent situation is always easier said than done. Dependent children and the lack of money or resources will keep a woman tied to a man (or a woman) who abuses her. Often, the cycle of physical and emotional abuse has a woman so demoralized that she feels like she deserves to be hit and that she can't make it on her own. And then there is the grim reality that for most victims of domestic abuse, leaving can be deadly: The woman who leaves her abuser increases her odds of being killed by him by 75 percent.

It is impossible to predict just who will become a batterer, but according to the National Coalition Against Domestic Violence, there are some warning signs that you should pay attention to. This applies to both male partners and lesbians lovers. Here's what to watch for:

He comes from a violent background. People who grow up witnessing abuse in their families are likely to mimic that behavior later on in life.

He has a hot temper and frequently uses force to solve problems. Someone who gets into fights, tortures animals, or punches walls when upset is likely to take out frustrations on his loved ones.

He abuses drugs or alcohol. Drinking and drugs can make an already violent person worse.

He is excessively jealous. A mate who always wants to know where you are or is jealous of everyone—even of strangers passing on the street—is trouble.

He is verbally abusive. Look out for a mate who cuts you down or calls you names such as "stupid" or "ugly."

He has low self-esteem. Abusers who feel bad about themselves often take it out on those closest to them.

He has little respect for women. A man who thinks women are second-class citizens may feel free to batter.

He has guns or knives.

He is possessive. Partners should feel comfortable with friends and family and not want to isolate you from loved ones.

He is controlling. Notice whether he tries to control you and expects you to follow orders.

You're afraid when he is angry.

He blames his behavior on you. "If you hadn't burned the dinner, I wouldn't have to smack you."

If you are indeed being battered by your spouse or lover, don't blame yourself. It's not your fault; he is the one with a problem. And there is help out there. Before things reach the violent stage again, it's a good idea to figure out a plan of action.

Hide extra cash and important papers such as birth certificates, Social Security cards, and your driver's license in a safe place where you can get to them in a hurry. (A sanitary-napkin box is a good spot.) Whatever you do, don't put them in your purse because your mate may take it away from you. If you can, hide a change of clothing with the papers.

Go through every room in your house and figure out the quickest escape route. Find out where the closest pay phone is, and target neighbors you can count on to help out in an emergency. In most cities, bus drivers will let you ride for free if you tell them you are in an emergency situation.

If you can sense that you and your mate are headed for another violent episode, consider calling emergency shelters in advance to see if they will have room for you and your children later on in the week.

Mentally rehearse your escape plans again and again until you can do them by rote. Being prepared is essential: If things at home get violent again, you won't be able to think clearly.

Emergency shelters can give you a safe, anonymous place to hide while you put your life back together. At the shelter, you can get counseling (usually free) for yourself and your children, as well as employment, housing, and legal information. Generally, a shelter's location is kept secret from the batterer so he can't find you.

Not so long ago, the law provided little if any relief for battered women. Today that is changing. Thirty-four states plus the District of Columbia have enacted "antistalking" laws that prohibit abusers from threatening bodily harm or repeatedly following or harassing women. Violations of these laws are considered felonies. Protective orders are another option; you have to petition the court to get a restraining order placed against the batterer. With a protective order, the abuser has to keep his distance from you. If he violates the order, he could go to jail. But be warned that for some batterers, a protective order is just a piece of paper.

Homicide

Guns are bloodying our streets—and our school yards. When third-graders start carrying guns to school, it's time for us to take a long, hard look at gun control. These days, it seems anyone can get a gun; in fact, a new handgun is produced every twenty seconds. According to FBI statistics, nearly seventy million handguns are now in circulation throughout the country. Firearms are responsible in the killing of more than 80 percent of African-American men under twenty-five; every year 1 out of 28 Black men will be killed by an unlicensed gun—compared to 1 out of 164 white. And instead of the Saturday-night special, people are now arming themselves with assault weapons, such as AK-47's, that were once seen only on the battlefield.

Our men and boys continue to suffer the greatest calamity in our homicide epidemic. Young Black males are nine times more likely to be homicide victims than are young white males. Of course, it's not just our men who suffer. Poverty and living in dangerous neighborhoods greatly increase the odds that women also will become murder statistics. Each year hundreds upon hundreds of women and children are killed in the cross fire of gang warfare. Still, in 80 to 90 percent of all African-American homicides, gangs and drugs are not the culprits. Too often our people are killed by folks they do know and maybe even love, usually during an argument.

The mounting death tolls won't subside until we learn to deal with our anger and resolve our conflicts without resorting to violence. Homicide doesn't have to be part of our communities.

According to Deborah Prothrow-Stith, M.D., coauthor of the book *Deadly Consequences: How Violence Is Destroying Our Teenage Population and a Plan to Begin Solving the Problem,* violent aggression is learned behavior. Simply put, children mimic what they see at home. If their parents use violence on them and on each other, it stands to reason that children will grow up thinking that fighting is the only way to solve their problems. Parents who demand that their sons "act like a man" raise men who never learn to walk away from trouble.

According to Dr. Prothrow-Stith, if we taught every single one of our children how to handle their angry feelings without violence, our national homicide and assault statistics would plummet 50 to 75 percent. Dr. Prothrow-Stith also notes that it will take a groundswell of support from our schools, churches, social-service agencies, law-enforcement officials, and the medical community to achieve that. Children who live in despair must be taught that there are other options beyond the violent confines of their inner-city battle zones.

Still, there is much that you can do, especially with children, on a one-on-one basis:

Check your own behavior. Are you quick to scream at or slap a child? Is your own violent behavior sending a negative message?

Pressure local police to bring community policing programs that work with local residents to your neighborhood.

Encourage your church to take a more active role in fighting violence and poverty. Contact social-service agencies for advice and help.

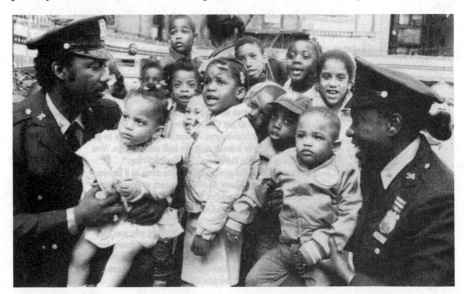

Police officers are most effective when they forge a bond with community members. *(Photo: New York Police Foundation)*

Teach your children the consequences of violent behavior; point out that violence only begets more violence and greatly decreases their chances of survival. Teach them that being cruel is not acceptable; remind them that all people have feelings.

Offer techniques that children can use to deflate anger such as counting to ten or walking away from a fight. If your child is a teenager, talk frankly to her or him about potential situations that could provoke anger; ask your child how she or he would handle the situation without becoming violent.

Urge your PTA to institute conflict-resolution programs in the schools. Your church should do the same.

Speak out about violence in the media through letter-writing campaigns.

Turn off the TV and shield young children from violent movies and TV shows. Don't allow your kids to become numb to violence. Explain to them that although cartoon characters pop up after being shot and actors go on to other roles after being killed in movies, real violence hurts, and when someone is bleeding, it's painful.

Help guide your children toward nonviolent role models. Explain to them that powerful people use their minds as weapons instead of guns.

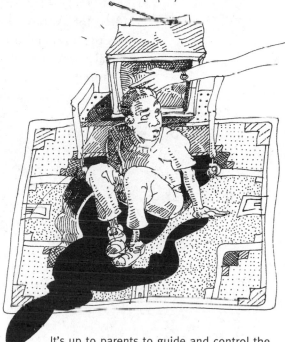

It's up to parents to guide and control the flow of violent images children take in.
(Drawing: Yvonne Buchanan)

For more information, pick up a copy of *Deadly Consequences,* in which Dr. Prothrow-Stith and others offer advice and help.

Protecting Yourself

To learn how to fight back, you'll need to take a self-defense class. Many sisters have found these kinds of courses very empowering, especially for women who have been attacked. Classes are offered in cities and towns from coast to coast through community centers, YMCAs and YWCAs, health clubs, colleges, rape crisis centers, or victims services agencies. (Be sure to look for self-defense rather than karate, which won't be as helpful in the event of an attack.) Model Mugging, a course in which women actually practice self-defense moves in the environment of a simulated attack, comes highly recommended. (Caution: Classes can be costly.) For more information on finding classes in your area, contact Model Mugging, 1251 Tenth St., Monterey, CA 93940, (408) 646-5425.

The very best way to defend yourself, especially if you haven't been trained in self-defense, is to avoid potentially harmful situations. The Center for Anti-Violence Education/Brooklyn Women's Martial Arts offers these general prevention tips:

Be alert and active.

Trust your instincts. They are usually correct.

Do not be afraid of making a scene, seeming "paranoid," or being "wrong." Denial frequently opens the door for trouble.

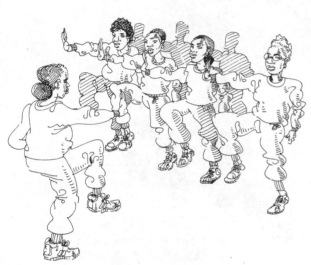

Examine your environments—home, workplace, frequently traveled routes. Figure out potential dangers, and think of ways that you can decrease them. Talk with others with whom you work or live, and think of ways to increase everyone's safety.

In public, be aware of how you are presenting yourself. If you are depressed or lost, try not to show it. Walk with your head up and eyes aware.

Beware of seemingly harmless questions. Attackers usually use a screening process to isolate easy targets.

Speak up if you are being bothered.

Yelling is one of the best defenses. It breaks the "victim role," attracts attention,

Learning self-defense can help combat violence and build confidence. *(Drawing: Yvonne Buchanan)*

and distracts the attacker. Yell "fire," which, unfortunately, will draw more people than yelling "help" or "rape."

Act in unexpected ways; attackers expect certain responses, and anything different may put them off for a few seconds—seconds you can use to your advantage.

Plan ahead. If you are going out or to a party and may be drinking, think about how you will get home, who you can stay with, or whether you have enough money for a cab or car service.

Think of ways to work with others in your neighborhood or workplace to prevent or deal with robberies and attacks. The best self-defense is collective.

Teach your daughters to be assertive so that they aren't easy targets.

Women tend to feel more secure when they're accompanied by a man, but that didn't help me when I was attacked. My husband, Jeff, and I were coming home at about eleven-thirty at night. We turned the corner onto our street, and two guys fell into step behind us. We thought it was weird, but we were on the side of the street closer to our house, so we didn't want to cross. We were pretty close to our house anyway, so I took out my keys. As soon we reached our building I started to unlock the door when Jeff let out a chilling scream. I spun around and found this young guy holding a gun on him, and next to him I came face to face with another gun, pointed at me.

I can't remember what went through my mind, if anything. I was terrified, but I somehow managed to get out my money when they demanded it. Jeff also took his money out of his wallet and dropped the money and his wallet on the ground to show that there was no more money in it. After grabbing the money they asked us to enter our building while they themselves walked off casually, without any hurry. They hadn't bothered to try to hide their faces either. I remember the one who held the gun in my face was really not much more than a kid, maybe eighteen years old.

Inside our apartment we called the police, and that's when I started crying. The police came right away. It turned out these two boys were on parole and had been going around mugging people in the neighborhood.

I tried to resume my normal life without completely freaking out. I was able to go to work, but I felt very uncomfortable coming home at night. Being wintertime, it was already dark after work. I became very jumpy when people walked behind me. After about three or four months I saw an ad for a self-defense class and decided to take it.

Learning self-defense helped take away my fear of walking the streets. We were taught how to observe our surroundings, to be more aware of dangerous situations and avoid them. The course also stressed walking down the street alert and with assurance. Too often women get tunnel vision, staring down at the ground while walking and looking vulnerable. I also learned to protect myself if need be. For example, women are usually taught to go for the groin, but most guys protect that area. It's better to strike the eyes, nose, knees, or— to do damage—the throat.

The class didn't get rid of all of my fears or make me feel invincible. I'm not going to walk through Central Park alone in the middle of the night. I wouldn't even do anything different in the same situation I was confronted with, but the class gave me a better sense of how to make judgments in a real-life situation. After taking self-defense, I moved on to karate, and I've

"Learning self-defense helped take away my fear of walking the streets."

—MARTHA SOUTHGATE, ENTERTAINMENT WRITER, BROOKLYN

been taking classes for almost two years. But I'm thinking about taking a
self-defense class again, because karate classes don't always translate in the
face of danger. And I don't want to live in fear.

Suicide

All too often we don't view suicide as violence, but it is: Violence against
oneself is violence.

The suicide of Leanita McClain in 1984 shocked the African-
American community. She seemed to be a sister who had everything to
live for: At thirty-two, she was already a columnist for the *Chicago
Tribune* and the first African-American member of the newspaper's edi-
torial board. *Glamour* magazine honored her as one of America's ten
most outstanding career women of 1984, and her writings were gaining
national recognition in publications such as *Newsweek* and the *Washington Post*. She had friends, respect, a loving family, and a new house in a
nice Chicago neighborhood that was a far cry from the projects where
she grew up.

Yet, despite the awards and the creature comforts, peace eluded her.
Just before swallowing a handful of pills on Memorial Day, 1984,
McClain wrote, "Happiness is a private club that will not let me enter.
As my dreams will never come true, I choose to have them in perpetual
sleep." (For more information about Leanita McClean, read the book *A
Foot in Each World: Articles and Essays by Leanita McClain*, edited by
Clarence Page, Northwestern University Press, 1986; or Bebe Moore
Campbell's article "To Be Black, Gifted, and Alone," which appeared in
Savvy magazine's December 1984 issue.)

Many people don't see suicide as a Black problem. If we can survive
four hundred years of whips and chains, the reasoning goes, why let the
blues get the best of us?

But while suicide continues to take a greater toll in the white community, the fact remains that we are not immune. Suicide poses the least
risk for Black women; we continue to kill ourselves at a slower rate than
Black men. But it is our young people that we should be the most concerned about: Between 1960 and 1984, the suicide rate among young
Black women aged fifteen to twenty-four nearly doubled, while the
number of young Black men who killed themselves nearly tripled.

We simply can't afford to ignore the reality of suicide. When feelings of
depression are overwhelming, death may seem like a welcome relief. If you

think someone you love is contemplating suicide, don't be afraid to take action. People who kill themselves are often undecided about whether they want to live or die. Your intervention can be truly lifesaving.

Pay attention to these warning signs:

Verbal warning. Up to 80 percent of people who commit suicide talk about it before they actually try to kill themselves.

Obsession with death. Someone contemplating suicide may read about it constantly or continually steer the conversation to death-related topics.

Suicide attempt. Those who attempt suicide once often succeed in a later attempt.

Unexpected gift giving. Someone who suddenly gives away valuables may be doing so in an attempt to settle her final affairs.

Changes in behavior. Sadness, loss of appetite, sleeplessness, and inability to concentrate may signal a deep depression that could lead to suicide.

If your loved one exhibits symptoms like these or tells you she is seriously thinking about taking her life, don't overreact. Express your concern, and listen attentively to what she has to say. Ask enough questions so that you can figure out whether she has a definite plan for killing herself. Acknowledge her feelings, and reassure her that what she is feeling may be temporary. Tell her help is out there. Don't make promises not to tell others; you may need to break your confidentiality to save your loved one's life. If necessary, stick with her until trained professionals can take over. And whatever you do, don't be afraid to seek professional help.

Female Genital Mutilation

In Africa about eighty million girls are experiencing a kind of violence that until recently was unheard of in this country. These girls and others in Asia, Europe, and Latin America are undergoing a procedure that is politely known as female circumcision, but that critics call female genital mutilation. It can be as mild as cuts in the clitoris or as extreme as the complete excision of the clitoris, both sets of labia, and the suturing or infibulation of the vagina leaving only a tiny hole for the passage of urine and menstrual blood.

Many Westerners are outraged at this barbaric custom, which is also found in the U.S. and in other countries where Africans have settled. It is said to be performed on young girls and adolescents for chastity, purification, cleanliness, and prevention of rape. Critics, however, believe this practice is yet another way to control women—to destroy their feelings by decimating their clitorises and to satisfy male sexual desires. Women who refuse to have their clitorises removed are shunned, considered unmarriageable and unchaste. But women who undergo the mutilation suffer from more than social stigma; many put their lives and health at risk. Health officials and feminist activists have found that complications of the procedure can cause extreme pain due to lack of anesthesia and lead to hemorrhaging, infection, blood poisoning, and even death. Women who undergo it may suffer from urinary-tract infections, painful intercourse, difficulty urinating, infertility, and complications during childbirth.

However, not all Black women believe that the practice is wrong. In fact, some women—most of them African—believe that Walker and other critics are looking at Africa and its customs through uncomprehending Western eyes. It is simply considered a rite of passage, like many others.

In recent years, though, some African women have spoken out about the practice. Aminata Diop, a Kenyan woman who refused to have her clitoris and labia removed—without sterilization or anesthesia—has become a touchstone in the volatile debate. And Soraya Mire, a Somalian woman who was genitally mutilated at age thirteen, has created a documentary called "Fire Eyes," in hopes of bringing the subject to the forefront.

To find out more about female genital mutilation, read *Warrior Marks: Female Genital Mutilation and the Sexual Blinding of Women* by Alice Walker, Harcourt Brace, 1993.

For More Information

ORGANIZATIONS: General Violence

PARENTS OF MURDERED CHILDREN, 100 E. 8th St., suite B-41, Cincinnati, OH 45202; (513) 721-5683. Provides support for survivors of homicide victims. Referrals to nationwide chapters of support groups and offers pamphlets.

NATIONAL ORGANIZATION FOR VICTIM ASSISTANCE, 1757 Park Rd. NW, Washington, DC 20010; (800) TRY-NOVA or (202) 232-6682. Provides information and refers victims to local programs; will assist victim directly if none available in their area.

NATIONAL VICTIM CENTER, 309 W. Seventh St., suite 705, Fort Worth, TX 76102; (800) FYI-CALL or (817) 877-3355. Referrals to local crisis centers or services nationwide; brochures available.

VICTIMS SERVICES AGENCY, 2 Lafayette St., New York, NY 10007; (212) 577-7700. National referral service, 24 hour crisis-counseling hotline, (212) 577-7777. Offers individual counseling and support groups for victims and their significant others, emotional counseling during police questioning, court appearances, and hospital exams.

ORGANIZATIONS: Rape and Sexual Assault

MINISTRIES WITH WOMEN AND FAMILIES IN CRISIS, Board of Global Ministries, United Methodist Church, 475 Riverside Dr., New York, NY 10115; (212) 870-3833 or 870-3600. This national program helps community groups and churches address problems of women in crisis, including domestic violence, rape/sexual harassment, drug and alcohol abuse, sterilization abuse, and women in prison.

NATIONAL CLEARINGHOUSE ON MARITAL AND DATE RAPE, 2325 Oak St., Berkeley, CA 94708; (510) 524-1582. Focuses on legislation to protect women's rights; compiles statistics, research, and the results of rape cases around the country.

NATIONAL COALITION AGAINST SEXUAL ASSAULT (NCASA), 912 N. Second St., Harrisburg, PA 17102-3319; (717) 232-7460. A national network of rape crisis centers and battered women's programs; can refer you to a local center.

WASHINGTON D.C. RAPE CRISIS CENTER, P.O. Box 21005, Washington, D.C. 20009; (202) 232-0789. Serves primarily women of color, counsels rape survivors, operates a 24-hour hotline, organizes staying-safe classes for children. The center has helped found other rape crisis centers around the country—ask if there's one in your area or for their book, *How to Start a Rape Crisis Center* ($5), and other brochures.

ORGANIZATIONS: Domestic Violence

CENTER FOR THE PREVENTION OF SEXUAL AND DOMESTIC VIOLENCE, 1914 N. 34th St., suite 105, Seattle, WA 98103; (206) 634-1903. Focuses primarily on education and resource information to religious communities. Call for brochures that discuss a religious response to domestic and sexual violence.

THE NATIONAL BATTERED WOMEN'S LAW PROJECT OF THE NATIONAL CENTER FOR WOMEN AND FAMILY LAW, 799 Broadway, room 402, New York, NY 10003; (212) 674-8200. Produces handbooks, public-education, and resource packets and serves as an information clearinghouse for advocates, attorneys, and policy makers on legal issues facing battered women. Call for a list of publications.

NATIONAL COALITION AGAINST DOMESTIC VIOLENCE, P.O. Box 18749, Denver, CO 80218; (303) 839-1852. Every state has an office that provides local information, resources, lists of support groups, and brochures.

WOMEN OF COLOR TASK FORCE OF THE NATIONAL COALITION AGAINST DOMESTIC VIOLENCE, contact Joan Dauphine or Karlene John, cochairs, P.O. Box 18749, Denver, CO 80218-0749; (303) 839-1852. Provides information on support groups and centers, a suggested reading list, and pamphlets on domestic violence.

WOMEN'S CENTERS: Contact them for guidance and referral to local services. If you have trouble locating one in your area, contact the Women's Action Alliance, 370 Lexington Ave., New York, NY 10017; (212) 532-8330; for comprehensive and up-to-date information on women's centers in the U.S. The Alliance can provide a name/address of a center over the phone, or write for a complete listing of women's centers.

WOMEN OF COLOR TASK FORCE AGAINST DOMESTIC VIOLENCE, P.O. Box 1743, Aurora, CO 80040; (303) 696-9196. Networks with women of color in other domestic-violence programs. Also working on starting an 800 line for battered women of color.

YWCA: Many local chapters house a women's center, have access to a shelter, or provide basic services such as referral to appropriate programs in your area—such as the YWCA Women's Support Shelter in Tacoma, Washington.

ORGANIZATIONS: Suicide

AMERICAN ASSOCIATION OF SUICIDOLOGY, 2459 S. Ash, Denver, CO 80222; (303) 692-0985. Maintains a directory of survivor groups across the country and a national list of crisis lines; call for one in your area. To purchase *The National Directory of Crisis Lines,* send $15 plus $2 for shipping. Also holds regular conferences.

AMERICAN SUICIDE FOUNDATION, 1045 Park Ave., suite 3C, New York, NY 10028; (212) 410-1111. Call for free pamphlets on suicide prevention, with tips on what to do if you suspect a loved one is contemplating suicide.

SUICIDE PREVENTION AND CRISIS SERVICE, P.O. Box 312, Ithaca, NY 14851; (607) 272-1616 (crisis line). Can provide referrals and crisis counseling.

Books: General Violence

Chain Chain Change: For Black Women Dealing with Physical and Emotional Abuse, Evelyn C. White, Seal Press (Seattle), 1985.

Deadly Consequences: How Violence Is Destroying Our Teenage Population and A Plan to Begin Solving the Problem, Deborah Prothrow-Stith, M.D., and Michelle Weissman, HarperCollins, 1991.

Violence Against Women and the Ongoing Challenge to Racism, Angela Y. Davis, Kitchen Table: Women of Color Press, 1987.

Books: Rape and Sexual Assault

Against Our Will: Men, Women and Rape, Susan Brownmiller, Ballantine Books, 1975. A classic.

I Never Called It Rape: The Ms. *Report on Recognizing, Fighting and Surviving Date Rape,* Robin Warshaw, Harper & Row, 1988.

Man Against Woman: What Every Woman Should Know About Violent Men, Edward W. Gondolf, Tab Books, 1989.

Sexual Assault & Child Sexual Abuse—A National Directory of Victims' Services and Prevention Programs, Oryx Press (4041 N. Central Ave., suite 700, Phoenix, AZ 85012-3397; 800-279-6799), 1989.

Still Loved By the Sun: A Rape Survivor's Journal, Migael Scherer, Simon & Schuster, 1992.

Stopping Rape: Successful Survival Strategies, Pauline B. Bart and Patricia H. O'Brien, Pergamon Press, 1985.

Surviving Sexual Violence, Liz Kelly, University of Minnesota Press (Minneapolis), 1989.

Books: Domestic Violence

Battered into Submission: The Tragedy of Wife Abuse in the Christian Home, James Alsdurf and Phyllis Alsdurf, Inter-Varsity Press (P.O. Box 1400, Downers Grove, IL 60515), 1989.

The Battered Woman's Survival Guide: Breaking the Cycle, Jan Berliner Statman, Taylor Publishing Co. (Dallas), 1990.

Battered Women's Directory, ninth edition, Betsy Warrior, 1985; lists shelters in the U.S., Europe, Australia, South Africa, and Senegal. Send $12 to Directory, Barbara Curuso, Drawer 62, Earlham College, Richmond, IN 47374-4095.

It Could Happen to Anyone: Why Battered Women Stay, Ola W. Barnett and Alyce D. LaViolette, Sage Publications (Thousand Oaks, Calif.), 1993.

Naming the Violence: Speaking Out About Lesbian Battering, edited by Kerry Lobel for the National Coalition Against Domestic Violence Task Force, Seal Press (Seattle), 1986.

Violent Betrayal: Partner Abuse in Lesbian Relationships, Claire M. Renzetti, Sage Publications (Thousand Oaks, Calif.), 1992.

What's a Nice Girl Like You Doing in a Relationship Like This? Women in Abusive Relationships, Kay Marie Porterfield, ed., The Crossing Press, 1992.

When Love Goes Wrong: What to Do When You Can't Do Anything Right—Strategies for Women with Controlling Partners, Susan Schechter and Ann Jones, HarperCollins, 1992.

Books: Self-Defense

Are You a Target? A Guide to Self-Protection & Personal Safety, Judith Fein, Torrance Publishing Co. (Duncan Mills, Calif.), 1988.

Back Off! How to Confront and Stop Sexual Harassment and Harassers, Martha J. Langelan, Fireside/Simon & Schuster, 1993.

Fight Back: Feminist Resistance to Male Violence, Frederique Delacoste and Felice Newman, eds., Cleis Press, 1981.

Free to Fight Back: A Self-Defense Handbook for Women, Marilyn Scribner, Harold Shaw Publishers (Wheaton, Ill.), 1989.

Her Wits About Her: A Collection of Women's Self-Defense Success Stories by Women, Denise Caignon and Gail Grove, eds., Harper & Row, 1987.

Practical Self-Defense Guide for Women, Paul McCallum, F & W Publications (Cincinatti), 1991.

Self-Respect and Sexual Assault, Jeanette Mauro-Cochrane, Tab/McGraw-Hill, 1993.

Sexual Assault: How to Defend Yourself, Dan Lena and Marie Howard, Fell Publishers (Hollywood, Fla.) 1990.

Books: Suicide

Healing After the Suicide of a Loved One, Ann Smolin and John Guinan, Fireside/Simon & Schuster, 1993.

30

Incest and
Child Abuse

In 1985 during an interview with a woman who had been sexually abused, talk-show host Oprah Winfrey said, without thinking, something like the same thing happened to me. At age nine Winfrey was repeatedly raped by a cousin and molested by a family friend; the abuse continued until she was fourteen. As a teenager she was also molested by her favorite uncle. Since revealing her own struggles with the aftermath of incest, Winfrey has become an activist for all incest survivors. She narrated a documentary called *Scared Silent: Exposing and Ending Child Abuse,* which aired on both network TV and PBS simultaneously. Winfrey was also instrumental in getting passed federal child-protection legislation that maintains a database of criminal offenders convicted of child abuse and other crimes; the database is made available to child-care providers.

Oprah Winfrey has become a touchstone for many women who are survivors; not victims, but survivors—a reminder that there is life beyond incest. She has also been a voice of candor about the prevalence of physical and emotional abuse in the Black community. The National Committee to Prevent Child Abuse (NCPCA) estimates that 2.9 million

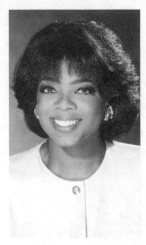

Oprah Winfrey has become a forceful activist for survivors of sexual abuse. (*Photo: Elledge/ Jensen; courtesy* The Oprah Winfrey Show*)*

children were victims of abuse or neglect in 1993—a rate of one every ten seconds. The same year saw a record number of deaths of children resulting from abuse or neglect (approximately 1,299, nearly half of whom were under one year old). About one in every three or four girls is sexually assaulted by age eighteen, and their offenders are known 85 percent of the time. And these statistics are falsely low: All forms of physical and sexual abuse are underreported. Counselors and other mental-health workers believe the numbers may be much higher.

Studies have shown abuse is more common in households and families that are forced to live with high amounts of stress. That makes all kinds of abuse a particular problem for us. African-Americans deal with the daily stresses that racism exacts on us. Other pressures such as unemployment, lack of adequate child care, and financial hardship add to the problem. A study conducted by Gail E. Wyatt, Ph.D., of UCLA found that 57 percent of Black women reported at least one incident of sexual abuse prior to age eighteen. In a 1992 survey of *Essence* readers, who tend to have higher-than-average economic and educational levels among Blacks, 43 percent reported some kind of sexual abuse during their lifetimes.

Despite these startling numbers, many folks in our community continue to deny the existence of physical and sexual abuse. Many whisper that it's "white people's nastiness." Others refuse to believe that, given the inhumane treatment our ancestors endured at the hands of white men, Black men would beat and rape Black girls. The silence is so ingrained that many Black folks criticized Winfrey, chiding her for discussing "her business in the streets."

But denying the existence of physical, emotional, and sexual abuse of children will not make it go away. In fact, silence only fuels the problem and leaves survivors feeling lost, confused, guilty, and painfully alone. The survivor of abuse carries lasting scars. Long after the abuse has stopped, she may find it difficult to trust people and may abort relationships out of fear of intimacy. She may abuse food, alcohol, or drugs in an attempt to numb herself to the pain that she feels, which may seem to have no origin. Some women are aware of the exact nature of the abuse throughout their lives, while others don't recall it until later. In either case, the great majority were not allowed to respond when they were little girls. They were made to be silent or keep a secret, to move on as though nothing was happening.

Reaching out for help is the only way a survivor can find a path into a consciousness that sheds light on what she may be experiencing on the surface as low self-esteem, self-doubt, or a general inability to "get it together." Admitting that the problem exists and working to stop it is the only way our community can make it go away.

Child Abuse

One of the biggest myths about child abuse is that the abuser is a stranger, some inhuman monster. The media generally highlights the most dramatic cases of physical child abuse, which usually means those ending in death. While it is true that in this country more than three children die of injuries inflicted by caretakers every day, there are more abused children who are living and ignored. And many abusers aren't monsters: They are men and women, many of whom were abused themselves, who are overwhelmed and crying out for help.

According to the NCPAC, in 1993 more than 250,000 cases of physical abuse and 477,520 cases of neglect were reported in thirty-seven states. These states reported 40,640 cases of emotional maltreatment. A disproportionate number—26 percent—of the victims were Black, and over half were female. Approximately one third of confirmed child-abuse reports involved caretakers who abused drugs and/or alcohol. And again, because all kinds of abuse is underreported, these estimates don't reflect the true picture.

The National Resource Center on Child Abuse and Neglect defines abuse as "the physical or mental injury, sexual abuse, negligent treatment or maltreatment of a child under age 18 by a person who is responsible for the child's welfare under circumstances which indicate that the child's welfare is harmed or threatened thereby."

Physical Abuse

Physical abuse refers to the use of excessive force that results in injuries. In the Black community, the line between physical abuse and proper discipline is often blurred. Many Black parents go to great lengths to discipline children, hoping to "raise them right" so that they can avoid worse punishment and abuse by whites who are quick to lash out at what they perceive as "unruly" or "uppity" Blacks. Others were raised being "slapped upside the head," so they discipline their children with physical punishment.

Studies have found that physically abused children generally cannot remember the reason they were hit. In many cases, the child ends up feeling confused because her behavior has been normal or the reason for the abuse was never explained.

"I was not a bad child."

—RENOIR DARRETT,
SCRIPT SUPERVISOR,
NEW YORK CITY

It was never with her bare hands. My grandmother used a cord that attached the waffle iron to the wall; it was always that. She would keep a list of what I had done wrong. I don't honestly remember what was on the list. As she would be beating me she would tell me what I had done wrong.

I was not a bad child, everyone knew that. I'd do something and she'd say, "That's going on the list," and nothing would happen. And then one day she would say, "Go get the ironing cord and go up to your room." And she'd go to her room and get the list and then come in and start beating me. Afterwards I was expected to get on with life. I had to take what was happening to me, and there was no room to even feel bad. So I didn't. I don't think I recognized it as what we called abuse until four or five years ago, through therapy.

What happened to me has affected every single aspect of my personality and my life. When I think of what I was like as a child before I moved in with my grandmother, it's like I'm looking at a movie of a totally different person. I was exuberant, I was lively, I really had a sense of the world as a safe place and of me as almost a central character. But that confidence and sense of freedom was totally eroded.

Not that I think any of this was good, but a few positive things came out of being abused. Because of what I went through I have more compassion for people. I listen more carefully, not just to what people say, but to what they're not saying. I can tune into people even when they're in denial. It's almost as if we have a code.

Neglect

Nearly 48 percent of abuse cases are classified as neglect. Neglected children are denied adequate food, clothing, medical care, or supervision. "Sometimes neglect is not being available. The child is left feeling devalued," says Julia A. Boyd, a Seattle psychotherapist and author of *In the Company of My Sisters: Black Women and Self-Esteem.* For example, parents who work long hours and spend little time with their children are neglecting the children's emotional needs. When heard with regularity, phrases like "I'm busy" communicate to children that everything is more important than they are.

Emotional Abuse

Emotional abuse is difficult to define and recognize. "There are no scars," says Boyd. It is defined by the American Humane Association as "continual or consistent criticism or neglect of emotional needs."

"What I call mother-abuse tends to be more emotional, but the symptoms of this abuse are very much the same as those of physical abuse," says Boyd. She describes mother-abuse as an intense combination of physical abuse and a barrage of verbal abuse to which the child is defenseless. Mothers are more likely to be the perpetrators of this type of abuse because they are generally in frequent contact with the children. This kind of verbal battering, whether it comes from the mother or father, erodes a child's self-esteem, often in radical ways. Because the child is told to love and respect the words of the mother, Boyd says, it is often difficult for her patients to speak freely about it.

"Women are often more hesitant to talk about mother-abuse than sexual abuse. Because I'm a Black woman and they are not sure if I'll be different from the rest of the community."

The aftereffects of child abuse are many, but most common is what Dr. Leonard Shengold describes as soul murder. "Soul murder is the perpetuation of brutal acts against children that result in their emotional bondage to the abuser and finally, in their psychic and spiritual annihilation." The mention of psychic and spiritual devastation is key. The soul murder of a child produces an adult who is angry and unable to trust and tolerate intimacy.

What to Do About Abuse

Many well-meaning parents may be abusing their children, not aware that their behavior has moved from spanking and scolding to physical and verbal abuse. It's a delicate balance. While some parents don't believe in hitting their children at all, others stand by the old saying "Spare the rod and spoil the child." Experts are also divided on this issue.

If you aren't sure whether your disciplinary measures are appropriate, check your behavior: When you scold or spank your child, are you simply trying to teach your child a lesson, or are you acting out of anger and frustration? If you feel your anger or emotions getting out of control, remove yourself from the situation. Take a walk or call a friend. For more detailed information on this subject, see chapter 28, "Loving Our Children."

In recurring or more serious situations, consider seeking professional help. Parents who are concerned about whether or not their discipline is too violent can contact Parents Anonymous (PA), 520 S. Lafayette Park Pl., suite 316, Los Angeles, CA 90057; (213) 388-6685. PA is a support group for overwhelmed parents, many of whom were abused themselves, who are trying to learn effective nonviolent parenting skills at free weekly meetings led by professionals.

If you are being abused, tell an adult you trust. For referrals to a place where you can get help, contact the National Coalition Against Domestic Violence, 1201 Colfax Ave., Denver, CO 80218; (303) 839-1852. If you were abused as a child, contact the Coalition for referral to a local support group in your area, or seek the professional help of a therapist. It is important that you get some kind of help— individual therapy or a support group—because the abuse you suffered may affect your life in ways that you are not immediately aware of. For example, many survivors find that they have an inability to maintain relationships or to trust people. For a complete list of helpful books and organizations, refer to the resource list at the end of this chapter.

If you suspect a child is being abused, you must report it to the child abuse and neglect or child welfare department in your area, which is listed in the phone book under the Department of Health and Human Services. You can recognize abuse in the following ways:

PHYSICAL ABUSE	NEGLECT	EMOTIONAL ABUSE
Physical Indicators:	Physical Indicators:	Physical Indicators:
unexplained bruises (in various stages of healing), welts, human bite marks, bald spots	*abandonment*	*speech disorders*
	unattended medical needs	*delayed physical development*
	consistent lack of supervision	*substance abuse*
unexplained burns, especially cigarette burns or immersion burns (glovelike), unexplained fractures, lacerations, or abrasions	*consistent hunger*	*ulcers, asthma, severe allergies*
	inappropriate dress	
	poor hygiene	Behavioral Indicators:
	lice	*habit disorders (sucking, rocking)*
	distended stomach	*antisocial behavior, destructiveness*
Behavioral Indicators:	*emaciation*	
self-destructiveness		*passive and aggressive behavioral extremes*
withdrawn and aggressive behavioral extremes	Behavioral Indicators:	*delinquent behavior (especially adolescents)*
uncomfortableness with physical contact	*regular display of fatigue or listlessness*	
arriving at school early or staying late as if afraid to be at home	*stealing or begging for food*	Source: American Association for Protecting Children
chronic running away (adolescents)	*reports that no caretaker is at home*	
complaints of soreness or discomfort in moving	*self-destructiveness*	
wearing clothing inappropriate to weather, to cover body	*dropping out of school (adolescents)*	

Sexual Abuse and Incest

Until fairly recently the definition of sexual abuse in an incestuous relationship required that a woman be penetrated. This narrow definition left many women confused and at odds with their own disturbing memories. Perhaps an uncle showed her pornographic material or exposed himself to her when she was a child, or another male relative fondled her breasts or genitals. Was this sexual abuse? The answer is, unequivocally, yes.

An estimated one out of six girls is sexually abused in an incestuous relationship, and that abuse can be physical or verbal in nature. The abuser can be a man or woman, but in the vast majority of instances, it's a man abusing a girl. Like sexual intercourse with a little girl, describing sex acts to a child, talking inappropriately about sexual relations with a child, masturbating in front of her, or fondling her capitalizes on the child's innocence and betrays her trust.

Experts understand that sexual abuse is about power and control. Says author and psychotherapist Julia A. Boyd, "After a certain age these men are actively making choices. It has nothing to do with sex; it's about power and control. It may also have something to do with the fact that they were abused themselves." But she adds that in a study of offenders and nonoffenders, when both groups were asked, "Were you sexually abused as a child?" for an almost equal number in each group the answer was "yes."

Abusers generally have low self-esteem, feelings of isolation and failure, and may be acting out their own sexual abuse under the influence of alcohol or chemical substances. But ultimately "we're talking about an act of choice," says Boyd. "The offender actively plans the abuse. They know what they're going to do. They have to figure out how and where. If it was okay, why do they tell the child not to tell anybody? Incest survivors are the best secret keepers in the world."

In the case of sibling incest, the victim is often younger and the abuser in puberty is using her for sexual experimentation. Many times survivors don't take sibling incest as seriously as parent/child incest, thinking, "Oh, we were just kids." But actually it can be just as damaging to the survivor. In all cases, the child may not divulge the existence of the abuse to anyone because of shame or threats. Even if she is too young to know precisely what is happening to her, she takes her cues both internally and from the abuser and knows that something is wrong.

The shroud of secrecy heightens feelings of shame.

If you suspect that a child is being sexually abused, you must report

"I thought people wouldn't believe me."

—Name Withheld, college student, Brooklyn

He was younger than me, but he didn't look his age. He was about thirteen when it started, but big—6 feet tall and about 165 pounds. I was a year older but barely 5 feet tall. It was like he was watching me, sizing me up when I would come over to baby-sit his little sister for his mother, my godmother. She didn't trust him to take care of the little girl.

I was reading one day, and all of a sudden he took me by the shirt, and the next thing I knew, I was on the ground. He said he was wrestling, but he started getting rough and kept telling me to shut up. I couldn't move because he had me by the wrists, and he put his kneecaps on the upper part of my thighs. He started smiling, and then he started tearing the jumpsuit my mother made. He grabbed my breasts really hard and said, "Do you like it rough?"

He threatened me when we heard his mother coming toward the door, and I pretended nothing happened. When his mother said I looked like I had been in a fight, I lied. When I got home and my mother wanted to know how I got the marks on my wrists and thighs, I told her I fell off a bunk bed. I took off the outfit and threw it down the incinerator. I thought it was my fault because it had a V in the back.

Through my teens, I kept going there. I didn't say anything about what he was doing to me because I was afraid to hurt the friendship between my mother and godmother. I wasn't important. I also felt so weak because this guy was younger than me. I didn't tell anyone because I thought people wouldn't believe me because I was overweight. So each time I went over there he would attack me. When my mother asked about the bruises on my breasts, I told her my bras were too tight.

It was on and off until I was seventeen or eighteen. Once I slept over at their house because his mother needed me to be there in the early morning to get his sister up and ready for school. I was asleep, and he came in and covered my mouth and was pulling my hair and trying to kiss me so hard that his braces cut my mouth. He was trying to enter me in my vagina and my anus. It was very painful, and he got angry because he couldn't get in. After he came on me he started bruising me and was saying, "Why didn't you let me do it?" The whole time I was telling him to get off. The next morning I thought it was a dream until I saw the stains and my gown hiked up.

To this day I feel like I did something to make him think what he did was okay. And if I'm with a guy and he wants to do something sexual, we do it because I'm afraid he might make me do it. I feel unattractive, and I don't like my body. I feel it's caused me too many problems, it's gotten me into trouble.

I know I need to talk to a therapist. I went to a therapist at my school, but I stopped because I was afraid. But I'm ready to talk to someone now.

your suspicions to the child protective services agency in your area. Child victims of sexual abuse can be recognized by the following:

Physical Indicators
Torn, stained, or bloody underclothing
Pain or itching in genital area
Difficulty walking or sitting
Bruises or bleeding in external genitalia
Sexually transmitted infection
Frequent urinary or yeast infections

Behavioral Indicators
Withdrawal, chronic depression
Speech disorders such as stuttering
Excessive seductiveness
Role reversal, overconcern for siblings
Poor self-esteem, self-devaluation, lack of confidence
Peer problems, lack of involvement
Extreme weight change
Suicide attempts (especially adolescents)
Hysteria, lack of emotional control
Sudden school difficulties
Inappropriate sex play or premature understanding of sex
Problems swallowing or going underwater
Distaste for physical contact, closeness
Promiscuity

Source: American Humane Association

For more information, read the book *Secret Survivors: Uncovering Incest and Its Aftereffects* by Sue E. Blume.

No woman survives sexual abuse unscathed. Survivors are affected in many ways. The extent of the damage depends on the length of the abuse, the reaction of adults she may have told, whether extreme violence was a part of the abuse, and other factors that are essentially unknown. Like the survivor of child abuse, the incest survivor experiences depression and low self-esteem. In addition, the incest survivor is more prone to have difficulty with sex, sexuality, and intimacy.

Survivors of incest may also experience anxiety attacks, visual flashbacks of the abuse, and body memories—physical recollections of sexual abuse. The survivor may experience unexplained pains in her vagina or pelvis or, if the abuse was oral, feel as though she is choking. The body memories occur because at the time of the abuse, the child was unable or not permitted to respond or cry out, resulting in emotional shutdown and repression. Flashbacks and body memories are triggered by things like a fragrance, the death of the abuser, or hearing others talk about their own abuse.

According to Claire Griffin, a psychotherapist who specializes in treating survivors of incest and violent crimes, if the abuse occurs before the age when language develops, the flashbacks and body memories are more severe because "the language to support the memory is not there."

Many survivors use drug and alcohol addiction to push down feelings associated with the abuse. Women are more likely to develop eating disorders. "Food is women's drug of choice," says Becky W. Thompson, Ph.D., author of *A Hunger So Wide and So Deep,* who has studied eating disorders among Black women. "When they need the drug, it's not going to get them arrested; it's cheap, and it's accessible." Many women eat to escape the overwhelming feelings the trauma of the abuse has left. Thompson argues that it is also a way for women to remain grounded in their bodies instead of spiritually leaving their bodies, which is what many girls do to escape the horror of the abuse.

Among the women Thompson interviewed, 61 percent were survivors of sexual abuse. One woman who gained 110 pounds said she did so because it was a way of "taking her breasts back." Whether she did this intentionally or not, it was clearly an act of defense. "Size becomes a protection from objectification because fat women are invisible," adds Thompson. Others wear loose clothing to hide their bodies in hopes of desexualizing themselves.

For Black women, acknowledging and talking about the abuse can be difficult because of sexual stereotypes that we are "loose" and "fast." These stereotypes are holdovers from slavery when white men created these myths to justify their rape of Black women. "There are so many stereotypes about Black women that the pressure is tremendous," says Boyd. "Knowing that people think we're always ready for *it* or that all Black women know how to do is have babies makes us afraid to disclose the abuse."

The media sensationalize the most severe cases of sexual abuse. This causes many women to minimize their own experiences. "We hear all the gory stories in the media, and we think, 'Maybe what was done to me wasn't so bad. I didn't die, I can hold a job.'"

But any woman who has been sexually abused in any way should get help. Fear of the flashbacks, body memories, and feelings of grief and shame may deter you from seeking help, but the energy it takes to keep everything in the place you tucked it away long ago will prevent you from fully living. Griffin says that recovery efforts can help women go beyond being survivors and "reclaim themselves and see that they can take that control back." The fact that you are here proves that you are strong. It may help to remind yourself that facing the past is emotionally intense, but it is not happening to you now. You can find your way out of the maze.

Now more than ever, therapists are sensitized to issues surrounding sexual abuse, and many activist organizations and support groups can provide services. For a more complete listing of organizations, articles, and books, refer to the resource list at the end of this chapter.

In addition to seeking professional help, Griffin recommends that survivors do the following.

Be gentle with yourself. You haven't done anything wrong. In fact, you are a strong person because you were able to survive.

Connect with others who are survivors. It's important to know you're not alone.

Tell friends and family members whom you trust and who care about you that you are doing work in this area. Bringing up painful memories can be very difficult, and loved ones can provide support when you need it.

Keep a journal in order to sort out memories that may be fragmented and sporadic. This way you can record your personal growth and find a way to express your anger and rage.

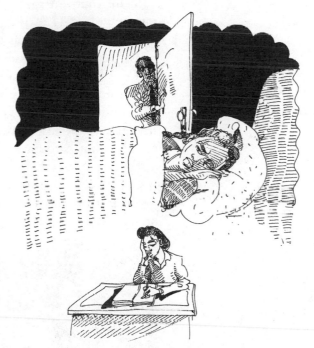

Keeping a journal can help sort through the anger and pain associated with memories of child abuse.
(Drawing: Yvonne Buchanan)

Know that it isn't necessary to confront the abuser. Sometimes it helps to express your rage at that person; at other times it makes matters worse. If he denies the abuse—as he did during the victimization—all your feelings of guilt, anger, and powerlessness will come up again.

If you suspect that a friend or family member is being abused or is a survivor, Boyd recommends that you open the door by asking whether she has been touched in a way that made her uncomfortable as a child. If a friend or loved one reveals that she is a survivor, Renee Fredrickson, author of *Repressed Memories: A Journey to Recovery from Sexual Abuse,* advises the following responses:

Always make your first response sympathetic to the survivor's feelings: "That must have felt awful," or "I'm sorry that happened to you."

It is okay to ask, "What do you need from me?" when you do not know what to say.

Stick with the topic of abuse until the person gives a clear indication that she wants to stop talking. If in doubt, ask, "Do you want to stop talking now?"

Share your outrage, compassion, and concern with appropriate comments.

After the survivor has told you the story of her abuse, you may want to ask her how she is feeling now.

You may have a delayed reaction to hearing this story, so be sure to notice and meet your own emotional needs in the next week or two.

Do not request further information without first responding compassionately to the disclosure. Especially avoid asking "How old were you?" or "How much younger were you than the abuser?"

Do not say anything positive about the perpetrator.

Do not ask, "Are you sure?"

Do not change the subject. Do not take this opportunity to disclose or speculate on your own abuse issues.

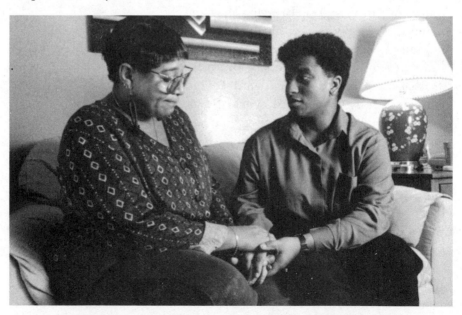

An understanding friend can provide compassion and concern. *(Photo: T. L. Litt/Impact Visuals)*

Do not get into your own feelings at the expense of the survivor. Keep the focus of attention on the survivor.

Do not hug or approach the survivor physically. If you feel it may be appropriate to hug or pat her, ask permission first. Remember that the survivor may not be able to say no even if she does not want to be touched.

When the Abuser Is a Woman

Statistically, mother-daughter incest is rare; in the vast majority of cases the abuser is a man and the victim is a little girl. More commonly, fathers abuse their daughters while the mother does nothing or even tacitly encourages the abuse, in many cases because she, too, was abused as a child. But in some instances, the abuser is a woman. The incest perpetrated by mothers is often insidious in that it is not overtly sexual. The mother often has an inability to view her daughter as separate from herself, and the abuse tends to be masturbatory in nature. It also takes place during daily activities such as bathing and dressing a child, which easily allows the abuser to mask her actions.

Vejan Smith was physically and sexually abused by her adoptive mother. "There were a lot of examinations and accusations that were coming from my mother of things that I didn't even know anything about because I was just a kid." Smith went into therapy when she was twenty-five because of severe anxiety attacks and revealed to the therapist that she was subjected to frequent and unnecessary enemas. The therapist identified this abuse as incest, but Smith "tucked it away and just went on with my life for five years."

Like most victims of incest, Smith repressed the abuse. "When you get into your thirties, you remember a lot of stuff," says Smith. "It wasn't until my early thirties that I started crying during sex and having really strange dreams.

"It's hard to hold in your mind these two opposites, that this person cared for me in her way and nurtured me in her way but then on the other hand what she did was wrong and sick."

In an attempt to integrate her anger toward her mother and the feelings of inadequacy and emotional fragmentation the abuse caused, Smith has begun to tell her story through video. Her first effort, *Mother's Hands,* depicts mother-daughter incest. The mother is shown washing dishes, cooking, cleaning, and performing seemingly domestic and nurturing work. The same hands turn to abuse a little girl. Smith used a doll for the abuse scenes.

Her second project, *Pain and Power,* is about the way incest survivors experience touch. "They can't be touched physically in a certain way," says Smith. "They can't be touched emotionally in a certain way because they were violated in such a way that it shut them down.

"You've got to find your healing. It's the only way you are going to survive. It doesn't matter how accomplished you are or how attractive you are. If you are that damaged, sometimes it doesn't save you. That's why it's really important that people get help."

For more information read *Betrayal of Innocence: Incest and Its Devastation* by Susan Forward and Craig Buck. Parts of this book and *The Courage to Heal* by Ellen Bass and Laura Davis deal directly with abuse of girls by women.

For More Information

ORGANIZATIONS

AMERICAN HUMANE ASSOCIATION, Children's Division, 63 Inverness Dr. E., Engelwood, CO, 80112-5117; (800) 227-4645 or (303) 792-9900. Provides resources for people in the public- and social-services field and does research on child welfare and protection.

AMERICAN BAR ASSOCIATION, Center on Children and the Law, 1800 M Street NW, suite 200 S., Washington, DC 20036; (202) 331-2250. Offers many publications and holds conferences on topics concerning children and the law.

INCEST HELPLINE, (212) 227-3000, gives referrals to victims and survivors of child sexual abuse.

INCEST SURVIVORS ANONYMOUS, P.O. Box 17245, Long Beach, CA 90807-7245. Write to find a local support group.

INCEST SURVIVORS RESOURCE NETWORK, Friends Meeting House, P.O. Box 7375, Las Cruces, NM 88006-7375; (505) 521-4260. Provides information packets on incest.

KEMPE CENTER FOR THE PREVENTION AND TREATMENT OF CHILD ABUSE AND NEGLECT, 1205 Oneida St., Denver, CO 80220; (303) 321-3963. Offers literature and educational materials and referrals to organizations.

NATIONAL CHILD ABUSE HOTLINE, (800) 422-4453. Provides crisis intervention, professional counseling, and referrals. Also has literature.

NATIONAL CLEARINGHOUSE ON CHILD ABUSE AND NEGLECT, P.O.

Box 1182, Washington, DC, 20013; (800) 394-3366 or (703) 385-7565. Serves as a major resource center for the acquisition and dissemination of materials on child abuse and neglect. Free publications catalog upon request.

NATIONAL COMMITTEE TO PREVENT CHILD ABUSE, 332 S. Michigan Ave., Chicago, IL 60604-4357; (312) 663-3520. Provides educational materials, referrals, and statistics.

NATIONAL RESOURCE CENTER ON CHILD ABUSE AND NEGLECT, 63 Inverness Drive East, Englewood, CO 80112; (800) 227-5242 or (303) 792-9900. Provides general information and statistics about child abuse. Sponsored by the American Humane Association.

NATIONAL VICTIMS RESOURCE CENTER, P.O. Box 6000, Dept. F, Rockville, MD 20850-6000; (800) 627-6872. Offers statistics, literature, and referrals.

PARENTS ANONYMOUS, 520 S. Lafayette Park Pl., suite 316, Los Angeles, CA 90057; (213) 388-6685. Provides support and assistance for parents in crisis; call for a local chapter.

PEOPLE AGAINST SEXUAL ABUSE, 26 Court St., suite 403, Brooklyn, NY 11242-1102; (718) 834-9467. Focuses on educational training and offers statistics, referrals, and literature.

SURVIVORS OF INCEST ANONYMOUS, P.O. Box 26870, Baltimore, MD 21212; (410) 433-2365. Call for a referral to a local support group.

VICTIM SERVICES AGENCY, 2 Lafayette St., New York, NY 10007; (212) 577-7777. Provides an array of services, including crisis counseling and advocacy, to victims of crimes.

BOOKS

Allies in Healing: When the Person You Love Was Sexually Abused As a Child: A Support Book for Partners, Laura Davis, HarperCollins, 1991.

Banished Knowledge: Facing Childhood Injuries, Alice Miller, Doubleday, 1990.

Betrayal of Innocence: Incest and Its Devastation, Susan Forward and Craig Buck, Penguin Books, 1988.

Chain Chain Change: For Black Women Dealing with Physical and Emotional Abuse, Evelyn C. White, Seal Press (Seattle), 1985.

The Courage to Heal: A Guide for Women Survivors of Child Sexual Abuse, Ellen Bass and Laura Davis, HarperPerennial, 1992.

Crossing the Boundary: Black Women Survive Incest, Melba Wilson, Virago Press (London), 1993.

Daybreak: Meditations for Women Survivors of Sexual Abuse, Maureen Brady, Hazelden/HarperCollins, 1991.

Double Duty: Help for Adult Children Who Were Sexually Abused, Claudia Black, Ballantine, 1990.

Father-Daughter Incest, Judith Lewis Herman, Harvard University Press, 1981.

For Your Own Good: Hidden Cruelty in Childrearing and the Roots of Violence, Alice Miller, Farrar, Straus, & Giroux, 1983.

Healing Words: Affirmations for Adult Children of Abusive Parents, Anthony Juliette, Ballantine, 1991.

In the Company of My Sisters: Black Women and Self-Esteem, Julia A. Boyd, E. P. Dutton, 1993.

Intimate Violence: The Causes and Consequences of Abuse in the American Family, Richard J. Gelles and Murray A. Straus, Simon & Schuster, 1988.

Lessons in Evil, Lessons from the Light: A True Story of Satanic Abuse and Spiritual Healing, Gail Carr Feldman, Crown, 1993.

Mothers of Incest Survivors: Another Side of the Story, Janis Tyler Johnson, Indiana University Press, 1992.

Outgrowing the Pain Together: A Book for Spouses & Partners of Adults Abused As Children, Elliana Gil, Dell, 1992.

Repressed Memories: A Journey to Recovery from Sexual Abuse, Renee Fredrickson, Fireside Books, 1992.

Secret Survivors: Uncovering Incest and Its Aftereffects, Sue E. Blume, John Wiley & Sons, 1990.

Soul Murder: The Effects of Childhood Abuse and Deprivation, Leonard Shengold, M.D., Yale University Press, 1989. (Scholarly.)

This Is About Incest, Margaret Randall, Firebrand Books, 1987.

Through the Fire: Personal Recovery Stories, Mary LeLoo, The Crossing Press, 1992.

Violence Against Women and the Ongoing Challenge to Racism, Angela Y. Davis, Kitchen Table Press, 1987.

31

HIV and AIDS

In 1981, when the first stories about AIDS appeared in the *New York Times*, most African-Americans took little notice. Many of us, preoccupied with the daily realities of making the rent, watching the kids, and getting food to the table, barely heard the reports of rare cancers and pneumonias that were suddenly and inexplicably attacking gay men. And, though some of us felt sympathetic, more simply didn't pay much attention, surmising that since we weren't gay men, this AIDS business had nothing to do with us. Others were hostile, thinking that the disease was divine retribution for sexual immorality and that sufferers brought AIDS on themselves.

We soon learned, however, that viruses have no prejudices. Gay, bisexual, and straight; white and Black; men, women, teenagers, and children; drug users and the clean and sober—all have been struck with the human immunodeficiency virus (HIV), the virus that causes AIDS. That fact struck home most powerfully in 1991 when basketball star Magic Johnson announced in a press conference: "Because of the HIV virus that I have obtained, I will have to retire from the Lakers." It struck again in 1992 when tennis great Arthur Ashe tearfully disclosed that he had contracted AIDS from a blood transfusion more than three years earlier. He died ten months after his announcement.

AIDS is ravaging the Black community. Among us, gay Black men have been hit the hardest, but the toll has also been great on Black women and children. The numbers of Black women infected with HIV are increasing rapidly: Black women account for 52 percent of all AIDS cases among women. AIDS is now the leading cause of death of Black women aged fifteen to forty-four in New York and New Jersey; and it is the fifth leading cause of death of Black women nationwide. Although women are often blamed for passing the virus to men, it is easier for a man to pass it to a woman during sexual activity, and once infected, women die more quickly from AIDS than do men. There are also more Black children infected with HIV than there are white or Hispanic: 55 percent of all youngsters under thirteen with HIV are African-American.

The disease is also taking Black lives internationally. In fact, African and African-diasporic people make up the bulk of those infected. The virus supposedly originated in Africa, though no one is sure how. In the motherland AIDS has always been primarily spread heterosexually, and the continent has been hit so hard that some areas are decimated. Experts estimate that some seven million people are believed to be infected with the virus in sub-Saharan Africa alone, and in countries like Zaire and Uganda numbers of orphaned children grow as the virus takes away their parents and even grandparents.

AIDS is killing far too many of us and will continue to steal away precious lives unless we all take the responsibility for learning about HIV—how to prevent it and how to care for those with HIV and AIDS. The most important thing each of us can do is protect ourselves. We must also become educated about HIV disease and make sure everyone we know understands what it is, how it is spread, and how to prevent it.

The Basics of HIV Disease

One of the reasons AIDS is so frightening is that many people still don't know what it is or how it is transmitted. We've all heard the myths: AIDS is the result of government experiments with biological warfare gone awry; you can get it from mosquitoes; all people with AIDS will die within a year.

None of these statements are true. While AIDS is a devastating, often fatal illness that is still a mystery in a number of ways, there are certain things we *do* know about it. It is time to separate fact from fiction.

What Are HIV and AIDS?

HIV stands for human immunodeficiency virus. It is the virus that causes AIDS.

AIDS stands for acquired immune deficiency syndrome. It is a collection of symptoms or diseases you can get as a result of HIV infection. When the immune system is compromised, it can't fight off diseases as it normally would. A person with an immune system weakened by HIV may develop *opportunistic infections*— illnesses an HIV-negative person generally wouldn't get.

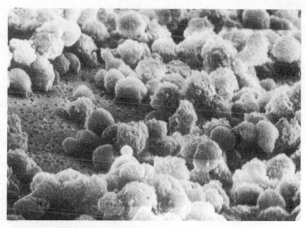

HIV on the surface of a white blood cell.
(Photo: Peter Arnold, Inc.)

Being HIV-positive is not the same thing as having AIDS. AIDS is actually the end stage of HIV disease—the most serious manifestation of HIV infection. An HIV-positive diagnosis is not a death sentence; in fact, many people live ten years or more with HIV.

How can a person be infected with HIV?

Though some would have you think that HIV is lurking around every corner, there are only a few, very specific ways a person can be infected with the virus. They are:

- Through unprotected vaginal, oral, or anal sex with an infected partner.
- By sharing injectable needles with an infected person or being stuck with an infected needle. This can happen through intravenous or IV drug use (when a user injects the drug into a vein), skin-popping (injecting drugs without hitting a vein), tattooing, ear piercing, or in the health-care setting.
- From an infected mother to her baby during pregnancy, birth, or breast-feeding.
- From a blood transfusion with blood that is infected.

The only way to be infected with HIV is by introducing infected blood, semen, or vaginal fluids into your body. You *cannot* be infected through casual contact (hugging, social kissing, shaking hands, sitting next to an infected person, etc.) HIV can survive only a few seconds outside of the body, so you can't be infected by using plates, towels, or any other object used by a person with HIV. You can't be infected by eating a meal cooked by an HIV-positive person or by being in the home of someone who's infected.

How can you tell if someone is HIV-positive?

You can't. A person can look and feel perfectly healthy and still be infected with HIV. Only an HIV-antibody test can determine whether a person is infected.

How does HIV destroy the immune system?

These are the steps:

1. The person is infected.
2. The body begins to produce antibodies to the virus.
   Antibodies are the body's natural defense against invading viruses and bacteria. The making of antibodies is called seroconversion.
3. Some people experience an "acute infection" stage during seroconversion. They suffer flulike symptoms—a sign that the body is reacting to the HIV infection by producing antibodies. Most people are not aware of this acute infection stage, however.
4. As HIV reproduces, it interferes with the proper functioning of the immune system. The exact process by which this happens is unknown, though there are several theories. One is that the virus kills the cells that orchestrate the immune response, T4 cells (also known as T cells or CD_4 cells). However, most researchers now believe that this explanation is too simple, and that HIV may destroy the immune system in several ways at once.
5. The person begins to develop symptoms.
6. As the virus causes more damage to the immune system, symptoms become more severe. The disease has progressed from asymptomatic HIV infection to symptomatic infection to AIDS.

Stages of HIV Infection

There are three general stages of HIV infection: asymptomatic infection, symptomatic infection, and AIDS. During the *asymptomatic* stage, the virus is actively reproducing in the lymphatic system (the system responsible for defending the body against infection and disease), quietly killing the T cells that are crucial in fighting disease and crippling the immune system in a number of other ways that are only partially understood. At this stage, however, the damage done to the immune system is still fairly minimal, so there are no real symptoms. Many HIV-positive people remain asymptomatic for a decade or more.

As the virus reproduces and mounts an intensified attack on the immune system, the body's defenses weaken and infections usually kept in check by normal immune function begin to appear. These signs of *symptomatic HIV infection* include:

- Vaginal yeast infections that won't go away, even with treatment
- Pelvic inflammatory disease that won't respond to treatment
- Other sexually transmitted diseases (genital herpes, genital warts, etc.) that don't respond to treatment
- Thrush (yeast infections of the mouth, throat, or esophagus)
- Swollen lymph nodes
- Fevers
- Persistent diarrhea
- Skin rashes, hives, lesions
- Fatigue
- Night sweats
- Chronic cough, shortness of breath, or tightness or pressure in the chest
- Vision problems

Any of these symptoms could be explained by a number of factors. It is important to remember that they are only signs of advancing HIV infection when symptoms are chronic, otherwise unexplained, or extreme, and they occur in a person who has been infected with HIV.

Once an HIV-infected person develops one of the twenty-seven AIDS-defining conditions (one or more of a number of bacterial, viral, and fungal infections; cancers; drastic changes in body weight or mental function; or a count of fewer than 200 T cells), that person is diagnosed as having AIDS. Though in the early years of the epidemic an AIDS diagnosis meant impending death, today, with better treatments for opportunistic infections, people often live for years after their AIDS diagnosis.

Gynecological Manifestations of HIV Disease

As with many other diseases, women with HIV have a number of symptoms that men do not. Unfortunately, it has taken too long for the medical establishment to recognize these gynecological symptoms as HIV-related. As a result, many HIV-positive women do not get the regular Pap smears or pelvic exams that could detect diseases like cervical cancer and pelvic inflammatory disease before they progress to an untreatable stage. Women should not die of these illnesses, which can be treated if caught in time, but they do. All women with HIV should know the possible gynecological manifestations of HIV disease and should get regular checkups to ensure diagnosing them early enough to treat them. They are:

Pelvic inflammatory disease. PID is the result of untreated infections of the upper genital tract (uterus, ovaries, and fallopian tubes) in women. It is most often caused by untreated chlamydia and gonorrhea, and its most frequent symptom is severe abdominal pain. (For more information on sexually transmitted infections, see chapter 12, "Reproductive-Tract Infections.") Women with HIV often have more severe cases of PID, are hospitalized for it more often, and are more likely to require frequent surgery to treat it.

Herpes simplex virus. Genital herpes, a disease distinguished by painful blisters or ulcers in the vagina or on the vulva or anus, affects HIV-positive women more than women who do not have HIV. Cases in HIV-positive women are more persistent, harder to treat, and more severe. HIV infection should be considered a possibility in all women with recurrent or persistent herpes.

Candida or yeast infection. Women with HIV commonly report severe, recurrent, and persistent vaginal yeast infections that do not respond to treatment. Again, HIV infection should be considered a possibility in all women with hard-to-treat, persistent, and/or recurrent vaginal yeast infections.

Human papillomavirus/cervical dysplasia/cervical cancer. Human papillomavirus (HPV) is believed to be the cause of most genital warts and cervical cancer (though each is caused by a different strain of the virus). Genital warts in HIV-positive women are usually more pronounced and harder to treat, which can be frustrating, but in themselves they are not life-threatening. Cervical cancer in HIV-positive women, however, can be deadly. The precursor to cervical cancer, cervical dysplasia occurs at an extremely high rate in women with HIV, and it progresses to cancer more quickly than in HIV-negative women. Cervical dysplasia can be detected by a Pap smear, and because it can lead to cancer so rapidly, it is suggested that women with HIV have Pap smears every six months.

The New CDC Definition: What It Means for Women

In January 1993, the Centers for Disease Control (CDC) expanded the AIDS definition to include invasive cervical cancer, pulmonary tuberculosis, recurrent bacterial pneumonia, and a T cell count of 200 or less. That means that a person who is infected with HIV and has any of the 27 conditions (including the four above) is considered to have "full-blown" AIDS.

While it is encouraging that cervical cancer made the list, it still doesn't acknowledge the fact that there are several other diseases, as listed above, that women get *before* they get cervical cancer that are indicators of decreasing immune function related to HIV infection. Why is this important? Without an official AIDS diagnosis, women are not eligible for Social Security benefits or a number of other services (like child care, meals, homemakers) that they may need. The new CDC definition ignores the most common manifestations of HIV disease in women, which can be debilitating and chronic enough to force a woman to quit her job. Without another change in the definition, women will continue to be forced into working longer than they should or living on less money than they are entitled to. What's more, cervical cancer is the *most severe* of the gynecological manifestations. It would make more sense to include dysplasia in the definition, since more women experience it. Though the new definition did help some women, the majority will see few benefits from it.

Women and HIV: Other Symptoms

There are several other diseases and symptoms that, though not part of the official AIDS definition, either occur more often in women with HIV disease or present particular problems.

Sexually transmitted infections (STI's) such as syphilis, chancroid, vaginitis, and gonorrhea tend to be more severe in HIV-infected women. They also make transmission of HIV easier. In other words, if you have any of these STI's, you are at greater risk of being infected with HIV. This is because these STI's may cause open sores, lesions, or vaginal irritation that make it easier for the virus to enter your bloodstream if you have sex with an infected person. These STI's are more likely to go undiagnosed in women, since the telltale signs may occur in the vagina where they can't be seen. Women are therefore at a particular risk for HIV infection if they have other STI's.

The Politics of AIDS for Black Women

The solutions to these problems are political. Black Americans are disproportionately poor and are therefore more often captives of an increasingly dysfunctional health-care system. Budgets for government-funded clinics were slashed in the eighties and in most cases have yet to be restored to their original inadequate levels. Clinics remain understaffed, waits are long, care is often hurried at best; at worst it can be incompetent and racist. We are still perceived by many in the health-care and social-service establishments as oversexed, irresponsible children who

Black People Get AIDS Too.

Call the S.F. Black Coalition on AIDS Help-Line: (415) 346-AIDS

No one should still believe the myth that Blacks don't get AIDS. (Courtesy: San Francisco Black Coalition on AIDS.)

can't be trusted to take care of ourselves. Consequently, we don't get the care and prevention education we need.

Black women and men are less likely to get routine preventive health care than whites, and when we do seek treatment for any illness, including HIV, chances are it will be when the disease has progressed to a less treatable or untreatable stage. With HIV disease, this can be fatal.

Add to this the fact that women of all races have been invisible in the epidemic. In the early eighties, almost all attention was focused on gay men. Because so many white gay men had contracted AIDS, many thought the virus had a gender and sexual-orientation preference—at one point it was even called Gay-Related Immune Deficiency, or GRID for short.

Once researchers figured out that AIDS was a sexually transmitted infection and that both men and women could be infected, women were singled out as potential "carriers" or "vectors" who could pass the virus to men or, worse yet, their innocent babies. Money was found to study HIV among prostitutes and pregnant women so that men and babies could be spared. Few people actually cared about what was happening to the women themselves. Until recently, there was precious little money available to study the virus's effects on the female reproductive system, how treatments for HIV disease differ in effectiveness in women, or whether women develop the same opportunistic infections that men develop. Women were actually excluded from a number of the clinical trials that test treatments for HIV and AIDS, and even today many of the trials sponsored by pharmaceutical companies require women to be surgically sterilized before they can participate. (Government-sponsored trials require that a woman be on "a reliable form of birth control").

I'm a forty-year-old African-American woman, and I'm HIV-positive.

I grew up in Colorado. When I was sixteen or seventeen I ran away to San Francisco and became an exotic dancer.

During this time I met my husband. He was beautiful, half Italian and half Black, and he played the saxophone. I didn't know who I was, but he knew everything. We were together fourteen years. He was my best friend.

I started to suspect that he was seeing another woman. He'd come home late at night, and I'd be there demanding to know "Where were you?" He started to get sick. Finally in 1984 we got in a big argument, and it came out that "the other woman" was a man. On the outside I was pissed. But on the inside I felt like it was my fault. "Maybe I'm too ugly. Maybe I'm too fat. Somehow I made him do it."

I was scared. He was getting sick, and we didn't know why. I didn't want to deal with the gay issue. I thought, "I gotta make him well. Then I can kick his butt." But he never got well. At first the doctors told me he had "gay cancer." Three months before my husband died, the doctor told me he had AIDS.

He went into the hospital, and the nurses wouldn't go into his room without a mask and gloves on. He'd be lying in his own feces and I'd hear them say, "I ain't going in there. He got AIDS."

I took care of my husband up until the end. I know if it had been the other way around, he would have been there to take care of me. I was with him on July 17, 1984, when he died.

I was devastated. To this day he's the best friend I ever had. I turned to drugs. When I decided to get clean, I was lucky that I had a job with great insurance. I entered a drug program in Beverly Hills—lots of movie stars getting clean. It saved my life.

On October 15, 1985, I picked up the paper and learned that Rock Hudson had died of AIDS over a week earlier. I remember thinking, "What a bummer. I really liked him." That same day my counselor called me in and said, "Your test came back positive. You have AIDS."

My first thought was to run to my group-therapy session. I cried and told them, "They just told me I got AIDS." I thought they would support me, but the stars freaked out. Suddenly everybody wanted to get out of the program.

I was locked in my room, fed on paper plates with a plastic fork, and told to pee in a chamber pot so no one would have to share a toilet with me. I had such low self-esteem that it didn't even occur to me to defend myself. One nurse said, "So how's it feel to have five months to live?" and I actually answered her politely. Lucky for me, my doctor intervened. Later on I learned to stand up for myself.

> "The same day Rock Hudson died, my counselor called me in and said, 'Your test came back positive. You have AIDS.'"
>
> —MONIA PERRY, LECTURER AND ACTIVIST, SACRAMENTO, CALIFORNIA

Through all I've suffered, I've become an incredible survivor. But I'll never forget what it feels like to hurt and be scared and feel alone. Even now loneliness is the hardest part of this disease. Since my husband died, I've never found anyone I could trust.

Now my focus is on young people. I know a lot of them are hurting. Now I can go out and talk to young people and Black people to educate them about AIDS. When I speak to young people in school, and to young guys and ex-gang members who come to play midnight basketball, I tell them that since I've been HIV-positive, I've learned to live to be the best person I can be each day. And to me, to survive is a victory.

Perhaps most tragically, many women—especially Black women—are at risk for HIV infection and don't know it. Sexism and racism conspire to keep a disproportionate number of us disempowered and impoverished, living in areas blighted by crime and drug use. Chances are greater that one of our boyfriends or husbands is shooting up and hiding it from us. Chances are greater that if we confront the men in our lives, we may be beaten for it. Chances are greater that we will be stuck—in a dangerous neighborhood, with a violent man, with drugs as the quickest

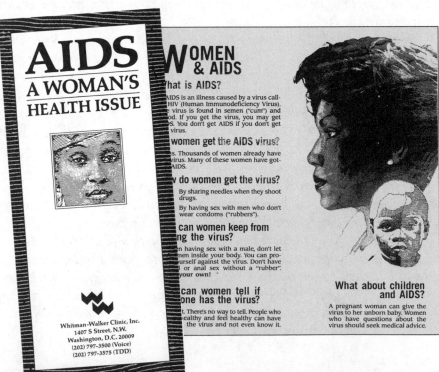

Many AIDS organizations can provide information, resources, and support. *(Courtesy: Whitman Walker Clinic.)*

and easiest escape from a life constrained by racial inequality. And more of us will be infected, only to learn of it when our husband or boyfriend or child becomes ill or dies.

Another deadly social reality —homophobia—also puts Black women at risk. Black gay and bisexual men, fearful of the blatant hostility the African-American community often displays toward them, sometimes have relationships with and marry women as a cover or to maintain their standing in the community—while they conduct clandestine gay relationships. Our community's inability to create a safe and accepting environment for Black gays only exacerbates the spread of HIV.

Things are slowly changing. Change is a process, however, and much remains to be done. HIV is now a part of all our lives, and we must act accordingly. This means educating ourselves, preventing transmission, fighting for more research, treatment, and social-service funding, and caring for those among us who are living with this disease. It also means determining our own risk, finding out our HIV status, and, if necessary, changing our behavior and the social situations that put us at risk. We do not have to be victims. We do have some control over this epidemic.

HIV Testing: What It Is, When to Do It

Today, when someone tells you he's been tested, you don't ask what for. You know. "The Test" carries with it all the fear you can imagine and all the hope you can muster. It's the HIV antibody test, and the results can change your life forever.

What is it? What does it tell you? When should you be tested? And where should you go? You should have the answers to these questions before you get tested for HIV, and you should never be pressured into being tested.

Being tested is frightening—don't let anyone tell you differently. But there are reasons to know. If you are positive, medication and holistic treatments can help the body ward off opportunistic infections and can prolong your life. Knowing your HIV status will impact your decision to get pregnant. If you are positive, you should not get pregnant because chances are you'll pass the virus to your child. Knowing the truth may also put an end to worrying and spur you to change behaviors that put you and your partners at risk.

If you think you've been infected, don't bury your head in the sand. Get yourself tested.

What Is "The Test"?

Commonly (and misleadingly) known as "the AIDS test," the HIV-antibody test determines your HIV status by identifying HIV antibodies in your blood. A positive test result does not necessarily mean you have AIDS.

When and why should you be tested?

Ask yourself the following questions:

What do I think I would do if I were positive? Would I want to harm myself? Or would I seek help and try to live each day as it comes?

Would knowing my HIV status help me practice safer sex?

Would finally knowing one way or the other relieve the stress of wondering about my status?

Am I pregnant or thinking of getting pregnant?

If you don't think a positive result would make you suicidal, and if knowing would put an end to worrying and spur you to change behaviors that put you and others at risk, you should be tested. If you are pregnant or thinking of getting pregnant, a positive test result might impact your decision to have the baby and would certainly mean that you should have prenatal care as early as possible.

Are you at risk?

You are at high risk of HIV if any of these statements apply to you:

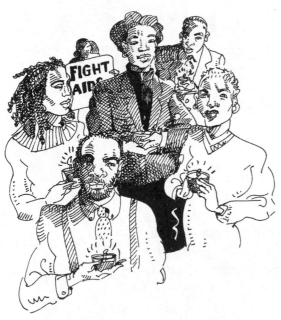

All of us must be AIDS activists.
(Drawing: Yvonne Buchanan)

- I have sexual intercourse without using a condom and spermicide.
- I have oral sex without using a condom, dental dam, or plastic wrap.
- I have unprotected sexual contact with someone whose sexual history is unknown to me.
- I have unprotected sexual contact with someone who has had sex with another partner or many other partners.
- I have unprotected sex with a man who has had unprotected sex with another man or woman.
- I have unprotected sex with someone whose drug history is unknown to me.
- I share needles for drug use.
- I had a blood transfusion between 1977 and 1985 or had sex with someone who had a transfusion during this time.

In October of 1991, I found out that I was HIV-positive. I had contracted an STD from a former boyfriend and was in the health clinic being treated. I was sitting there feeling really stressed out, and I saw a sign on the wall that talked about AIDS. I just decided, "I may as well get tested for that, too."

Two weeks later a counselor called me. He sat me down and told me my test was positive. I didn't really understand what that meant. He tried to explain things, to tell me where to get help, but I wasn't hearing him. I think I was in shock. I said thank you and abruptly left the office. I went straight home, and then it began to sink in. I'm not a crier, but I cried.

I'm not sure where I got it. It could've been the guy that gave me the STD's. He was very promiscuous, sleeping with other women even while we lived together. I called him and told him about me and encouraged him to get tested. Eventually he called me and told me that he was positive, too. Another of my former boyfriends was a bisexual. He told me about his bisexuality while we were seeing each other, but I didn't mind. It didn't interfere with our relationship. Even after we broke up, we remained friends. I was there for him until he died of AIDS last July. Another guy that I'd had an intermittent relationship with also told me that he was positive. It would seem logical that the bisexual man gave me HIV, but it really could've been any of these three guys.

The hardest thing I've ever had to do was tell my mother that I have HIV. We are close, like sisters. I'm from a small family, and I'm an only child. So it's like my mother and I breathe the same air. I took the coward's way out and called her on the phone. I said, "I have something to tell you that's important. I'm HIV-positive." She was just quiet. I really can't even remember what we said after that. After the initial shock, my family has been very supportive.

I'm also "out" about being positive at work. It's no problem at my job since I work at an agency that does AIDS work, and others there are positive. But I'm only out with my family and in the AIDS world. Part of me really wants to go public, to take a leadership role and speak out about women and AIDS. But I'm not ready yet.

Last year I got involved in a support group for Black women with AIDS so I could try to deal with some of my issues. The first time I went was difficult, because I didn't know anyone. But now it's great. We meet at a community organization and talk about everything—fear of becoming very ill, husbands, boyfriends, children. Sometimes we cry, other times we just hang out. We also share treatment information and talk about our symptoms.

I haven't had anything serious. I have some skin rashes, and at first I had

> "The hardest thing I've ever had to do was tell my mother that I have HIV."
>
> —NAME WITHHELD, ADMINISTRATIVE ASSISTANT IN AN AIDS ORGANIZATION, HARTFORD, CONNECTICUT

yeast infections over and over. But now I take acidophilus twice a day and the yeast problem's over. I've taken a holistic approach to caring for myself. About the time I was diagnosed, I had started to make some changes in my diet. I read books and researched nutrition and holistic care. Now I don't eat beef, and I eat much less meat. I eat more brown rice, grains, fresh fruit, and vegetables and drink lots of water. I also take garlic twice a day, blue-green algae, and vitamins.

I have changed since I found out about this. I would never have called myself a patient person, but I've learned how to be patient. I've learned to accept people for who they are—idiosyncracies and all. It doesn't matter anymore. I can't remember the last time I was angry with someone. I may fuss here and there, but I haven't been screaming angry in a long time. I've also learned to understand what faith can do. I understand the power of nurturing the spirit.

If you answered yes to any of these statements, you should seriously consider being tested.

What happens when you are tested?

First, you should be counseled about what HIV is, your risk, and what your plan of action would be if you learned you were positive. *Everyone should get counseling both before and after the test. It is your right.* You should also give your fully informed consent before you are tested. *No one should be tested without giving fully informed consent. It is unethical and illegal to do so.*

After you are counseled, a blood sample will be taken. The blood will be tested for antibodies to HIV using the ELISA test first. If this test is negative, you do not have HIV at this time. You should be tested again in six months to be sure. If you change partners, you should be retested.

If the ELISA test is positive, a Western Blot test, which is more specific, will be done. If both the ELISA and the Western Blot are positive, you do have HIV.

Where can you be tested?

You can be tested at a public health clinic, at a doctor's office, or in a hospital, but there are some important considerations when deciding where to be tested. First, most public health clinics offer both confidential and anonymous testing; doctor's offices and hospitals tend to offer confidential testing. The difference is crucial: With anonymous testing, you are identified only by a number—no one has your name, and your results can't be connected to you by name, nor will they be in your medical records. You may have to wait longer for your results, however.

A confidential test will have your name on it, and the results will be in your records. Be sure to weigh which is the best choice for you.

When should the test be taken?

An HIV-antibody test should be taken a minimum of two to six months after your last possible exposure to the virus. The vast majority of people will produce antibodies within two months of exposure.

Treatments for HIV Disease and AIDS

There are many reasons to get tested, but one of the best ones is the possibility of early treatment. There are several treatment options for people with HIV, and the earlier they are begun, the better. All medical treatments must be prescribed by a doctor.

Antivirals: The First Line of Defense

Antivirals are drugs that affect the virus itself. They work by interfering with the virus's reproduction in some way. Most research has shown that they slow down the progression of HIV disease, though recently their effectiveness has been debated.

AZT (zidovudine or Retrovir) is the most commonly used antiviral. Most people with HIV begin taking AZT as their first antiviral. It is also the most controversial. It was once thought that taking AZT early on, before becoming symptomatic, was highly beneficial. However, the thinking has changed. HIV mutates very quickly in response to antivirals, and starting AZT early may mean that it will be less effective later on in the progression of the disease. AZT is also highly toxic: It can cause very serious side effects ranging from anemia, nausea, and headaches to bone marrow and liver damage. About half of those who try AZT will not be able to tolerate it. AZT therapy is usually begun when a person's T-cell level drops to 500.

DDI (didanosine or Videx) is an antiviral used to treat people who cannot tolerate AZT. It may also be used in combination with AZT. The full scope of long-term effects of DDI are unknown, though it can cause pancreas and nerve damage.

DDC (zalcitabine) is closely related to DDI and has similar side effects. It is usually used in combination with AZT or alone in patients who can't tolerate AZT.

D4T is a recently approved antiviral that is used for people who have tried all the other antivirals and have either stopped having success with them or become intolerant to them.

Acyclovir (Zovirax) has been used to treat herpes for some time, and researchers are now looking at it as a booster for AZT.

Preventing Infections

The other major class of drugs used to treat HIV disease are the antibiotics and antifungals used as preventive measures or treatment for opportunistic infections that attack the body because HIV has lowered immunity. There are many of these; the following is a list of the most common ones and the infections they are used to prevent or treat.

Aerosolized pentamidine is used to prevent Pneumocystis carinii pneumonia (PCP), which is caused by a protozoan. PCP was a major cause of death early in the epidemic, but it can be controlled by taking aerosolized pentamidine or Bactrim as a preventive method.

Bactrim, a sulfa drug, is also used a prophylaxis and treatment for PCP.

Clotrimazole (Mycelex), fluconazole (Diflucan) and *ketoconazole (Nizoral)* are antifungal medications used to treat yeast. Mycelex is a topical cream used locally for vaginal yeast infections; Diflucan and Nizoral are taken orally for thrush and esophagal yeast infections or when vaginal yeast does not respond to local treatment.

Acyclovir (Zovirax), mentioned earlier, is used to prevent and treat herpes outbreaks. It is also a treatment for cytomegalovirus (CMV) infection, which damages the eyes.

Megace is a treatment for wasting syndrome, in which people with AIDS lose a significant percentage of their body weight very quickly and without trying.

There are also a number of antibiotics used to treat bacterial infections in people with HIV; among them are *clarithromycin* and *azithromycin*.

Paying for HIV Treatments

Most pharmacies in major cities carry these drugs, though they are often extremely expensive. If you have insurance, check your plan's prescription-drug policy. You may have to pay up front and get reimbursed by the company (in which case you might want to charge the drugs if you have credit cards and pay the charged amount when you get reimbursed). Your plan may require only a small copayment, or it may pay the entire amount.

If you are on Medicaid, any nonexperimental drugs are covered in full when you fill your prescriptions at a pharmacy that accepts Medicaid reimbursement. If you don't have insurance coverage for prescription drugs but your income is too high to qualify for Medicaid, you can apply for help under the Federal AIDS Drug Reimbursement program. This program covers only a few drugs, however. Applications can be obtained through your state department of public health, or through AIDS service agencies. Your doctor may also be able to enroll you in a program to get medication for no charge.

Nonmedical Alternatives

Many people with HIV make use of a number of supplemental therapies to treat their symptoms, including acupuncture, Chinese herbal medicine, massage therapy, homeopathy, relaxation techniques, yoga, t'ai chi, visualization, and chiropractic. While there are varying reports of success with each of these methods, it is important to remember that they should be considered *supplemental* and *complementary*; they should not replace drug therapy. Talk to other HIV-positive women and women with AIDS about what works for them. And then research any treatment method thoroughly and decide whether it's right for you.

There are some conditions for which supplemental therapies seem to work best, however. Acupuncture can bring great relief from the pain of peripheral neuropathy, a condition in which people with HIV experience tingling, numbness, and pain in the extremities. And anything that reduces stress or helps your peace of mind is a good idea, as long as it doesn't interfere with other treatments or cause complications. Eating healthy food, exercising in moderation, and getting plenty of rest can also have a positive effect on the immune system.

Preventing HIV Infection

There is at least one good thing about HIV: It is preventable. We know what puts people at risk and how to avoid that risk. If everyone practiced safer sex and got into recovery and off drugs altogether, the numbers of new HIV infections would drop. To learn how to have sex safely, see chapter 27, "Sexuality and Having Sex Safely."

For More Information

ORGANIZATIONS

AIDS COALITION TO UNLEASH POWER (ACT UP), Women's Action Committee, 135 W. 29th St., 10th floor, New York, NY 10001; (212) 564-2437. An activist group.

THE BLACK LEADERSHIP COMMISSION ON AIDS, 105 E. 22nd St., suite 711, New York, NY 10010; (800) 573-2522 or (in New York) (212) 614-0023. Promotes organized leadership and education on AIDS-related issues within African-American communities.

NATIONAL ASSOCIATION OF PEOPLE WITH AIDS (NAPWA), 1413 K St., Washington, DC 20005; (202) 898-0414. Provides information about treatment and health care as well as referrals for people with AIDS.

NATIONAL MINORITY AIDS COUNCIL, 300 Eye St. NE, suite 400, Washington, DC 20002-4389; (202) 544-1076. Provides referrals and assistance to minorities.

NATIONAL RESOURCE CENTER ON WOMEN AND AIDS, Center for Women Policy Studies, 2000 P St. NW, suite 508, Washington, DC 20036; (202) 872-1770. Publishes *The Guide to Resources on Women and AIDS.*

WOMEN RESOURCING WOMEN, 12734 S. Morgan St., Chicago, IL 60643-6612; (312) 928-8031. Leads workshops around the country to provide information, support, and resources for poor women and women of color living with HIV.

SOME SELECTED LOCAL GROUPS THAT SERVE WOMEN AND PEOPLE OF COLOR

In New York

BROOKLYN AIDS TASK FORCE, 22 Chapel St., Brooklyn, NY 11201; (718) 499-0352. The Brooklyn AIDS Task Force provides prevention and risk-reduction information and counseling as well as support services and referrals.

IRIS HOUSE, 2271 Second Ave., New York, NY 10035; (212) 423-9049. A center for women living with HIV.

MINORITY TASK FORCE ON AIDS, 505 Eighth Ave., 16th floor, New York, NY 10018; (212) 563-8340. Works to increase and give out HIV/AIDS-prevention information, counsel people living with AIDS, and advocate for people of color living with AIDS.

WOMEN AND AIDS RESOURCE NETWORK (WARN), 30 Third Ave., suite 513, Brooklyn, NY 11217; (718) 596-6007. Referrals and counseling for women and their families.

In Washington, D.C.

WHITMAN-WALKER CLINIC, 1407 S St., NW, Washington, DC 20009; (202) 797-3500. This facility offers information, resources, and medical services, including HIV testing in several locations. For information on testing call (202) 332-EXAM.

MAX ROBINSON CENTER, 3845 S. Capitol St. SE, Washington, DC 20032; (202) 562-1160. This program is part of the Whitman-Walker system and provides HIV/AIDS services and resources geared toward African-Americans.

In Atlanta

SISTERLOVE, 1432 Donnelly Ave. SW, Atlanta, GA 30310; (404) 753-7733. Provides education, prevention, and support services for women at risk for and living with HIV/AIDS.

In Chicago

CHICAGO WOMEN'S AIDS PROJECT, 5249 N. Kenmore, Chicago, IL 60640; (312) 271-2070. Provides support services, a therapy clinic, and education for women with HIV.

KUPONA NETWORK, 4611 S. Ellis, Chicago, IL 60653; (312) 536-3000. The Kupona Network's Imani Women's Program serves Black women through support groups, prevention education, and case management.

In Texas

OVER THE HILL INC., 2001 S. Freeway, Fort Worth, TX 76104; (817) 922-9955. A staff of predominately Black women provides education, testing, and counseling.

In the Bay Area

RAFIKI SERVICES PROJECT OF THE BLACK COALITION ON AIDS, 1042 Divisadero St., San Francisco, CA 94115; (415) 346-5860. Provides training for volunteers to give emotional and practical support and housing for people with HIV/AIDS. Also offers prevention information.

In Los Angeles

AIDS PREVENTION TEAM, a Project of the Black Gay and Lesbian Forum, 1219 S. La Brea Ave., Los Angeles, CA 90019; (213) 964-7820. Provides HIV/AIDS education and client services, prevention, early intervention, and treatment options geared specifically to African-Americans.

RUE'S HOUSE, 1166 W. 39th Pl., Los Angeles, CA 90037; (213) 295-4030. Shelter for women and children with AIDS.

Hotlines

CDC NATIONAL HIV/AIDS HOTLINE, (800) 342-2437; (800) 243-7889 (hearing-impaired TTY/TDD). Toll-free hotline providing confidential information, referrals, and educational materials to all.

CDC NATIONAL AIDS CLEARINGHOUSE, (800)-458-5231, (800) 243-7012 (hearing-impaired TTY/TDD). Questions answered; provides free publications mailed confidentially; and resources on clinical trials, AIDS-in-the-workplace policies, and prevention.

PEOPLE WITH AIDS COALITION, (800) 828-3280. Questions answered exclusively by people living with HIV/AIDS; advice regarding treatment, support groups, benefits, and financial assistance.

PROJECT INFORM, (800) 822-7422. Latest treatment information for people with HIV/AIDS.

BOOKS

AIDS: The Women, Ines Rieder and Patricia Ruppelt, eds., Cleis Press, 1988.

The Invisible Epidemic: The Story of Women and AIDS, Gena Corea, HarperCollins, 1992.

No Time to Wait: A Complete Guide to Treating, Managing and Living with HIV Infection, Nick Siano, Bantam Books, 1993.

When Someone You Love Has AIDS: A Book of Hope for Family and Friends, BettyClare Moffat, NAL Penguin, 1986.

Women, AIDS, and Activism, ACT UP/NY Women & AIDS Book Group, South End Press (Boston), 1990.

Women and AIDS, Diane Richardson, Methuen, 1988.

32

Our Work, Our World

Many American Blacks have never seen the earth in its natural, whole state, because too many of us live in overcrowded, noisy, dirty urban areas or in rural locales that have been marred by polluting industries. A 1987 study gave this phenomenon a name—environmental racism—pointing out that two-thirds of African-Americans and Latinos live in areas with one or more uncontrolled toxic-waste sites. In 1992 a report by the Environmental Protection Agency confirmed that people of color suffer disproportionate exposure to dust, soot, carbon monoxide, ozone, sulfur, sulfur dioxide, and lead, as well as emissions from hazardous-waste dumps.

Existing in these conditions takes its toll on us in many ways. Living on top of one another, we become angry, and spending day after day in unkempt, polluted areas, we lose respect for the earth. But the greatest toll may be on our health: Blacks suffer disproportionately from environmental illnesses—from unexplained skin rashes to asthma to cancers.

The state of the smaller, more immediate environment where we spend the majority of our waking hours—the workplace—also affects the quality of our lives. For many of us, work can be profoundly rewarding and satisfying—even if we don't make a lot of money. But far too many of our people work in dangerous, unhealthy environments, enduring long hours, low pay, unfulfilling jobs, and unsanitary conditions.

In her 1968 autobiography *Coming of Age in Mississippi,* Anne Moody described the horrifying experience of working in a Southern chicken factory:

> The chickens had been moving very slow in the beginning. Now the rate of speed was doubled. I stood there with sweat running down my face and legs. It was so hot, I felt as though I would faint. The chickens were now moving as fast as I could blink my eyes. I was on the end of the trough which pulled the insides out. There were five of us at this spot. I stood there reaching up and snatching out those boiling hot guts with my bare hands as fast as I could. But I just wasn't fast enough. The faster the chickens moved, the sicker I got. My face, arms, and clothes were splattered with blood and chicken shit . . .

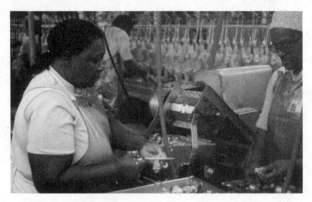

A woman working bare-handed at a poultry-processing plant is exposed to infections and is at risk for crippling injuries. *(Photo: Courtesy R.W.D.S.U., New York)*

On September 3, 1991, a parallel to Moody's chilling experience made headlines. A fire at Imperial Food Products, a chicken-processing factory in the town of Hamlet, North Carolina, killed twenty-five people and injured some fifty others—mostly African-American women. Deaths occurred because, of the factory's nine exit doors, six that could have been used as escape routes during the fire were securely locked: The employer was trying to make sure employees did not slip out these doors with chicken parts to take home.

Neither our macroenvironment—the air, land, and water—nor our microenvironment—the workplace—should be a living hell. To make the worlds we live and work in clean, safe, and comfortable requires that we become well informed and pull together to take collective action.

Environmental Racism

Industries that produce and use dangerous chemicals have problems locating their plants in this country. It's not surprising that the NIMBY—Not In My Backyard—sentiment exists. Better-off and better-organized communities come together to keep polluting industry out.

But many Black communities, especially those that are economically depressed, have trouble keeping industry out of their backyards. When

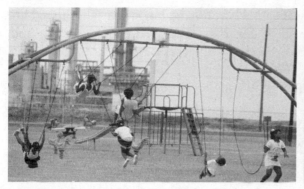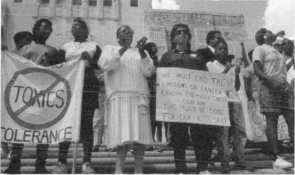

Left, children playing next to a polluting industrial plant. Right, a group protesting environmental racism.
(Photos: Sam Kittner; courtesy Greenpeace Media)

folks are poor, undereducated, sick, tired, and politically unsophisticated, they are often no match for a wealthy company that needs a home for its manufacturing facility. And in many cases the plant is not only unopposed but is invited in by under- and unemployed townspeople desperate for work.

This select locating of dangerous industries in Black and generally poor communities is called environmental racism, and it means that we are disproportionately exposed to toxins from hazardous-waste landfills, garbage dumps, incinerators, smelter operations, paper mills, chemical plants, highways, crumbling paint in dilapidated housing, chemical spills, and unsanitary water.

This has led to ill health in a number of understudied and poorly understood ways. Experts know that toxins in the environment can lead to health problems, but it has long been difficult to specifically prove that living in X polluted area causes Y negative health effect—such as watery eyes, skin rash, bronchitis, asthma, tumors, miscarriage, birth defects, and cancer. For one thing, it's hard to estimate the concentration of toxins once they've been released into the air and water and onto the land, much less link them directly to a particular illness. For another, pollution is relatively unregulated, and manufacturers are often left to police it—a fox-guarding-the-chicken-coop scenario.

Nonetheless, we know that environmental contaminants infect our bodies in one of three ways: They can penetrate through the skin, can be consumed in products we drink and eat, or they can be inhaled into and infect our lungs. In our neighborhoods we are threatened with exposure to a number of toxic substances, but lead is one of the most common and most dangerous. (See below.)

Until recently, the mainstream environmental organizations offered little in the way of help for problems that concerned people of color and employed few of us on their staffs. While they seemed to be off saving whales and seals, Blacks, Native Americans, Latinos, and Asian/Pacific Islanders were living in unhealthy conditions and complaining of mysterious health problems. In fact, a few years ago, civil rights organizations and environmental groups created by people of color accused large "green organizations" such as the National Wildlife Federation, the Sierra Club, the National Audubon Society, and the National Resources Defense Council of "being isolated from the poor and minority communities that were the chief victims of pollution." The organizations themselves agreed that they had a poor record of hiring and promoting employees of color.

So, as always, African-Americans looked out for themselves:

In 1982 the residents of predominately Black Warren County, North Carolina, organized a campaign of civil disobedience to protest the siting of a toxic landfill in their community.

The United Church of Christ's Commission for Racial Justice organized the National People of Color Environmental Leadership summit in 1991 for more than six hundred people of color and offers information and support for communities fighting environmental racism.

Harlem residents formed West Harlem Environmental Action in response to the sewage plant, bus depots, and highways that are marring their community.

Welfare mothers in Milwaukee came together as the Welfare Warriors to fight lead poisoning.

Concerned Citizens of South Central Los Angeles organized public meetings and distributed flyers to successfully prevent a solid-waste incinerator from locating in its community.

No community should sit by and allow companies (including the government) to pollute its environment. For help getting your community organized, contact the United Church of Christ Commission for Racial Justice, 475 Riverside Dr., suite 1950, New York, NY 10015; (212) 870-2077.

Air Pollution

Air pollution is highest in industrialized nations. In the United States some 110 million people live where the levels of air pollution are considered harmful by the federal government. Air pollution has damaged the ozone, a protective layer that covers the atmosphere, causing much worry among scientists.

An estimated 8 percent of Americans suffer from lung diseases that are aggravated or caused by our polluted air. African-Americans suffer from lung diseases such as lung cancer and asthma in disproportionate numbers. In fact, when University of Southern California researchers studied the bodies of Los Angeles youth of color (who had died of violence and other nonmedical causes), they found that 80 percent had abnormal lung tissue. In Los Angeles and other large cities where Blacks reside, toxic emissions from automobiles and industry pollute the air, and the poor and people of color are most likely to be affected and infected. We are especially vulnerable to damaging our delicate lungs because many of us smoke too much, eat poorly, and lack exercise – which predisposes us to all kinds of health problems, including lung disease.

For more information on preventing and treating asthma and lung cancer, see chapter 7, "We Are at Risk."

Cancer Alley and Other Toxic Areas

An eighty-five-mile stretch of Louisiana, along the Mississippi River between Baton Rouge and New Orleans, has the dubious distinction of being known as Cancer Alley. Communities of poor Blacks live among the hundreds of oil refineries, chemical plants, paper mills, and other industries that spill waste into the water, dump it into the ground, or release it into the air. These brothers and sisters must endure minor irritations such as watery eyes, itchy skin, and runny noses; major health problems such as cancer (which, along with mortality, is higher than the national average); not to mention the noise, ugliness, and odor that are a direct or indirect result of the surrounding industrial processes. In many cases, our people were there first and industry came later, invading communities where residents were too beaten down to keep them out.

The South should be our birthright, a gift from our ancestors who toiled there as slaves. But along with Cancer Alley in Louisiana, other parts of the region are also polluted. For example, the largest hazardous-waste landfill in the United States is located in Sumter County, Alabama, in the heart of the nation's "Black belt." This site holds almost 25 percent of the nation's commercial hazardous waste, and waste is trucked in from nearly every state and shipped in from several foreign countries. The people of Emelle, the town where Chemical Waste Management is situated, are 80 percent Black, and many can't even get jobs at the facility that profits from the poison and pollution.

Nonetheless, in Louisiana, North and South Carolina, Texas, Alabama,

Mississippi, and other states, communities are fighting back. For more information and assistance contact the Gulf Coast Tenants Association, P.O. Box 56101, New Orleans, LA 70156; (504) 949-4919; or the National Toxics Campaign, 1168 Commonwealth Ave., Boston, MA 02134; (617) 232-0327.

Fighting Back

If you live in an area where traffic is heavy or where polluting industries have located, don't be afraid to ask for help: Groups of people of color all over the country will work with you to clean up your environment. If there's no such group in your area, start your own. Sometimes Black folks are concerned about an issue but think there is little they can do to stop it. But show your friends and neighbors that they can make a difference if you all stick together and fight back. You may feel a sense of urgency about the subject, but be patient with the groups of people you are trying to educate; make sure they are given the chance to understand what's going on.

Pat Bryant of the New Orleans Gulf Coast Tenants Association, which has fought against environmental racism in many communities, offers these suggestions:

Be cautious when shopping for a new home. Find out what kind of industries are presently or were formerly operating in that area and what kind of residues they might have left behind. (Most area universities have laboratories that will test soil samples for toxins, or contact the EPA.)

Often we have little choice about the neighborhoods we want to move into. If you find yourself in a neighborhood threatened with pollutants, organize your community to fight back. Look into public policy regarding pollutants in your area. For example, are there federal regulations, congressional laws, or state ordinances regarding pollution and the local industry? Get sufficient documentation of what the government is supposed to be doing to prevent pollution and educate your community about this.

Try to determine whether the community's health is being affected by pollution. It's best to call a community meeting and get folks to speak out about any health problems. Then encourage friends and neighbors to get health screening to determine if there are any chemical poisons in their bodies. Though it's difficult to prove that the pollution is causing any kinds of illness, you must go through this process.

With information in hand, your group can begin to agitate and for-

I live on the southeast side of Chicago, in a community I call a toxic donut. West of us is a steel mill, south of us is a landfill, northeast of us we have incinerators and some more steel mills, and northwest of us we have Metropolitan Sanitary District, a sewage-treatment plant that smells like decomposed bodies. We also have Sherwin-Williams paint company, P&M chemical company, and many others around us. We sit in the center and we're surrounded with all of this.

Anyway, I heard through the media that our area had one of the highest rates of cancer. I knew we had a lot of people that had had cancer within our community. My husband had died of cancer. I have a respiratory problem. A lot of my neighbors had died of cancer or were in remission from cancer, and I wanted to know what was going on. So I started doing some research. I called the city health department and got in touch with a Black man there. I ended up making numerous calls to New York, and finally one organization told me to call the Environmental Action Foundation in Washington, D.C. A young toxicologist there gave me a lot of information.

I know a little bit about organizing, but not writing proposals and getting money; I wasn't aware of that. So, one guy who knew I was using the little money that I had, running here and running there, asked me would I like for him to write a proposal so I can get some money. I told him "yeah." He gave us the name of organizations and foundations to contact and how much money to ask for. That's how we got funded and started to get organized within our office.

Then we started protesting and complaining. The first thing was I went before the state legislature. There was a community adjacent to us to the south. They had never had city water, they only had well water that was highly contaminated with extremely high levels of cyanide. They had benzene, zinc, and all the rest of the junk up in it. They were never able to drink their water, and they had been living there for over twenty-five years. I went before the state legislature to complain about it, and one of the state representatives said it was time to do something for those people. That community got a sewage system and the clean running water after being over there over twenty-five years!

The next thing we did was protest out here at Chicago Housing Authority for them to remove the asbestos from our apartments. We had that done. Then we went to the local schools and ended up getting the asbestos removed from there.

At the same time, we got people in our community—sixteen blocks each with 132 apartments and one block with more—to fill out health surveys

> "I'd be a fool if I knew I was being poisoned and I sat up and accepted it. That's crazy."
>
> —HAZEL JOHNSON, FOUNDER AND CEO, PEOPLE FOR COMMUNITY RECOVERY, CHICAGO

that we had gotten from the Environmental Action Foundation. Plus, we had forms from the Illinois EPA that asked about the air. That helped us prove to the city and the state that there was a need for a health clinic, because a lot of people were on fixed incomes and couldn't pay the high costs for medical service. And we got the health clinic.

We also held demonstrations. One lasted for over twelve hours in front of landfills owned by Chemical Waste Management; we turned fifty-seven trucks around that day. Everybody was out there—over five hundred people and the media. We had Greenpeace and all the adjacent communities around our area participating. We had decided if it takes for us to go to jail, we would just go to jail. We were praying together. After all the media left, Chemical Waste Management decided to have us arrested for trespassing. Seventeen of us went to jail.

Two weeks before we went to court Chemical Waste Management's incinerator had an explosion. So when court time came they didn't appear in court, and the judge just threw it out. That incinerator has been closed ever since.

I'd be a fool if I knew I was being poisoned and I sat up and accepted it. That's crazy. But I'm also not going to move out of my community. I like it here. I'd rather stay and have this place cleaned up, not only just for me but for everybody.

I remember one of the media asked me, how can a minority group like you buck up against a multimillion-dollar corporation. I told him you never know what you can do until you try it.

---

mulate demands to put to local politicians about cleaning up your environment. If the politicians do not respond, make sure part of your new group's effort includes registering voters—this should get the attention of local politicians.

Don't forget about the power of the press. Contact your local newspaper and TV and radio stations about the pollution in your community.

What You Can Do to Keep the Earth Clean

We all have to do our part to clean up our planet and keep it healthy and pollution-free. Greenpeace, The Take It Back Foundation, and Norris McDonald, president of the Center for Environment, Energy and Commerce recommend:

Try to reduce your impact on the earth. Don't get locked into the American consumerism grind; learn to live more simply. If you don't really *need* a second car or TV or many other products, don't buy them. Don't order every publication you hear of; instead see if you and a neighbor or two can share a magazine or newspaper subscription. Have your name removed from mailing lists by using a postcard or a company's own postage-paid reply forms. Write and photocopy on both sides of the paper and save junk-mail envelopes to reuse.

Recycle your garbage by separating glass, paper, and metals and setting them out for curbside sanitation pickups. If your community or workplace does not have a recycling program, contact your local government officials or speak with your employer and ask that recycling be put in place. Make the effort to buy only recycled products and materials (like glass, aluminum, steel, paper, and cardboard) that can be recycled. Take used motor oil and car batteries to gas stations or recycling centers rather than throwing them out.

Purchase a sturdy reusable shopping bag so that you won't have to bring home extra plastic or paper bags or boxes from stores. Don't buy aerosols; their containers create more waste and they harm the environment. Buy foods in bulk, and avoid disposable plates and utensils. Use ceramic plates, cloth napkins, sponges, and silverware instead. If you drink coffee or tea often, carry a cup with you so that you won't have to use paper or Styrofoam cups.

Organize a car pool in your neighborhood and/or among fellow workers to cut down on pollution, or if possible, try to use public transportation, or walk or ride a bicycle.

Maintain the appliances used in your home. Don't ignore leaks; fix them. Seventy-five percent of leaks are in apartment buildings, particularly in toilets. Gallons of water are wasted this way because it ends up going to wastewater treatment plants that have to use electricity to treat the water. Insulate your attic to reduce your utility bill. Put door sweeps and weather strips on doors to keep in heat. Clean the filter on your refrigerator and furnace, and keep your car's tires in good condition and properly inflated.

Instead of throwing out old clothes, office furniture, or equipment, donate them to a local organization or church that collects them for the needy and homeless. Conserve water, especially hot water, turn off lights, hang clothes out to dry instead of using the dryer, and use heat and air conditioning conservatively. Avoid pesticides and toxic house-cleaning aids, and don't use disposable diapers.

Radon and You

Radon is a gas that you can't see and maybe you've never heard of. But though little known and invisible, it's deadly: Exposure to radon decay is the second leading cause of lung cancer. Radon occurs naturally when radium, an element found in soil, releases it as a radioactive gas. It seeps into homes from the soil through water, walls, basement floors, pipes, insulation, and drains and is found in millions of homes throughout the country.

Radon poses special risks to African-Americans because we suffer in disproportionate numbers from lung diseases. We smoke more than white people, and cigarette smoking combined with exposure to radon is a deadly combination.

Since you can't see, smell, or taste radon, you have to test for it to find out whether your home is affected. You can purchase a do-it-yourself radon test kit at hardware and retail stores. Make sure they are marked as meeting EPA requirements and that you follow the directions to test for radon levels in your home. There are also EPA-qualified trained contractors who can do these tests for you.

If you have a high level of radon in your home, the methods of reducing your exposure are not expensive. Sometimes it is as easy as fixing holes and cracks in the building structure; other times it may take more work, but it shouldn't cost more than other home repairs.

For more information, call (800) SOS-RADON. Ask for the booklets "A Citizen's Guide to Radon: The Guide to Protecting Yourself and Your Family from Radon" and "Consumer's Guide to Radon Reduction."

Get the Lead Out

Lead can be found just about everywhere. It gets in the air through industrial emissions, tobacco smoke, paint dust, and the burning of solid wastes. (Car exhaust also contains lead, although that became much less of a problem when the United States phased out leaded gasoline.) Industry and paint chips contaminate the soil with lead, and when crops are grown in soil containing lead, poison can enter the food supply. Lead can also contaminate food through lead-glazed pottery, lead crystal, and food sold in cans soldered together with lead. (Lead-soldered cans are banned in the United States, but imported foods are sometimes sold in lead cans.) When the soil contains lead, that lead can contaminate ground water. And though the use of lead in plumbing is banned, it still contaminates the drinking water in old homes.

Black people are at particular risk of lead poisoning. We are more likely than whites to live near highways or industry where emission of lead fumes is a problem. Many of us live in homes containing lead paint or send our children to schools or day-care centers that contain it. Even if the paint has been removed, the soil around the building is probably contaminated with lead. That soil and the dust that arises from it can be highly toxic. The water pipes in these old urban buildings may also be lined with lead.

Lead poisoning is most dangerous to children; they absorb far more lead than adults exposed to the same levels. Because children play in the dirt and often put their fingers and hands in their mouths, it's easy for children to ingest lead—especially if they are exposed to flaking chips of lead paint. Studies show that childhood exposure to lead can cause mental retardation, reduced IQ, reading and learning disabilities, impaired growth, hearing loss, reduced attention span, and behavioral problems.

Your child can be tested for lead contamination with a simple blood test. Speak to your doctor or contact your local department of public health. In the meantime, try to reduce your family's exposure to lead, especially children and pregnant women:

If you live in a house built before 1950, leave the paint alone if it is in good condition or has been painted over with lead-free paint.

If you have to remove the paint, demand that your landlord either do it or hire a contractor certified to do lead-abatement work. Or do the work yourself (your local department of health can provide guidelines). Pregnant women and small children should leave the house while this work is being done, and all dust should be cleaned up afterward with an industrial vacuum.

Have your drinking water tested for lead. For more information contact your local Environmental Protection Agency.

If you drink tap water, let it run for a minute or two first each morning. If your water is a problem, bottled spring water might be a better bet.

Avoid imported canned goods.

Avoid cooking in ceramic ware, and don't use ceramic dishes or old china with a damaged glaze to serve hot or acidic foods, including coffee and tea. Don't use lead-crystal containers to store any food.

For more information, contact the National Health Law Program in Los Angeles, (310) 204-6010, and ask for a copy of "Lead Poisoning: What It Is and What You Can Do About It." Or contact the Alliance to End Childhood Lead Poisoning, 227 Massachusetts Ave. NE, suite 200, Washington, DC 20002; (202) 543-1147.

Our Work

Work has always been a part of Black women's lives—whether we got paid for it or not. African-Americans spent two and a half centuries under the harshest conditions working for no pay, producing wealth for whites with little more than pain to show for it. We have been free for just a little more than half of the amount of time we were enslaved and free from legal discrimination for only a quarter of a century. Miraculously, many of us have managed to secure satisfying and rewarding work, but far too many others of us are still toiling under harsh conditions as maids, hospital employees, farm and factory workers, and word processors.

Regardless of our status, however, Black women have always been fighters, and sisters have long been on the forefront of the labor movement. In that tradition, it's important that as Black women we know our rights and make sure that we are not being abused.

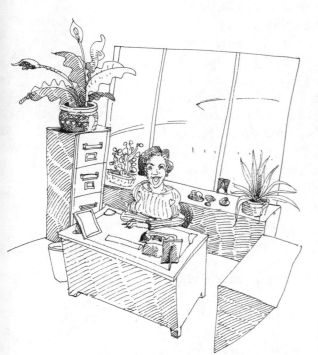

To feel comfortable on the job, we must make our work areas reflect a part of ourselves.
(Drawing: Yvonne Buchanan)

Workplace Hazards

Every year hundreds of thousands of workers die from work-related illness, and tens of thousands more die due to accidents. New cases of occupational diseases in the United States are estimated to range from 125,000 to 350,000 per year. For millions of others of us the toll is more subtle, but serious nonetheless: Quite literally, our jobs make us sick. For example, Imperial Food Products, where so many Black women burned to death or died of smoke inhalation, was never inspected during its eleven years of operation. Few workers in the poultry industry have union contracts. In North Carolina some twenty thousand people are employed in the industry, and they are three times more likely to be injured on the job than other workers in the state; one in four is injured at work every year. Their most common injury is carpal tunnel syndrome, a painful and often debilitating injury to the wrist caused by repetitive motions in the slaughterhouse (see below). By law the folks who work in the poultry industry can be fired by employers for any reason at all. Paying $5.30 an hour, Imperial Foods was considered one of the better-paying employers in rural North Carolina; problem employees were easily replaced.

I was a station cleaner, one of the people out there at night with the uniforms on, washing the walls and tracks, sweeping the platforms, and emptying garbage. We worked in a team with three, five or seven other people. I hate to make it a racial thing, but a lot of us down there were nonwhite; it was Blacks and Latinos. Every now and then you'd see a white guy someplace, but whites didn't want to be down there.

I was picking up a lot of feces behind a lot of homeless people who had a lot of problems. You're talking about people lying around on benches; one woman had gangrene in the legs and the stuff was dripping all over the place, and they'd send me down to clean up behind her. I didn't know the long-term effects of whether I could bring this stuff home to my kids. I didn't know what kind of effects this would have on my children or on me.

They gave us respirators. They handed you the respirator and said, "Here, utilize this." They never told you you had to be fit-tested, never said the filters had to be cleaned, and they never told you the conditions under which you don't use your respirator. If you go into one of those subway bathrooms where there are no windows, and you put this industrial-strength cleaner in there, you can choke to death!

They would send me out to clean graffiti and tell me to pour it in the bucket and slop it onto the walls, but they never said how much, and they never let me know what was in the chemical. Consequently, I was using a graffiti remover with the gloves they used to give us that only rolled down to the wrist. When I would raise and lower my arms, the chemicals rolled up under the gloves. My hand was all burnt up with pus running out of it, because the chemical I was using was industrial-strength and had acid in it. My hands had all kinds of sores. I had to go to a specialist to have it taken care of.

They kept giving me more chemicals to use that made me sick. The stuff was making me sleepy, I would go home, and I mean I would just fall out. I didn't realize that this was the chemical doing this to me. A lot of the chemicals they were using required ventilation. The Transit Authority seemed to think that a train coming by every twenty minutes, that's ventilation. We also had to use chemicals that would make you itch, some had acid that could eat through your work boots, some would irritate your eyes and make them red. We had a chemical out there one time that was causing respiratory failure. It cleaned like hell, but people were falling out all over the place.

After I made my year, when they could no longer just fire me, I started making noise all over the place about health and safety. I was directed toward the director of the union's Safety Committee. Whenever I had a prob-

"I started making noise all over the place about health and safety."

—JULIA MCMILLON, RECORDING SECRETARY FOR N.Y.C. TRANSIT WORKERS LOCAL 100, NEW YORK CITY

lem he would tell me how to go about straightening it out. I started asking questions, I wanted to be taught certain things. I didn't want to die.

After a year of complaining I learned about the OSHA [Occupational Safety and Health Administration] laws, the Department of Labor, and where to go with my complaints when management wouldn't cooperate. I went out there and I organized the cleaners to go down to the attorney general and complain about the fact that we didn't have an infectious-waste policy. We went down to the attorney general, and we testified that we were never given chemical-safety training. Then we ended up in court. Transit couldn't deny it; they didn't have an infectious-waste policy or chemical-training program.

Anybody in a situation like I was in should go to your union, first thing. If not you can go to any library and find OSHA regulations that everybody has to adhere to. You can also go to the Department of Labor or, if necessary, to your attorney general. There are places that will hear the cries of the worker, but it takes time. When we went to the attorney general we went down at nine o'clock in the morning, and we didn't get out until two-thirty in the afternoon, and that was after we'd already put in a full day's work. But if your life is worth anything, you've got to go through these measures.

Stress at the Workplace

Nearly everyone—even those of us who love our jobs—have experienced stress at the workplace. It may be a result of too much to do in too little time. Personal and family problems may be pressing and taking their toll all day long. Your work conditions may be unpleasant, making you feel anxious and irritable. The environment may be too noisy, cold, hot, dark, crowded, or uncomfortable; you may be forced to use poor equipment or perform repetitive hand motions. You may be having trouble with other employees who are racist, sexist, or just plain hard to take. Or it may be your boss who is the problem. The whole structure of your workplace may be unfair, discriminatory, or dangerous. You may feel a sense of powerlessness and lack of control at work; you may feel underpaid and unappreciated. All of these problems can cause stress.

Some stressful situations you can't change without changing jobs, but there are ways to lessen your day-to-day stress.

Examine your work setting. Act through your labor or employee organization to alter stressful working conditions such as poor lighting, inadequate ventilation or temperature control, noise, and insufficient sanitary facilities. Or, if you can, alter your work setting yourself. Do you feel out of control because you can't locate what you need when you need it? Try cleaning up and reorganizing your work area.

Assess your skills. Feeling like you're "in over your head" causes stress. Talk to your employer about getting additional job-related training such as through a trade school, adult education class, or seminar. Some employers will be impressed by your honesty and enthusiasm.

Talk to someone about problems you're having on the job. Many companies have employee-assistance programs, which operate in the strictest of confidence. The EAP can provide counseling or refer you to resources outside of the company.

Feel at home in your work space. Let your job setting reflect the joy and happiness you do have in your life. Surround yourself with photos of loved ones, drawings, pictures, cloth, and knickknacks that reflect your identity as a Black woman.

Make sure you take your breaks. Try to get away to a quiet place where you can relax and unwind far from your work responsibilities. Aerobic activities such as walking, stretching exercises, and meditation are good ways to bust stress.

If you feel burned out in a job that you don't feel you can leave, create a more equitable balance in your life. Invest more of yourself in family, social, and spiritual activities so that your job doesn't have such an overpowering influence on your life.

Combating Workplace Discrimination

Laws protect us from discrimination at work. Title VII of the 1964 Civil Rights Act reads:

(a) It shall be an unlawful employment practice for an employer—

(1) to fail or refuse to hire or to discharge any individual, or otherwise to discriminate against any individual with respect to his compensation, terms, conditions, or privileges of employment, because of such individual's race, color, religion, sex, or national origin, or

(2) to limit, segregate, or classify his employees in any way which would deprive or tend to deprive any individual of employment opportunities or otherwise adversely affect his [or her] status as an employee, because of such individual's race, color, religion, sex, or national origin.

However, using legal protections as recourse against job discrimination may be a long, stressful, expensive process. Based on interviews with employers and employees, Darien A. McWhirter, author of *Your Rights at Work,* offers this general advice:

Keep a record of everything. All employees should keep a daily logbook or diary noting who ordered them to do what, along with a record of accomplishments and complaints.

Keep your mouth shut. Everything people say really can be used against them in court. If you need to talk, speak to a family member, trusted friend, or therapist—outside of the work setting.

Talk to an attorney early. Get legal advice, for example, from your company grievance committee, union representatives, the Equal Employment Opportunity Commission, the NAACP Legal Defense Fund, or other nonprofit organizations before doing something dramatic like resigning.

Keep pay records. You may need to prove what you're earning.

Ask questions. The more you know and understand, the better off you'll be. And remember that laws change constantly.

Keep up with deadlines. The major cause for malpractice lawsuits against lawyers is that they waited past the deadline to file a lawsuit. If you are filing a lawsuit, make sure your attorney files the necessary paperwork on time.

Do not accept legal advice from anyone other than your own attorney. Well-meaning friends and coworkers may do more harm than good.

Tell your attorney everything that might be relevant. This will help you once you get into court or help you avoid it.

Examine your own behavior. Instead of getting a lawyer and going to court, would it be easier to confront your supervisor with the discrimination you're seeing or feeling? Are you avoiding confrontation because it's unpleasant or scary?

Sexual Harassment

Who could forget the 1991 spectacle of the Clarence Thomas Supreme Court hearings? Calm, cool, and firm, Professor Anita Hill dragged the shameful act of sexual harassment into the forefront. Even as people all over the country sat mesmerized, watching the drama unfold, millions of women of all colors pondered their own firsthand brushes with harassment in the workplace. In fact, 50 to 85 percent of women are expected to experience some kind of employment-related sexual harassment; some will even be sexually assaulted. Twenty to 90 percent say they have been sexually harassed at work. In a 1990 U.S. Defense Department study 64 percent of military women said they have experienced abuse.

Equal Employment Opportunity Commission guidelines state that sexual harassment is a form of sex discrimination that violates Title VII of the Civil Rights Act of 1964. According to the act's definition, "unwelcome sexual advances, requests for sexual favors, and other verbal or physical conduct of a sexual nature constitute sexual harassment when submission to or rejection of this conduct explicitly or implicitly affects an individual's employment, unreasonably interferes with an individual's work performance or creates an intimidating, hostile or offensive work environment."

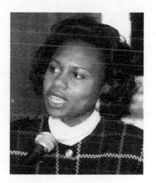

Professor Anita Hill sparked a national debate on sexual harassment in the workplace. *(Photo: Globe Photos, Inc.)*

Sexual harassment has nothing to do with how a woman looks or what she wears. It's not about sexiness and attraction; it's about power and control. Sexual harassment crosses lines of race and class. It works to remind women who may see themselves as able to achieve economic independence that they are and will always be sex objects as defined by men.

Sexual-harassment charges have tended to go unreported for many reasons. Women fear the consequences of coming forward. They often blame themselves for inducing the harassment. They may worry about being blackmailed; they may feel that reporting it won't stop it and may cause them loss of their jobs. They know that most of the time the majority of people who won't believe their claims are other women. Sisters have come up with a variety of savvy and creative ways to combat harassment using humor and common sense. However, you may need to take other measures. If you are continually confronted with unwanted remarks, jokes, or physical contact of a sexual nature, advise the person that you find the behavior offensive. If it continues, follow this strategy checklist adapted from *Stopping Sexual Harassment: A Handbook* by Camille Colatosti and Elissa Karg:

1. Prepare yourself. Before you begin to fight sexual harassment, get copies of anything in writing about the quality of your work. During an investigation, the employer may claim that you were fired because your work was poor.
2. Confront the harasser.
3. Put it in writing. Write a note telling the harasser to stop. Date it and keep a copy.
4. Keep a record. Write down any incident, including date, time, place, and witnesses. Write down your response word for word. If

you have to defend yourself, evidence will be crucial because it's your word against his.

5. Get support. Victims of sexual harassment feel isolated. You can break the isolation by talking to coworkers and friends. And by taking coworkers into your confidence, you may end the rumor mill, get emotional support, and find witnesses.

6. Get witnesses. If an incident of sexual harassment occurs when someone else is around, have her or him describe what happened in writing, then sign and date the statement.

7. Research your options. Exhaust in-house channels. If there is a union, contact the representative. If that person doesn't take your complaint seriously, form a women's committee. You can also talk to someone in human resources or the EAP.

8. Get outside help. Contact your local Human Rights Commission office, your local chapter of the ACLU, or your local city, state, or county antidiscrimination unit. You can also file a claim with the Equal Employment Opportunity Commission, but they may take longer to process your case (contact numbers listed below).

For more information, call any of the following support networks:

9 to 5, National Association of Working Women, 614 Superior W. Ave., suite 852, Cleveland, OH 44113; (800) 522-0925. Counselors who answer this hotline can help put you in touch with people in your local area who can help you.

CLUW (Coalition of Labor Union Women), 1126 16th Street, NW, Washington, DC 20036; (202) 296-1200, ext. 210. This organization, with representatives from more than 60 unions, specializes in helping union workers and can direct you to union help in your local area.

Equal Rights Advocates, 1663 Mission St., suite 550, San Francisco, CA 94103; (415) 621 0505. Provides information and legal advice and can refer you to groups in your local area.

Equal Employment Opportunity Commission, 1801 L Street NW, Washington, DC 20507; (800) 669-4000 to file a claim or (800) 669-3362 for written information. (Although the Hill-Thomas debate brought to light the ineffectiveness of this agency, we must make it work for us.)

You can also read: *The 9 to 5 Guide to Combating Sexual Harassment* by Ellen Bravo and Ellen Cassedy; *Step Forward: Sexual Harassment in the Workplace: What You Need to Know* by Susan L. Webb; *Stopping Sexual Harassment: A Handbook* by Camille Colatosti and Elissa Karg (this book is designed as a handbook for union workers); or *When No Means No: A Guide to Sexual Harassment By a Woman Who Won a Million-Dollar Verdict* by Cheryl Gomez-Preston with Randi Reisfeld.

Repetitive Strain Injury

Repetitive strain injury (RSI) or chronic musculoskeletal-system disease, also known as carpal tunnel syndrome, occurs when nerves and tendons in the hand are inflamed and swell due to damage caused by fast, repetitive work. Many workers—those in the meatpacking industry or those who work on computer keyboards, for example—suffer from RSI, because their jobs require them to constantly repeat the same motions, like cutting meat or striking a keyboard, for long hours at a time.

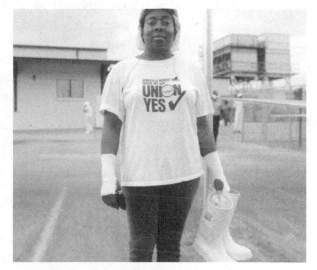

You can tell if you have the first signs of RSI: If you feel any pain or tingling sensations in your fingers, hands, arms, or neck; or, if your hands begin to swell or seem to have more aches and cramps than normal, talk to a doctor immediately. A physician should be able to tell you how advanced your injury is and how to care for it. Doctors may prescribe physical therapy, cortisone injections, or the use of wrist splints to ease the pain. In severe cases surgery is performed, but it is always best to use surgery only as a last resort.

Fast, repetitious work with the hands can lead to repetitive strain injury. *(Photo: Courtesy R.W.D.S.U., New York)*

You can make efforts to avoid RSI by rearranging your workplace:

If you work on a computer keyboard, adjust your computer screen so that it is about two feet to an arm's length away from you and just below your line of sight.

Keep your wrists straight—not bent upward or downward—and your forearms parallel to the floor at all times while typing. Your elbows should be bent at right angles. If possible, have forearm rests attached to your chair.

Make sure you have an adjustable chair that can be lowered or raised so that your knees can be kept bent at right angles and your feet can be kept flat on the floor. It should also have a backrest that can be adjusted to support the small of your back.

If possible, schedule your workday so that you are not continuously performing the same motion. If you have lots of typing to do, try to break up the time you have for doing it.

Do stretching exercises every fifteen minutes or as often as possible. Wiggle your fingers, flex your hands, move your wrists around, and stretch your forearms.

Work with your union to have management invest in tools that are shaped to the contours of workers' hands.

If your company has a union, ask union representatives to lobby for the following:

Redesigned equipment so that workers won't place undue stress on their hands and arms while working

Training of employees in proper and safe use of equipment

The development of worker/management committees that will look for the latest designs in safe equipment

Improved medical care for sufferers of repetitive strain injuries.

For more information, read *Repetitive Strain Injury: A Computer User's Guide* by Emil Pascarelli, M.D., and Deborah Quilter.

For More Information

BOOKS: Environment

Design for a Livable Planet: How You Can Help Clean Up the Environment, Jon Naar, Harper & Row Publishers, 1990.

Dumping in Dixie: Race, Class, and Environmental Quality, Robert D. Bullard, Westview Press (Boulder, Colo.), 1990.

Fifty Simple Things You Can Do to Save the Earth, EarthWorks Group, G. K. Hall (Boston), 1991.

Toxic Wastes and Race in the United States: A National Report on the Racial and Socio-Economic Characteristics of Communities with Hazardous Waste Sites, United Church of Christ Commission for Racial Justice (New York), 1987.

Turning Things Around: A Woman's Occupational and Environmental Health Resource Guide, Lin Nelson, Regina Kenen, and Susan Klitzman, National Women's Health Network (Washington, D.C.), 1990.

Unequal Protection: Environmental Justice and Communities of Color, Robert Bullard, ed., Sierra Club, 1994.

We Speak for Ourselves: Social Justice, Race and Environment, Robert Bulland et al., The Panos Institute (Washington, D.C.), 1990.

BOOKS: Work

The Minority Career Guide: What African Americans, Hispanics and Asian Americans Must Know to Succeed in Corporate America, Michael F. Kastre, Nydia Rodriguez Kastre, and Alfred G. Edwards, Peterson's Guides (Princeton, N.J.), 1993.

Reproductive Hazards in the Workplace: Mending Jobs, Managing Pregnancies, Regina Kenen, Haworth Press (Binghamton, N.Y.), 1992.

Success at Work: A Guide for African-Americans, Anita Doreen Diggs, Barricade Books, 1993.

A Troublemaker's Handbook: How to Fight Back Where You Work—and Win! Dan La Botz, Labor Notes (Detroit), 1991.

Volunteer Slavery: My Authentic Negro Experience, Jill Nelson, The Noble Press (Chicago), 1993.

Work, Sister, Work: How Black Women Can Get Ahead in Today's Business Environment, Cydney Shields and Leslie C. Shields, S & S Trade, 1994.

ORGANIZATIONS: Environment

BLACK ENVIRONMENTAL SCIENCE TRUST (BEST), P.O. Box 3000, Boulder, CO 80307-3000; (303) 497-8680. A clearinghouse for information on environmental issues.

CENTER FOR ENVIRONMENT, COMMERCE AND ENERGY, 122 C St, NW, suite 701, Washington, DC 20001; (202) 393-3303. This group's membership arm is the African-American Environmentalist Association.

CENTER FOR THIRD WORLD ORGANIZING, 1218 E. 21st St., Oakland, CA 94606; (510) 533-7583. Provides assistance and training for low-income and people of color organizers and organizations.

CITIZENS CLEARINGHOUSE FOR HAZARDOUS WASTE, P.O. Box 926, Arlington, VA 22216; (703) 276-7070. Provides assistance in the fight against hazardous and toxic waste and other environmental problems.

CITIZENS FOR A BETTER AMERICA, P.O. Box 356, Halifax, VA 24558; (804) 476-7757. A research organization for environmental and equal rights.

CLEAN WATER ACTION, c/o David Zwick, 1320 18th St, NW, Washington, DC 20036; (202) 457-1286. Citizen action organization working for strong pollution controls and safe drinking water.

EARTH ISLAND INSTITUTE URBAN HABITAT PROGRAM, 300 Broadway, suite 28, San Francisco, CA 94133; (415) 788-3666. Coordinates environmental protection projects and supports a program to develop multi-cultural urban environmental leadership.

ECO-JUSTICE WORKING GROUP OF THE NATIONAL COUNCIL OF CHURCHES, 475 Riverside Dr., Room 572, New York, NY 10115; (212) 870-2385. Educates and promotes activities leading to better environmental and social justice.

ENVIRONMENTAL ACTION FOUNDATION, 6930 Carroll Ave., 6th fl., Takoma Park, MD 20912; (301) 891-1100. Environmental research and education organization that operates the Energy Project, a resource and information clearinghouse.

ENVIRONMENTAL DEFENSE FUND, 257 Park Ave. S., New York, NY 10010; (212) 505-2100. An advocacy group staffed by lawyers, economists, and scientists.

GREENPEACE USA, 1436 U St. NW, Washington, DC 20009; (202) 462-1177. High-profile environmental group whose sister foundation, Greenpeace Action, utilizes grass-roots lobbying.

GULF COAST TENANTS ORGANIZATION, P.O. Box 56101, New Orleans, LA 70156; (504) 949-4919. Assistance in problems dealing with hazardous waste.

INSTITUTE FOR LOCAL SELF-RELIANCE, 2425 18th St. NW, Washington, DC 20009; (202) 232-4108. Assists grass-roots groups and small businesses with an emphasis on recycling and reducing consumption of raw materials.

LEGAL ENVIRONMENTAL ASSISTANCE FOUNDATION, 1115 N. Gadsden St., Tallahassee, FL 32303-6237; (904) 681-2591. Provides legal and technical assistance to deal with toxic pollution.

MINORITY ENVIRONMENTAL ASSOCIATION, P.O. Box 2097, Sandusky, OH 44871; (419) 625-3230. Advocacy organization for jobs, contacts, and training.

NATIONAL COALITION AGAINST THE MISUSE OF PESTICIDES (NCAMP), 701 E St., SE, Suite 200, Washington, DC 20003; (202) 543-5450. Promotes awareness of problems caused by pesticide use and offers alternatives; maintains library.

NATIONAL TOXICS CAMPAIGN, 1168 Commonwealth Ave., Boston, MA 02134; (617) 232-0327. Works for stronger laws against chemical contaminants.

NATURAL RESOURCES DEFENSE COUNCIL, 40 W. 20th St., New York, NY 10011; (212) 727-2700. Provides research and education on environmental concerns.

PUBLIC CITIZEN HEALTH RESEARCH GROUP, 2000 P St. NW,

Washington, DC 20036; (202) 833-3000. Provides information and education on environmental issues and workplace safety.

SOUTHWEST ORGANIZING PROJECT, 211 10th St. SW, Albuquerque, NM 87102; (505) 247-8832. A community-based grass-roots organization to promote leadership development and citizen participation on environmental and workplace safety issues.

UNITED CHURCH OF CHRIST COMMISSION FOR RACIAL JUSTICE, 475 Riverside Dr., suite 950, New York, NY 10015; (212) 870-2077. Provides referrals and technical and legal resources for combating pollution.

TAKE IT BACK FOUNDATION, 533 Swarthmore Ave., Pacific Palisades, CA 90272; (310) 459-2377. Promotes recycling and waste reduction through education and advocacy.

URBAN ECOLOGY, P.O. Box 10144, Berkeley, CA, 94709; (415) 549-1724. Deals with the design of cities relating to the environment and also focuses on recycling and transportation.

U.S. PUBLIC INTEREST RESEARCH GROUP (USPIRG), 215 Pennsylvania Ave. SE, Washington, DC 20003; (202) 546-9707. Grass-roots membership works to pass legislation for clean, healthy environments.

WORK ON WASTE, 82 Judson St., Canton, NY 13617; (315) 379-9200. Publishes weekly newsletter focusing on incineration and dioxin.

GOVERNMENT AGENCIES: Environment

ENVIRONMENTAL PROTECTION AGENCY, Public Information Center, 401 M St. SW, Washington, DC 20460; (202) 260-7751. Answers environmental questions.

NATIONAL RESPONSE CENTER; (800) 424-8802. Transfers reports of environmental problems to the appropriate agency for response.

U.S. NUCLEAR REGULATORY COMMISSION/OFFICE OF PUBLIC AFFAIRS, Washington, DC 20555; (301) 504-2240. Answers questions about nuclear energy.

ORGANIZATIONS: Work

AFL-CIO, 815 16th St. NW, Washington, DC 20006; (202) 637-5000. Support and advocacy for labor.

COALITION OF LABOR UNION WOMEN, 1126 16th St., NW, Washington, DC 20036; (202) 296-1200, ext. 210. Furthers the role of women in the labor movement and the workplace and will assist in finding union support for individuals.

COMMITTEES ON OCCUPATIONAL SAFETY AND HEALTH, c/o NYCOSH, 275 Seventh Ave., 8th floor, New York, NY 10001; (212) 627-3900. Trains and educates people about safety on the job.

9 TO 5, NATIONAL ASSOCIATION OF WORKING WOMEN, 614 W. Superior Ave., Suite 852, Cleveland, OH 44113; (800) 522-0925. Advocates for working women for rights and respect on the job; offers advice and support on workplace issues.

NATIONAL COALITION OF INJURED WORKERS, 12 Rejane St., Coventry, RI 02816; (401) 828-6520. Coordinating point for injured workers' groups; will refer individuals to the closest source for help.

GOVERNMENT AGENCIES: Work

OCCUPATIONAL SAFETY AND HEALTH ADMINISTRATION (OSHA), U.S. Dept. of Labor, 200 Constitution Ave. NW, Washington, DC 20210; (202) 219-8148. Answers questions about job-related problems.

OCCUPATIONAL SAFETY AND HEALTH ADMINISTRATION (OSHA) NOTIFICATION SERVICE; (800) 321-OSHA. Refers callers with job-related problems to the appropriate local office; provides emergency service on weekends.

WOMEN'S BUREAU CLEARINGHOUSE, U.S. Dept. of Labor, 200 Constitution Ave. NW, Washington, DC 20210; (800) 827-5335. Information and publications related to pregnancy discrimination, sexual harassment, and family medical leave; also supplies a working family resource kit.

Index